THE COMPLETE INTERVIEW TRANSCRIPTS

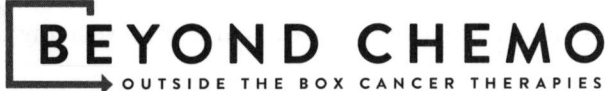

BEYOND CHEMO

OUTSIDE THE BOX CANCER THERAPIES

640BD00248

TABLE OF CONTENTS

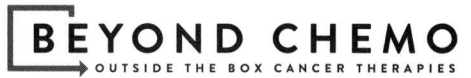

EPISODE 1: BEYOND CHEMO

Why Your Mainstream Treatment Just Isn't Enough (PLUS: Six Proven Treatments to Reverse Cancer)

A MESSAGE FROM DR. STENGLER

The reason I put together Outside the Box Cancer Therapies is to get credible information out to the public so that people with cancer, loved ones of people with cancer, and those with a history of cancer can improve their chances of survival and quality of life.

You know, right now in the world of medicine it's fragmented when it comes to cancer. That's why we need integrative oncology. That's the best of conventional and holistic natural therapies to get the best results.

You know, people are tired of not being offered credible and well-studied natural therapies, such as nutrition, targeted supplements, intravenous nutrients and other scientifically validated treatments.

Too many people are undergoing conventional cancer therapy and they feel like they're treated like a number, kind of like cattle. Instead of the valued people they are as part of God's most prized creation.

Most of us, including myself, have had experience with family members going through standard, conventional therapy the good and often too much the bad and the ugly.

People deserve better than this. Fortunately there's a revolution going on in medicine with the public demanding natural and holistic therapies, especially for cancer and I believe this series will expedite this progress.

So my goal is to strike a balance. I interviewed top doctors around the country seeing patients on a daily basis with cancer wanting the best for the patients. I mean if you need some conventional treatment, you get it. But always integrating the natural treatments which can only help a patient do better.

You might wonder—okay. You may wonder why most Americans haven't heard about many of the therapies being discussed in this series. While I'm not a conspiracy theory junkie, but there's a kind of suppression in medicine today, especially in terms of cancer, where the public is told that anything other than chemotherapy, radiation, surgery and other conventional treatments is dangerous and not scientific. This is pseudo-science and a complete myth.

You know, there's a ton of scientific research demonstrating the validity of the treatments discussed in this series that support the immune system and the buyers' ability to prevent and treat cancer.

Natural treatments are a fraction of the cost to most conventional therapies and have a lot to offer.

The types of treatments offered by these integrative doctors is a game-changer for those wanting to take charge of their health and to greatly reduce the risk of getting cancer, or those who have a history of cancer and want to reduce their risk of relapsing as well. It's for those who are not satisfied with the often poor results achieved by conventional oncology.

I chose to be a naturopathic doctor for many reasons. First, as a young kid, I was very much into athletics, so I was very competitive. Any one time of the year I'd be playing multiple sports and had to be the best in hockey and the best in swimming and the best in badminton and basketball and track and field. My mother drove me around a lot. [Laughs] So I was very much interested in using like diet and nutrition to enhance my performance. And later on I became interested in nutritional supplements. As a kid, I used to walk down with my little allowance and go to the one small health food store I lived in, less than 10,000 people, and you know I'd buy B vitamins and multivitamins and I'd get the free health magazines and take them home and read them. So I was very much into it. So it started off just having almost like an intuitive appreciation for nutrition and holistic therapies.

To me, it just made a lot of logical sense. Our bodies were designed to interact with these things. And as I got older and seeing you know people get sick and have health problems, I was interested in medicine. Originally, I was gonna go into chiropractic as a lot of ex-athletes do. And then I started thinking over the future as much as I like chiropractic I thought, "Wow, someday I'll be married and probably have kids, and if my kids get sick I'll have to be able to offer more treatments if I want to take care of them." And I thought about naturopathic medicine where as a naturopathic medical doctor I'd learn both types of medicine. Learn regular medicine with lab tests, physical exams, diagnostic images, pharmaceutical medications, minor surgery, and then integrated with that nutritional herbal therapies, homeopathy, nutritional IVs, natural hormones, you know psychological approaches, body works, just many different natural therapies.

I thought wow, that makes the most sense being trained with both and having a balance. So that's what got me going.

You know I've been practicing over 21 years. So when a patient comes to me with cancer, I basically assess where they're at. I mean some patients come in, they've just been newly diagnosed; they're still going through other lab tests. So we're trying to gather all the information. So I look at it from two aspects.

One is what's going on from a conventional standpoint. Being trained in both types of medicine, I want to know what type of cancer they have, what regions of the body are affected, you know what their bloodwork is showing in a general sense. But then I dig much deeper. I'm trying to find out why they were predisposed to getting this cancer, and I go through all the different categories. And dig deeper. We look at things which would interfere with proper immune system function and cellular health. So it could be things like toxins. Toxins you get like parabens from cosmetics, toxins from heavy metals made from the water or other things people have been exposed to.

And so we look at the root causes of you know why they have problems. Nutritional deficiencies. You know the immune system can't work optimally if you have nutritional deficiencies. So we look at all these different categories for that patient based on their symptoms, their exposure, and the lab tests we run figure out where the weak points are and then hone in on those to optimize their immune system, help them fight cancer more effectively. That's kind of the first phase, and then we initiate also just direct natural anti-cancer therapies. And so we use things like the high-dose intravenous vitamin C shown in several studies now to improve quality-of-life scores, people undergoing chemotherapy and radiation, and length of life. So it's a win-win really. I'm one of the first to really integrate intravenous ozone therapy combined with intravenous vitamin C; it's kind of a unique treatment. They're both in this category called oxidative treatment. Cancer cells do not like oxygen; they're anaerobic. And so when we introduce oxidative treatments into the system, it's excellent for their anti-cancer effects.

And then we use immune-boosting supplements. You know years back I published research in books on the most well-studied nutritional supplements. So I focus with patients on using supplements demonstrated in human studies to have anti-cancer properties to be safe and can be used with conventional therapies. So that's a large part of my focus. And then with any holistic approach, see how a person is doing with their stress, you know try and help them with all the stress they're under. And if people are diagnosed with cancer, you know their stress level is gonna be up. So any ways we can help them with that, whether it be counseling, referrals to ministers, things like that, and using supplements to help keep their nervous system more calm, help to balance out their stress hormones.

I think the general public would like to know my practice it's very well balanced. When patients come in, we're using physical exams, we're using very modern scientific lab testing where the blood tests, urine test, stool tests, and identifying what are the root causes of their health problems currently or what they're gonna be predisposed to having. We actually do more testing than your typical medical doctor does, so we've very much into science.

It's just typically our treatment methods differ a lot. So instead of just focusing on pharmaceutical treatment and surgery, we're focusing on nutrition, nutritional supplements, maybe natural hormones, intravenous nutrient therapies, body work. We have an osteopathic doctor, acupuncture. So we focus more on those treatments because, A, they treat the root causes generally much better than conventional treatment. They're much safer for sure and we just see better results. Then if people need pharmaceutical treatment or specialists, we still incorporate those things, whatever is best for the patient. But they'll see that our treatment hierarchy differs greatly than conventional medicine.

So if a patient comes in they've been diagnosed with breast cancer and they've only been offered chemotherapy and radiation, what I tell the patient is they're only being recommended a partial comprehensive treatment plan. In my opinion, it would be negligent to only offer a patient chemotherapy or radiation, just as if a patient came in to see me and I thought they were having a heart attack and I didn't send them to the hospital; that would be negligent. So it kind of works both ways, you gotta have a balance. And so I'd also mention to them you know the side effects of the different chemotherapy or radiation they're being offered, how modern scientific studies have shown how we can greatly reduce the likelihood of those side effects or treat them with natural medicine. And so we can help their quality of life. We also show them data showing that people that get conventional medicine only versus people who get conventional medicine plus natural therapies—

Studies are very clear these people that do both treatments have better quality of life scores and longer length of life, so why wouldn't you do them? Well you only wouldn't do them if you don't know about it, if you're ignorant of the information. And unfortunately, even though the research is out there and it's been published, your average oncologist seems to show not much interest in it and so people aren't aware of these studied treatments.

In terms of cancer, we consistently see we're helping people, and so that's why we keep working with people with cancer. So recently for example in the past years I've been treating a patient who has breast cancer that spread to her brain. You know she's had different rounds of chemotherapy, so we've been able to help her with the side effects. She doesn't have any you know major side effects from her treatments. And with the combination of the treatments, surprising to her specialist, she actually goes to MD Anderson for treatment, goes back and forth, she believes and I believe and her oncologist isn't sure but you know she isn't showing any more lesions in the brain or cancer anywhere else, and that's a very difficult thing to do. And so we see these things, and it matches up to what the studies have shown.

People that do the combination of treatments do much better. I have a man you'll see in the series who's had prostate cancer for ten years. Now, he declined to do any conventional treatment; he's done natural treatment only. There's no signs of cancer spreading; it's still contained, and his quality of life is phenomenal. Another patient I've been working with the last couple of years she had very aggressive breast cancer and very high-dose chemotherapy as a treatment she was given. And her oncologist even said last week at her followup visit, it's been again about two years, just shocked. You know she did not have lasting side effects like most people have like the neuropathy or nerve pain, numbness and so forth. Her hair has come back about 80 percent. Her energy is better than before she was even diagnosed with cancer. So we just consistently see we're helping the quality of life with people. We seem to be matching up to what the studies show, longer length of life, and yeah, people are very happy with the results.

My worldview is that people are made in the image of God, which means we're highly valued, more than the plant and animal kingdom, although they should be treated with respect too, and so that everyone should be treated with dignity and respect.

And so when I see people, no matter what backgrounds they are, even what faith backgrounds they have, they're valuable to God and to their family, and you don't want to see people suffering. And I try to help them also because maybe I'll be a good witness to them too for my faith. So in a general sense, that's my motivation in terms of when I see people in the clinic. And that's why if you talk to my patients, they'll tell you I tend to spend more time with them if they're having problems even outside of clinic appointments. I make sure they're taken care of. And so we try to go that extra step, and our motto here at the clinic is to treat every patient as an MVP.

Basically, for the average person when you're diagnosed with cancer, you see an oncologist and usually you're given very few options. Usually it's surgery and chemotherapy and/or radiation or maybe some experimental drugs. And usually there is not much flexibility. I have a lot of patients telling me that they feel like a number in a medical system. You know you get these treatments, yeah, you're gonna feel sick and all that. A lot of people tell me they feel like they're in a factory and treated like you know lower animal life, so to speak. And I just think it's critical you get integrative care. You see a holistic doctor who can incorporate the types of things we talk about in our series so that first you feel like you're being cared for, you're valued, and you're reducing the side effects of the conventional treatments, and you're increasing the potential for being cured or for a longer length of life. And so I think it's just critical that people go outside the box or else a lot of people are just very disappointed in terms of how they're cared for and the results.

THE TRUTH ABOUT THE CANCER INDUSTRY

— MIKE ADAMS —

The cancer industry like any other industry is a for-profit industry and so as a result it needs repeat customers, it needs repeat business, and it needs to make sure that people need cancer treatments. That's their profit model; it's the whole business model. As a result they don't want people to prevent cancer or even have the knowledge of how to prevent cancer. They don't want people to cure cancer and reverse cancer. Even though those solutions are readily available they are deliberately withheld from the people, from patients. For example, cancer centers don't tell patients that vitamin D alone can prevent 78 percent of cancers. They don't tell African-Americans that their dark skin pigmentation blocks the creation of vitamin D in their own skin and that's why cancer is more severe or aggressive in Black men and women.

They don't tell people that chemotherapy causes cancer. It actually causes cancer cells to spread throughout the body and this has been backed up by literally dozens of mainstream published science studies that chemotherapy causes cancer; it causes cancer to spread. Why is chemotherapy used? Because it results in repeat business. Chemotherapy shrinks a tumor but spreads the cancer stem cells causing more tumors 2 or 3 years later, which brings the person back to the cancer center for more repeat business. To really understand why natural cures and even cancer prevention is suppressed you just have to get a grip on the idea that these corporations, they aren't compassionate, they aren't interested in helping humanity, they don't have a humanitarian mission even though they may fake like it to get you into their clinic to poison you with their chemotherapy. They are interested in profit.

Profit requires repeat revenue and repeat revenue requires keeping people sick and making sure they don't prevent or reverse cancer and that is the truth about the cancer industry. Now the mainstream media is funded in large part by drug companies that sell cancer treatments and even profit from cancer the disease, you know medical imaging device manufacturers and so on. About 70 percent of the revenues to the mainstream media today come from drug industry advertising so the media has no incentive to tell the truth about this because then they would offend their primary source of revenue: the drug companies. If the truth came out it would be absolutely shocking to consumers because it's a racket. The cancer industry, which involves the non-profits, the ACS, the NIH, all of these government organizations that fund cancer industry research using taxpayer money

This whole system is a racket that does not want people to get well, to be healthy, or to reverse cancer. In fact, when people turn to turmeric or juicing or other natural means that reverse cancer the cancer industry says, "No, you didn't reverse it. It's just in remission. That must be a coincidence," they say. In truth people are curing cancer right now every day and they're doing it with medicinal herbs, with superfood nutrients like turmeric root, or with juicing and fasting, changing their diet, changing their lifestyle, getting more sunshine, getting more vitamin D. People are reversing cancer every day. They're curing cancer every day and yet the cancer industry falsely says that there's no such thing as a cancer cure. The truth is there is no such thing as a cancer cure that the cancer industry wants you to know about but there are dozens of cancer cures that exist outside that status quo system and these cancer cures are readily available.

Some of them are dirt cheap or free, for example sunshine and water, fasting; these are all free and other cancer cures are at very low cost, high efficacy, high safety, low cost and they don't poison you, they don't make your hair fall out, they don't make you lose muscle mass. They don't poison your heart, brain, and kidneys like chemotherapy does but the cancer industry doesn't profit from those things. They can't make money off sunshine. They can't make money if you generate your own vitamin D and prevent cancer in your own body and that's frankly why this kind of alternative information is becoming so incredibly popular because people want solutions to cancer and they don't want to poison themselves and they know that big pharma is a racket, they know they've been lied to this whole time, and they know there must be better options available and there are and that's what this is all about. If you really want to solve cancer you have to look at what causes it.

Now keep in mind that the cancer establishment wants you to believe that disease is a spontaneous creation, that it is disease without cause. Now that is a wildly unscientific idea but that's the idea pushed by the cancer industry. They say, "Well there's nothing you could've done about it. The food you eat doesn't matter," they say, "It just happened. It's just bad genetics. You just spontaneously generated cancer for no reason." Nonsense. That's completely quackery and any doctor that pushes that false theory frankly should have their medical license revoked. It's total nonsense. Every case of cancer has a cause. Every disease has a cause because a disease is an effect and we live in a universe of cause and effect. So if you don't believe in cause and effect then you know you're not living in the real world but cancer can be prevented by changing the inputs. In other words, if you remove the causes of cancer you don't get the effects of cancer tumors. It's very simple. So what are the causes? This is the key question: what causes cancer in our world today?

And to a large extent it is exposure to toxic chemicals and these pollutants invade our food supply, they're in medicines, they're in the environment, and they're in personal care products that people put on themselves; they give themselves cancer every day. You know the average American exposes themselves to over 200 chemicals before they leave the bathroom in the morning you know with the deodorants and the shampoos and the fragrance and all these things that they put on themselves. They're giving themselves cancer with all these chemicals and then they wonder, "Whoa, all of a sudden where'd this cancer come from?" Well you're giving yourself cancer. And if you're eating cancer-causing foods you're eating cancer in essence and these foods can include fried foods and trans fatty acids, hydrogenated oils, glyphosate saturated products, which include genetically modified foods that are soaked in glyphosate, but even wheat products can contain glyphosate as well. That's an herbicide also sold as Roundup® by Monsanto. These are carcinogenic chemicals and there are many others as well.

There's atrazine, which is a chemical hormone disruptor; it's called a chemical castrator. Atrazine interferes with normal hormone function, even at very low levels of exposure such as parts per trillion concentrations circulating in your blood and you can get that from eating 1 meal at a restaurant that uses food ingredients, which are heavily saturated with pesticides, herbicides, and agricultural chemicals. So these chemicals have a powerful physiological effect that destroys the normal cell division function of the human body. They are physiological terrorists you might say. They go into your body and they rip apart your normal physiology at a cellular level and they cause then cell division to become very confused because that's based on intracellular and intercellular communication. Cell division is something that the body knows how to do when you're not contaminated with toxic chemicals but the more chemicals you have in your body then the more cell division becomes out of control and that's what a cancer tumor is out of control cell division where the cell doesn't understand its role of specialization and limiting its growth and division. Instead that cell wants to become an entire body, an entire you, and this is why by the way a lot of cancer tumors that have been allowed to grow for a very long period of time are found to contain hair and teeth and fragments of bones and fragments of—of nerve systems. A cancer tumor is trying to become a whole body inside you because it hasn't—the shut-off signal isn't working correctly so it's a miscommunication between your body's cells. That miscommunication is causes in many cases by these toxic chemicals that are found in food and cosmetics and personal care products. Heavy metals are also linked to cancer as well. Lead for example has a very strong link with bone cancer. Cadmium is linked to various types of cancers as well.

Heavy metals are like bad minerals so what they do is they occupy the—the places in your body where minerals would normally go, healthy minerals, uh, such as for example zinc or copper or magnesium. You know these—these metals—and by the way some of these can be toxic in high concentrations, you can have too much copper, but you also need a little bit of copper, you need a little bit of zinc, and you need quite a lot of magnesium as it turns out but calcium is another mineral that you need quite a bit of. Well lead can come in and displace calcium and mercury can displace zinc and there are affinities from these elements. And so toxic heavy metals, which occur in food and medicine and pesticides, they then get into your body and interfere with normal mineral functions in your body and minerals basically function as physiological catalysts for, uh, protein synthesis and DNA repair and other functions within the body, metabolic functions and so on, even neurological functions.

Uh, even just to beat your heart you have to have calcium and magnesium. To move water into every cell in your body you have to have potassium. Potassium can be invaded or replaced by cesium 137, a radioactive isotope for example that also causes cancer in a different way. Heavy metals in essence encourage your body to generate cancer over time and although eating lead today, right now won't cause cancer tomorrow over time with the accumulation of these heavy metals you can absolutely have cancer tumors growing, especially if you have these other factors coming in, which is vitamin D deficiency, immunosuppression, as well as exposure to toxic chemicals in foods, pesticides, herbicides, cosmetic chemicals, artificial fragrance, laundry detergent. This is where people bathe their clothing in toxic, cancer-causing chemicals. It's the fabric softeners, the dryer sheets, and the detergent that people put in their laundry. You know there's warning recently about kids who are doing this YouTube challenge where they eat Tide laundry pods.

They eat them and doctors are warning like crazy. Oh my god, these Tide laundry pods, they're full of toxic chemicals. You could do serious damage. You could threaten your life by eating them. But wait a minute, why isn't anybody talking about you're bathing your clothing in this stuff. If it's so toxic to eat why are you wearing it? You know people don't even think about this but laundry detergent, typically detergent, is toxic. It's full of cancer-causing chemicals, which is why it's dangerous to eat Tide laundry pods. It's also dangerous to wash our clothes in it frankly and it's dangerous for all the fish downstream when you do your laundry and you have that dirty water drain out of the washer. So you—you've got to think about all these things. Cancer is caused by chemical exposure, heavy metals exposure, stress, and lack of nutrition.

So if you don't have the anti-cancer foods and the anti-cancer nutrients and you do have exposure to cancer-causing heavy metals and chemicals plus stress, lack of sleep, emotional distress, depression, and so on, you will grow cancer. It has a cause and if you want to prevent it you've got to look at those causes and you've got to take those away so that you're not generating cancer in your body. The good news in all of this is that there are powerful anti-cancer foods readily available just at any grocery store. For example turmeric is number 1 probably in my book. Turmeric, you know the orange root similar to ginger but a little different chemical make-up, there are documented cases. One was written up in the British Medical Journal of a woman who cured cancer using curcumin, which is an extract from turmeric root. So if you're eating turmeric or you do what I do, I put a heaping teaspoon of turmeric powder into my smoothie every day, you're getting that curcumin and you're getting other chemical constituents of turmeric root by the way, which also have anti-inflammatory effects.

And of course cancer goes away when you eliminate inflammation and you have anti-cancer foods. And by the way, inflammation is 1 of the underlying causes of many types of cancer and is being recognized as such by the medical literature. So inflammation of neurology, inflammation of joints and muscles, but also inflammation of the entire immunological system and endocrine system; you can actually have endocrine inflammation, which is aggravation of the endocrine system by exposure to pesticides. So by calming this systemic inflammation what you do is you allow your body to express its own natural anti-cancer blueprint. In other words, you're born with the genetics to overcome cancer and to live a life that's free of cancer, but in order for those genetics to be expressed you have to calm the inflammation in the system that's caused by exposure to junk foods, fried foods, heavy metals, pesticides, toxic GMOs and all these other things so turmeric is key to accomplishing this.

In terms of nutritional supplements I think vitamin D is the key to cancer prevention. It's fascinating. Vitamin D, which is actually kind of a hormone and is generated in your own skin and then absorbed through your skin and it circulates through your—your kidneys and it—there are receptor sites for vitamin D on your heart and your liver and other organs throughout your body, prostate, breast tissue, and so on. Vitamin D should be called the anti-cancer vitamin because it activates your immune system to fight off cancer. In fact, if you're vitamin D deficient you're almost guaranteed to grow cancer tumors at a certain rate. It might be very slow, you might never be diagnosed with cancer because it might take 30 or 40 years to grow those tumors, but if you're deficient enough and you have exposure to these other chemicals you will grow cancer tumors rapidly and this is why most people in North America tend to grow cancer tumors in the winter months because they're vitamin D deficient.

And the official government recommendations on vitamin D, which I think are like 800IU per day are just almost designed to keep you deficient. Most people would benefit from taking anywhere between 4,000IUs and 10,000IUs a day. Check with your naturopathic physician but I personally take between 4,000 and 10,000 a day and at that level it's a very potent anti-cancer effect and it's very affordable. And again it's aiding your body in activating itself to carry out its own anti-cancer potential. It already knows what to do. Your body does it automatically and you just have to give it the right nutrition. You've got to activate your immune system cells; vitamin D does that. In terms of anti-cancer medicinal herbs and supplements I'm a big believer in many of the medicinal mushrooms such as Reishi for example or Chaga. There are many in Chinese medicine as well, TCM, Traditional Chinese Medicine.

It's—it's crucial though, when you turn to medicinal mushrooms and you're looking for answer to cancer don't make the mistake of thinking that you don't have to change the causes of cancer and that you can just turn to Reishi mushrooms or Shitake mushrooms, which are also very potent, and that you can ignore everything else in your life. Remember you did something that gave you cancer. You probably did your laundry in toxic, cancer-causing chemicals. You probably ate cancer-causing foods. You probably didn't eat all organic. You probably put cosmetics on your skin that are full of cancer-causing chemicals. You probably didn't take vitamin D, you were deficient, and on and on. So there are many things that have happened that gave you cancer. So don't think that you can just take Reishi mushrooms or Shitake mushrooms and your cancer problems are solved. A lot of people want that secret pill, they can just slam a pill and think, "Oh, that's medicine. It's going to solve my problem for me." That's not how it works.

Beating cancer means taking responsibility for your diet, for your exercise, for your time in sunshine, eliminating the toxins in your life, maybe doing juicing for 90 days, clean out your system, get rid of the toxins, do a sauna sweating to eliminate more toxins. There are many, many things that you can do. Do a liver cleanse; do a kidney cleanse. You've got to take responsibility for your health and then the medicinal mushrooms can actually have a very powerful impact. But if you just try to depend on some external thing like, "Oh, I'm gonna add this pill to my diet, I'm going to take green tea or I'm going to take Astaxanthin or I'm going to take mushrooms," and you think that alone is going to cure your cancer while you're continuing to live a lifestyle that gave you cancer in the first place? Forget it. That's not going to work. You cannot simultaneously continue to eat cancer and use cancer-causing products and then think that this anti-cancer food alone is going to counteract all those things; it doesn't work that way. You've got to clean house top to bottom.

You need to rethink your whole life, rethink what's in your pantry, what's in the kitchen, in the bathroom. What are you wearing? What are you putting on your skin? What are you washing your hair with? What are you washing your clothing with? What kind of water are you drinking? What are the heavy metals in your food and water? Are you poisoning yourself with arsenic from a home water well for example? These are big deal questions and if you really want to solve cancer you've got to go down the whole list and check of all those check boxes and eliminate every cause of cancer while you're taking anti-cancer foods and supplements; that's the key. Most people frankly aren't willing to go that far. They'd rather go to a cancer clinic and just have an oncologist tell them, "Ah, we'll pump you full of toxic chemicals, it's called chemotherapy, you'll live another 5 years," and for some reason that's good enough for them when if they did all these changes they could live another 20 years without the suffering, without the toxicity, you know without their hair falling out, without them losing their minds and hearts from heart damage from chemo and all these other things.

It's just a question of personal fortitude. How much do you want to live? What kind of life do you want to lead? Do you want to lead a life of suffering while pretending to have a cancer treatment? Yeah, go visit an oncology center. They'll poison you for profit gladly and they'll—you'll be back in 2 or 3 years if you're not dead by then and you can pay them more money and they're—they'll be happy to poison you again for more profit. Or you could choose to take care of yourself and love yourself and start healing by changing all these things in your life that gave you cancer in the first place. If you really love yourself you'll go on that healing journey. Chemotherapy is really medical violence against humans whereas healing and juicing and anti-cancer foods are a form of self-love.

If you love yourself you'll start to explore natural solutions and you'll find ways to heal because they're readily available by the way.

These aren't big secrets. You know the cures for cancer already exist. They're all around you. You just have to have the wisdom to recognize it and the courage to start pursuing those things and frankly a lot of people don't have that wisdom or courage or they've just given up. Don't give up. Your body can heal. Your body can heal from almost anything but it's gonna take the right foods and the right nutrients and superfoods and lifestyle habits and you know vitamin D and sunshine and all these other things in order to make that a reality.

UNDERSTANDING INTEGRATIVE ONCOLOGY

— DR. PAUL ANDERSON —

Dr. Stengler: Hi, everyone. We have a really important video today for you. And today, I have a special guest, Dr. Paul Anderson. He's the co-author of *Outside the Box Cancer Therapies,* and Dr. Anderson, great to have you with us.

Dr. Anderson: It's great to be here.

Dr. Stengler: Well, it's a very important topic, the term, integrative oncology, has been around for a number of years now.

Dr. Anderson: Mm-hmm.

Dr. Stengler: People don't necessarily understand what it is. Would you mind telling the viewers what that all entails?

Dr. Anderson: Certainly. The idea behind integrative oncology is actually that you don't throw out anything good, but you look for the best of, uh, all worlds, as it were.

Dr. Stengler: Yeah.

Dr. Anderson: And so, you can have, uh, treatments, for example, from your standard hospital therapies, such as radiation, or chemotherapy, or surgery. And in some cases they are the very best thing for somebody, but then there's a lot of other things that have been left out of that mix. Uh, many, many natural therapies, many things that really border on—

What you would might get in a hospital if they were up to date on the latest research. They might even be giving it to you there, but you might have to go to somebody outside. So, integrative oncology really tries to take the best of both worlds, and mix them together so that the patient gets the best treatment that they can.

Dr. Stengler: Right, absolutely. Well, tell the viewers a bit about your background. I mean, I know, obviously, you have a clinic in Seattle. You train doctors around the country on this topic and other topics, too, so yeah, tell the viewers more about yourself.

Dr. Anderson: Sure. About, um, almost 42 years ago, I entered medicine, so I'm maybe older than I look. But I started out working in laboratories, and uh, which was a lot of fun, and there was a lot to do. And I got a really good kinda backside view of the, uh, standard medical community. And uh, that was very, very enlightening, and also, after a number of years, I became a little bit bored with it, and decided to go back and finish medical school.

And decided, uh, I might not do so well if I went to a real standard, kinda straight medical school, so decided to become a naturopathic medical doctor. So, about 25, 26 years ago, I went back and started to, that process.

Um, and one of the reasons, really, that I did that was I wasn't really thinking about integrative oncology back in those days, as maybe none of us were thinking of it in that way.

Dr. Stengler: Right.

Dr. Anderson: But really integrative medicine, uh, because I had seen the good that standard medicine could do, and I had also seen that there must be other things that we could add in. And so, becoming a naturopathic medical doctor really was the best avenue to do that.

So, that's what I've been doing ever since, and as you mentioned, the last ten years I spent, uh, in research in integrative oncology, and a couple of other areas, and I've been teaching other physicians about that ever since.

Dr. Stengler:	Yeah, that's great. Um, what have you found in terms of advances in integrative oncology—It seems like the field really has just exploded—
Dr. Anderson:	Mm-hmm.
Dr. Stengler:	In the last five to ten years. Is that what you're seeing in all your research?
Dr. Anderson:	Yes. I would say that the biggest thing that we've seen is, uh, a coming together of really two things. One is a, a little bit more acceptance by the standard oncology community that, you know, maybe we should be looking at other things. Doesn't mean that they're embracing everything—
Dr. Stengler:	Yeah—
Dr. Anderson:	But it means that, well, you know, we know what we know, and maybe there's other things we should know. So there's that, and then, uh, there are things such as a, a research project I was involved with uh, that, uh, will probably get to in a moment, but um, that the National Institute of Health funded to help, um, just see, you know, does any of this stuff actually work?
	You know, they really just, they, they have all this anecdotal evidence for years and decades. So, um, I think that the coming together of the standard oncology community saying maybe—
	Maybe we should look at some of these things, and then some research money available to look at some certain therapies or certain ways of doing oncology. That together, I think, starting about ten years ago, really in a sense exploded what went on with integrative oncology.
	Um, there's certainly much more to do, much more to learn, but I, I think it's those two things coming together.
Dr. Stengler:	Well, the good thing about you, you've been involved from both levels and still are. You know, you see patients, you've seen patients for many years, but you go to the next step, and have proven a lot of these therapies with well designed studies, and to get acceptance into the mainstream medical

community, we gotta have those studies, so we need people like you doing those.

So tell us more about, uh, one of the studies you're involved with. I think you're alluding to maybe the *[unintelligible]* did, you did with Bastyr, um, Center, but tell the viewers about that.

Dr. Anderson: Sure, the, um, original study that I was involved with was through Bastyr University in, in uh, Seattle Washington, and it was called, uh, Bastyr Integrative Oncology Research Center, so we shortened it to BIORC, which is a funny name, but that's what we were.

And the National Institute of Health through our collaboration actually, which was very, very important, with the Seattle Cancer Care Alliance, which includes University of Washington and Fred Hutchinson Cancer Research, etcetera, uh, we had two, uh, pr-principal investigators, PIs. One was from Bastyr University, uh, and one was from the Fred Hutchinson Center.

And so, it was truly a collaborative effort. And I think initially, um, eh, so the NIH funded it, for us to do this, uh, patient centered, so it wasn't in petri dishes. It was with real—

Dr. Stengler: Yeah.

Dr. Anderson: People with cancer. Um, and they funded it—I, I think just thinking, well, we have no idea what will happen here. You know, this could be a total bust or it could show us something. And uh, so—

I became involved with that in the very early stages of it, and the reason that I became involved was that they wanted to add intravenous therapies, and that was a specialty of mine from before. And so, we, uh, collaborated, the principal investigators and myself, and we set up an actual, uh, cancer IV research center, on top of the, the rest of it.

So, one of our goals in that was to see just from the point of view of survival, if you did integrative oncology vs. you just did standard oncology. And you matched the groups, between the, the same type of cancer and the same basic gender, age, etcetera, and integrative oncology, same cancer, same basic age, was there any survival difference that we saw. Did people actually live longer if they did integrative oncology?

Dr. Stengler: Right.

Dr. Anderson: And it was a good place to start, really. W-what happened, as often happens with research is when we added in the IV therapy center—

Um, that was added onto a very well integrated s-system, so we had naturopathic doctors, we had, uh, acupuncturists, we had nutrition, we had mind, body, uh, psychiatry people, we had a little bit of everything available to people.

And then the IV therapies were offered to people who had, uh, uh, stage four, so the highest stage of cancer possible. And through that, we started with sort of one or two therapies, and then we were able to expand them over time, and I know we'll talk later about the specifics of that, but that was a very exciting time, because we were actually able to track people and their lifespan and outcome through that.

So, it was very important, I believe.

Dr. Stengler: Oh, absolutely. So, if you had to summarize the outcome of that study, it was quite a landmark study, go ahead and summarize that.

Dr. Anderson: So, I can kinda summarize what, what we saw over that time. Um, looking at match data from, uh, well, the best match data we could use would be the SEER, which is a long acronym, but—uh, so SEER later would be standard oncology outcomes, for say, a stage four cancer patient with colon cancer.

Dr. Stengler: Right.

Dr. Anderson: And they would tend to live a certain amount of time after diagnosis with standard therapy. And they, they have thousands, tens of thousands sometimes of data points, so they're pretty good data to look at.

We had smaller numbers, but we would take and say, "Okay, let's say we had a colon cancer patient, and they did the standard of care—

But they wanted to do integrative oncology, would they live longer or not? In some of the cases, such as certain breast cancer cases, uh, ovarian cancer cases, colon cancer, and then there's a few others that we looked at, as well, uh, matching it to that SEER data, we actually have, uh, longer lifespans, and in some cases, much longer lifespans by adding integrative oncology.

And I think that this actually surprised the, uh, people, uh, who were funding the studies. See, I don't think they really thought that we were gonna come up with anything good.

Dr. Stengler: Yeah.

Dr. Anderson: What was the, uh, general response from the mainstream medical community, just a lot of surprise.

But what was the kind of feedback you got?

As you know, working with, you know, any other doctors, doesn't matter what kind of doctor it is, uh, you know, we all, we all have our ideas and our biases, and all that. In oncology, we—what we found because we're working with university-based doctors and people in, you know, very deep research, uh, in cancer, there was the normal spread that we usually see, all the way from very unaccepting, to you know, thinking that there, there can't be anything right here, I don't want to spend patients to you. I think this is all just, you know, uh, not good.

To people with mildly open minds who said, "You know, I'll send a couple of patients, and if, if you don't harm them, maybe I'll send you some more." Uh, all the way over to, you know, one that—I actually saved the e-mail, because it—I, I never thought I'd get an e-mail like this.

They were very skeptical, and they were, uh, at the university, and the medical oncologist, and they, they actually—

Had kept e-mailing me about, "Well, what about, you know, you're gonna do this IV therapy with my patient, and they're on this chemotherapy. That really worries"—you know, for good reason. And I would send back, and I would send research, and I would say, "Well, for that chemotherapy, you know, the only research is positive. Did you know this research existed?"

They'd often not respond, and then they'd send the patient, but I sent the research. After about the third or fourth time, they said, "Well, do you have this summarized anywhere?" And, and I said, "Well, no, but I can," and so I put it together in a long summary, which we eventually published.

And I sent it to them, and they, the e-mail back from this very high place medical oncologist was, "This data's overwhelming. I didn't know any of it existed, and I am now—feel very safe sending patients to you." So, we, we actually had a lot of patients from certain oncologists.

Dr. Stengler: Now, with doctors like ourselves trained in both types of medicine, conventional medicine, lab tests, and diagnosis, and physical exams and all that—

And then also, with the training in holistic medicine, nutrition, or *[unintelligible]* medicine, IV therapy, all these types of things. Let's tell the viewers a little bit more about the differences and similarities with conventional oncology and the way we do things holistically. Often, I—we talk about in our book about the reductionist approach to conventional oncology vs. more the holistic approach. Could you expand on that for the people?

Dr. Anderson: Yeah, I think, um, kinda boiling that down, the—if you look at modern, let's just say modern North American medicine, which is pretty much all about the same, it became reductionist, uh, in a way to find the best answer as quickly as possible to the problem, you know, because you go back, you know, 80, 100 years, you, you have lots of people dying from pneumonia, or you know, other—

Other, other things that not many people die from nowadays—

Dr. Stengler: Yeah.

Dr. Anderson: So, the reductionist approach would say, "Well, let's just find what causes pneumonia, and what we can kill pneumonia with." You know, and that's great. That is perfect, right?

Dr. Stengler: Yeah, has its place.

Dr. Anderson: It's, uh, it, it really works well, you know, if you, if you have an overwhelming strep infection or something, there's great ways to shut that down, and that, that's what, that's where the reductionist approach works.

And, and I would say probably in your and my practice, if we have somebody who's going to die of something, we would do the same thing, right?

Dr. Stengler: Right, sure.

Dr. Anderson: You know, That's what we do, right? Uh, so it's not that there's a war between the two things. It's just that the, the view is different based on what type of a problem the person has. When you get to more of a multifactoral, integrated disease or, uh, disorder, a reductionist approach will get you to one answer for one piece, that doesn't address anything else that's wrong with them.

And I think that the hope, um—

Uh, in fact I, you know, if you read back into any of the history, the hope in cancer was it was more like pneumonia, you know, where if we could just find one answer or one thing to kill it, it, we would be great, right?

Dr. Stengler: Yeah.

Dr. Anderson: Uh, and then, what they say is it's—this is a very, very complex problem, and it affects all the body parts differently, and it, you know, at one stage, it does one thing, and the other—so I think reductionism in that sense, it's great for designing specific drugs, but we all know specific drugs don't cure cancer.

So, a more integrative approach, or what we might call holistic, etcetera, the idea there is we honor the reductionistic point of view to find the little bitty answers, and then we take a step back, and say, "What's gonna be the best thing to treat all the other pieces of the patient that aren't getting treated?" Because as we know, you know, a strep throat, most of the time, you can cure with an antibiotic. Cancer, for the most part, you're not gonna cure with one therapy. There's lots of other things that need to be involved.

Dr. Stengler: Right—

Dr. Anderson: Yeah.

Dr. Stengler: So, in the holistic model, for example, um, we wanna help the immune system, and that can involve the gut, it can involve psychological factors, it can involve nutrients you may be low in. Uh, toxins you've been exposed to—

Dr. Anderson: Right.

Dr. Stengler: So there's just so many factors that could set up the environment for cancer—

Dr. Anderson: Right.

Dr. Stengler: And so, it makes sense, and what we're finding is a more holistic approach in general—

Dr. Anderson: Mm-hmm.

Dr. Stengler: You're gonna get better results.

Dr. Anderson: True.

Dr. Stengler: Um, and like you said, there are certain cancers where just kind of a one-focus treatment could work well, but in general, it usually takes more than that. Um, one of the good things we're finding out about, uh, the integrative approach, and the mindset, more the philosophy, I'd say, would be this quality of life issue.

Dr. Anderson: Mm-hmm.

Dr. Stengler: You know, there's certainly a lot of people out there now who have cancer, and it's being managed as a chronic disease, and so, quality of life in recent years has become more important, even in conventional oncology, as well, I think.

Dr. Anderson: Yes. Very much.

Dr. Stengler: And uh, we, we place a very high priority on that, in integrative oncology. Why don't you speak to that?

Dr. Anderson: Yeah, I think—and I, I do think that's something that, as we're having a discussion a minute ago about, you know, the sort of the two world views of reductionism vs. integrative, it-it's—it's not—I think now, and you and I have both practiced long enough to kind of see an evolution of the thinking around this.

Uh, you know, I think 15, 20 years ago, it, it was more of a very focused kind of reductionistic thing, and if you lived long enough to worry about quality of life, then they would, you know, and I think back in those days, probably you and I both got those referrals of, "Okay, well, you don't appear to have cancer anymore. We don't have any idea what to do with you now. Go to, go see one of these guys."

Dr. Stengler: Yeah.

Dr. Anderson: Uh, so that's kinda how we got our start. Um, I think that the idea now is as, as you mentioned, dealing with cancer as a chronic illness, as opposed to a death sentence.

And in many cases, by having a true integrative approach, where maybe there is a very useful, surgical procedure, or a very useful, focused radiation procedure, or a very useful, you know, focused chemotherapy, it's gonna do it's piece. But the whole rest of the person has to be taken care of.

Dr. Stengler: Yeah.

Dr. Anderson: So, having the ability to then step back and say, "Okay, well, what is it that would make your quality of life as excellent as possible, and also, potentially, keep the cancer from going anywhere, right?"

Dr. Stengler: Mm-hmm.

Dr. Anderson: So, then it's truly treating you like a chronic disease, and as you said, you know, that involves everybody's system, every part, you know, and, and sometimes, you know, even e-extending to the, to the family, and the, you know, the interactions with friends, and work, and everything else. You know.

Dr. Stengler:	Right.
Dr. Anderson:	And it goes pretty far.
Dr. Stengler:	Right.
Dr. Anderson:	So, I think that, um, that has been the thing that, uh, if-if you want to look at it as the more traditional oncology world, and then the integrative oncology world, that's been one of the places where, where we're meeting more, more, I think quickly, because there's a realization that, wow, you know, if I'm a medical oncologist, I'm-I'm really, really good at—
	At, uh, chemotherapy administration, etcetera. But I might not be that great at, you know, what do I do to fix your immune system after I give you the chemotherapy? I might not be so great about—
Dr. Stengler:	Right.
Dr. Anderson:	You know, gee, you have all these digestive problems, wha-what do I do about that? You know? And even in that literature, in that end of uh, oncology now, they're, they're writing more and more about it. You know, it'll take decades before they catch up, but still—
Dr. Stengler:	Yeah.
Dr. Anderson:	You know, so I think in the world of integrative oncology, the—one of the biggest benefits is that we can bridge that gap, when people don't have to wait a generation or two for everyone to learn how to do it.
Dr. Stengler:	We've got several modules coming up with you on these different, you know, areas of integrative oncology. Um, everyone's aware of the traditional, conventional therapies, chemotherapy, radiation surgery, and, and some other ones. Um, let's give the viewers a flavor of all the different tools that we have to help enhance the immune system, help to fight the cancer—
	Help to improve the quality of life. Give some of the categories of the different, you know, methods—
Dr. Anderson:	Sure.

Dr. Stengler:	You and I use in practice.
Dr. Anderson:	Sure. Yeah, I think that one of the most exciting things, and this is actually something that drew me to, uh, uh, when I kinda made that shift from being in the regular, medical system to looking at finishing medical school in a little more standard medical school, or becoming a naturopathic medical doctor, I like the idea of having more tools, and you know, back then, 25 or more years ago, there, there, there were very strict limits on what the standard medical doctor could do.
Dr. Stengler:	Yeah.
Dr. Anderson:	So, uh, and, and you and I maybe had the same experience, but what that led to was in the world of oncology, it allows us to have the training and background and experience to deal with things such as—one of the things I think is the most important is, is your digestive system. Because we think of it as, okay, it processes food—
	That goes through. But really, large portions of your immune system live in your digestive system. Large portions of your nervous system live there. It, it's, it's so critical, and it's always been treated, I think, you know, not as, uh, doesn't get as much respect as it deserves.
Dr. Stengler:	Yeah.
Dr. Anderson:	And that's an area that we work very hard with people with cancer on. So, that, that's one big area. And digestive can be anything from the, the diet that you eat to, um, maybe even the way that your foods are prepared.
Dr. Stengler:	Mm-hmm.
Dr. Anderson:	To, um, things that boost immunity in the gut or heal it after certain therapies, etcetera. So, diet and nutrition is probably the biggest core that we have.
Dr. Stengler:	Yeah.
Dr. Anderson:	Um, the other thing that I have found, and I think we've learned, you know, more in the last ten years than we did in the previous 15 or 20, is there's just more and more

interest around the world in studying some of the natural agents that would help immunity or healing—

Dr. Stengler: Yeah.

Dr. Anderson: So, I think that the ability to use some of these natural plant medicines that can, uh, do much more broad, uh, benefit and effect in a pa- in a patient is really a benefit to us.

So, you know, once you stu—kinda get the patient involved in the, the digestive system's so important, and it might take a lot but we're—

Gonna get that healed up and working, and then using some of the plant medicines—

Dr. Stengler: Mm-hmm.

Dr. Anderson: And some, some of the more, I think, basic things, you know, like uh, diet and nutrient therapy, so beyond what you eat, we, we may add nutrients and, and we might do that orally, we might do that, uh, through intravenous therapy, we might do it through any number of things.

Dr. Stengler: Right.

Dr. Anderson: And then there's other, um, I think, you know, some people call them, say modality, or, or technical things. Uh, which will actually be kinda showing some things from our clinics, but uh, hyperbaric oxygen therapy, which you know, used to be considered, "Oh, you can't ever do that in cancer," and now, you know the more we learn, the more we learn if you do it correctly, it's actually a benefit in cancer and healing, uh, hyperthermia, healing, literally heating people up.

Dr. Stengler: Yeah.

Dr. Anderson: It's uh, you know, it's, it's, it's a really wonderful way to get the, the body, the chemistry and the immune system back involved in, you know, fighting and healing.

And I, I think that's another thing that, you know, our, um, our conventional colleagues understand, but they're just, they're trying to find a way into, and that is they know that, you know, when you give certain chemotherapies that actually shuts off a lot of immune function, and so they would like it to turn back on afterwards.

Dr. Stengler: Right.

Dr. Anderson: Getting it to turn on is, has always been the big question mark. So these things, like, uh, hyperthermia, and hyperbaric oxygen, and some of the intravenous therapies, and some of the oral things. And actually, uh, simply, although never easy, healing the gut, and getting the digestive system working is, is huge.

Dr. Stengler: Uh, Dr. Anderson, maybe just in the remaining minute or two here, is there a case example or two you'd like to share with the viewers, um—

You know, in the series, we're giving people hope, but we're giving them, you know, real hope. So, any cases that come to mind for you recently?

Dr. Anderson: Mm-hmm.

Dr. Stengler: Yes, I think that, um, the, there's, uh, there's probably so many that I, you know, that I could share. One is, uh, a lady, and we actually write about here in the introduction to the book, um, who came into the research center, actually, and so this was a number of years ago.

And, uh, she was, uh, diagnosed, uh, they thought she had just a, um, a, a non-cancerous problem in her abdomen. They went in, uh, with a scope, and were gonna just do a quick surgery and send her home—

And you're gonna be all better. So, imagine going under anesthesia, thinking that—

Dr. Stengler: Yeah.

Dr. Anderson: She wakes up to the news, "Well, we got in there, and it wasn't what we thought. It was—there was cancer everywhere." Right?

Dr. Stengler: Mm-hmm.

Dr. Anderson: Uh, which, it—and I met her not long after this happened, and that was just not the news she was looking for, and she was about 84, turning 85. Um, and uh, so they said, "Well," and, and we see this all the time, which is very reasonable, "Here's the problem. You're 84, 85 years old, we can give you chemotherapy, but it would kill you. You know, that just would not be a good idea for usto do that."

And it, and there was too much cancer, that sur-surgery wasn't gonna be an option. It was just too, too far gone. And uh, so, she said, "Well, what do I do?" And they said, "Well, you know, go, uh, you know, you've lived a long time, go get your affairs in order and all those things." This really didn't make her happy at all, right? And her, her daughter and her were sitting there—

Listening to all this. So, she went back to a different doctor, and they said, "Well, no, really we can't treat you. There's, there's no good treatments." Um, and so, she, she was very persistent. You know, you don't live 84, 85 years without being a bit persistent, and uh, and she was actually in quite good health up to that point.

And she kept pushing, and so finally, they said, "Well, there's this research project going on, and there—I don't know what they're doing there, and it's, it's, it's integrative oncology, and so I don't know, you know. Uh, but maybe they can do something for you, 'cause it, they say that what they're doing is low toxicity and all this."

So, she came in, we talked to her, and we said, "Yeah, we, you know, we, we don't know if we can help you, but uh, this is what we're going to do," and um, she was traveling from, you know, moderate distance, so we, we couldn't have her come in every day in that, in that setting, we actually had a really nice thing, if you could come in three or four days a week, you could get acupuncture every day, and all this other stuff.

Dr. Stengler:	Oh, okay.
Dr. Anderson:	She, we—she just couldn't do that. It was too far away. So, we set up, uh, IV therapy with her, um, that was one of our original IV therapies we were doing, which happened at that time, for her, it was high dose vitamin C. We did

all the testing to see if it would be appropriate, and it was, and safe, and so we started working with her.

About three weeks in, um, and we have a lot of abdominal cancer. There's, there's particular signs that the person knows when it's active. Um, about three weeks in, she says, "You know, I might be making this up. I'm feeling better, and I can eat now. And I wasn't able to eat before. I was throwing up."

And I said, "Well, maybe that's in your mind, maybe not." You know, and so, I said, "Let's keep going a few more weeks." And so, she kept going, and she about six weeks in, she says, you know, "I don't have any trouble digesting and I feel better than I felt the last two years."

And you know, she's telling me all this, and meanwhile, her primary care doctor had said, "Well, you know, you're probably—

"Not gonna make your next birthday." Right, it's, I mean, 'cause she did have a lot of cancer, to be fair.

Dr. Stengler: Yeah.

Dr. Anderson: And, uh, so she just kept getting healthier and, and we adjusted her dose and her timing and all of this, and, and then um, I was gone, uh, out teaching somewhere, and she saw a colleague, and the colleague said, "Well, you're doing so good, just stop." Okay. So, she stopped, and she called me about three or four weeks later, and she says, "All of my symptoms are back."

And I said, "Well, I know, it's 'cause we haven't seen you." She said, "Well, they told me to stop." I said, "Well, maybe that wasn't the right idea." So I said, "Come back in," and so, we, we worked with her, and about three weeks in, all of her symptoms were gone again.

So, we were, we were so, both impressed but also intellectually curious. We sent her back to get more imaging, so *[unintelligible]* one image. And the interesting thing was the imaging didn't change at all. There was still the same amount of cancer—

Dr. Stengler:	Okay.
Dr. Anderson:	Just didn't have any symptoms from it. And, um—
	So, we, we adjusted her therapy over time, and spread it out to kind of a maintenance, you know, once you get a good effect, if it, if the therapy's—
Dr. Stengler:	Right.
Dr. Anderson:	Working, get maintenance. And uh, so she, uh, she would call her doctor every year on her birthday, and say, "Well, I made another birthday," you know. So, so she was about 85 when I first met her. Um, she celebrated her 90th birthday in our office, and she had, that was the only thing she was doing. She would come in once every about five weeks for an IV.
	She had absolutely no signs or symptoms from the cancer. Um, and I, I spoke to her on the phone a while back, and she's 93, and she's still with us, and she's, she's quite, you know, mentally clear, everything, and she, she will pass away from something—
Dr. Stengler:	Yeah.
Dr. Anderson:	But it hasn't been cancer yet. So, she, she was sort of a, she got a lot of people's attention, uh, because it was the, it was literally the only thing we did, and she, it was not appropriate for her to have chemotherapy or—
Dr. Stengler:	Right.
Dr. Anderson:	So—
	It was a sort of, this is an experiment with one variable, you know, and it worked great. So, she was sort of on one end of the spectrum, and, and uh, and still is, actually on that end of the spectrum.
Dr. Stengler:	Yep. Well, this has been great information with Dr. Anderson on integrative oncology, And so, Dr. Anderson, thank you, that was really good, inspiring.
Dr. Anderson:	Thank you.

THE DANGERS OF "BETTY CROCKER TEXTBOOK" ONCOLOGY

— DR. JAMES FORSYTHE —

Dr. Stengler: Well, hi, everyone! I'm really excited today. I'm here in Reno, Nevada, with the most well-known integrative oncologist in America, probably the world: Dr. James Forsythe. And we're gonna talk about his experience in treating tens and tens of thousands of patients with a variety of different types of cancers using integrative oncology, which this series is all about. So Dr. Forsythe, so great to have you—

Dr. Forsythe: Thank you, Mark.

Dr. Stengler: —on the show.

Dr. Forsythe: It's a pleasure being with you.

Dr. Stengler: And you've got a beautiful clinic here.

Dr. Forsythe: Thank you.

Dr. Stengler: Outstanding! And so we want to get into integrative cancer treatment with you today, of course, being you're the premier expert, in my opinion. But tell us a bit more about your background. I mean, you're a very interesting guy. You're a medical oncologist. You're Board Certified in Internal Medicine.

Dr. Forsythe:	Yes.
Dr. Stengler:	You're Certified in Homeopathy. I mean, I don't know of anyone else has those types of credentials and, of course, decades and decades of experience. So, yeah, tell us more about your background.

*All right, Mark. Thank you. Well, I grew up in Michigan.

I was really raised pretty much by a single parent, and in those days there wasn't much support on her, and so we were pretty much on the poor list. We did live in Chicago for a while, and Massachusetts, and then we moved to California. My dad was a stock broker, but he was out of the picture at that time. But I did my schooling in Hollywood. And one of the high points of my high school career was playing tennis with Ricky Nelson. So we were on the championship tennis team.

But I got a full scholarship to U.C. Berkeley and was a premed student, and I went through four years with a 3.6 grade point average at Berkeley in physiology/biochemistry. And they were nice enough to give me a full-ride scholarship for my first year of medical school. And then I went to UCSF across the Bay from Berkeley and spent four years there.

But in my senior year, Mark, I ran out of money, and the Dean's Office called me in, and they said, "You're not gonna make it. Did you think about maybe going into a Ph.D. program or something else? But your funds don't look like they're gonna carry you through." So I said, "Well, let me think about that. Let me try some other avenues." So I joined the Army, and I was the only one in my class, believe it or not, in 1963 and '64 to join the Army.

The Army was nice enough, they paid for all my debts. They paid me as a Second Lieutenant. But I did owe them five years for all that niceties. And so fortunately, they put me in an internship on the Presidio, and beautiful area: Letterman Army Hospital at the time, rotating internship. And then the Vietnam War was starting up, and I said, "I really don't wanna go over there. I don't even really know where it is."

So I said, "I think I'll be a pathologist for—it's good training for any subspecialty really, and it gets—that's more schooling for me." So I went into a pathology residency at Tripler Army Hospital in Hawaii for several years, became a pathologist, and then I was transferred to the 82nd Airborne site in Fayetteville, North Carolina, home of Fort Bragg, and there was Chief of Pathology at the hospital, and with the Airborne unit—the Special Forces Unit.

From there, I got shipped to Vietnam in 1969, Mark, and in Vietnam, I was the Head Forensic Pathologist of the country and also the Head of Tropical Medicine; set up four labs throughout the country mainly diagnosing all the cases of malaria in our troops and trying to do prophylactic prevention as well. When I got back, I decided, you know, I'm not really a pathologist at heart. I like people medicine.

So I went into an internal medicine residency in San Francisco Children's Hospital and got my degree in Internal Medicine.

And then from there went directly into an oncology fellowship, which was a new subspecialty of internal medicine at the time. I had never really heard the word that much. And there were only a few drugs out there, and they hadn't even started their boards yet when I went into my fellowship. Anyway, spent two years in my fellowship, and then graduated with a degree in Medical Oncology. And from there, Mark, I practiced in San Francisco for a few years, said, "This isn't for me"—the bridges, living in Marin County, doing eight hospitals—I said, "I'm gonna die by the time I'm 50 if I keep this up."

So we had a place at Tahoe, and I loved Reno. It's a small town. They had no oncologist, and so I've been here for actually 44 years, believe it or not.

Dr. Stengler: Wow.

Dr. Forsythe: And most of the time, Mark, I was doing straight conventional oncology—textbook oncology; we call it sometimes "Betty Crocker Textbook"—and it's a guessing game, Mark. I found that out after many years that, although well-meaning, most oncologists are guessing every time they prescribe a set of drugs. They don't really know. But thanks to the Human Genome Project, we now are able to know what we're giving and have accuracy.

You know, by the early '90s, I was starting to see long-term results that really weren't very favorable. We were seeing patients—a five-year survival rate was not that great. I couldn't believe it. So I start—began reading articles in the alternative and conventional literature and seeing that this was the case throughout the country in oncology where the survival rates were two percent.

And a large study came out in the *Clinical Journal of Oncology* in '04, one of their main journals, Mark, that showed in America a five-year study of over 150,000 patients—a retrospective study—

Dr. Stengler: A large study—yeah.

Dr. Forsythe: —that showed a 2.1 percent survival. I said, "What the—

Dr. Stengler: Oh, it's crazy, huh?

Dr. Forsythe: "What baseball manager would hire a batter with a two percent batting average?" That's not very good.

Dr. Stengler: You get better results with placebos, right?

Dr. Forsythe: And in Australia a parallel study was 2.3, so very similar statistics. So it was an accurate study, and the Australian study I believe had about 70,000 patients. So I said, "I gotta do"—because in Nevada, we are fortunate to have naturopathic boards and homeopathic boards. I said, "In order for me to do what I wanna do with natural therapies, I'd have to be boarded in that subspecialty," and then the medical boards would leave you alone.

Because a conventional doctor really can't give natural therapies.

Dr. Stengler: Yeah, they've got standards of care, drugs and surgery they're pretty much *[unintelligible]* that model.

Dr. Forsythe: Yeah, and it just doesn't work with their boards. So I did train at the British Institute of Homeopathy, and in a couple years I got my boards, and then I was off and flying. So since the year 2000, I've done about four outcome-based studies. This is survivalship studies, Stage 4 cancers, adults only—that means over 16 years of age—all types of cancer—blood diseases, solid tumors and so on—all takers—in other words, anyone—and my first study was for Nature's Sunshine out of Utah, and I did the Paw Paw study, which is a product from the Paw Paw tree, indigenous to the southeastern United States. And that came out favorable, and it's being used worldwide now, as you probably know, Mark.

Dr. Stengler: Now, take us through. So someone comes to your clinic. Obviously, you talk to them, get their history. Take us through the testing and then the treatments. Because like you said, the best way for medicine, no matter what your field, is to be specific to the individual. Everyone is a little bit different—their genetics and everything else.

Dr. Forsythe: Right—it's not one-size-fits-all.

Dr. Stengler: Exactly—so take us through that—those steps that make it so successful.

Dr. Forsythe: The AMA and the FDA would like to have one-size-fits-all. Makes it easier—the Kaiser System—where you take Betty Crocker off the rack and you follow the menu. Same for breast cancer adjuvant therapy. Remember, they're gonna get three drugs: they're gonna get a taxane, an alkylator like Cytoxan, and a taxane, taxotere Taxol. So it's for everyone, and no matter—they have no—they're guessing, and they're well-meaning. They really do wanna help that patient, Mark.

But they're not using the most advanced science to do it.

Dr. Stengler: So as an oncologist, though—this is very important. As an oncologist, you want to use science. You want to be evidence-driven.

Dr. Forsythe: Yes.

Dr. Stengler: There's a lot of unscientific things going on in oncology today, not necessarily in a sinister way—people are intentionally doing that—they're just kind of tunnel-vision and locked into a system. Is that an accurate assessment?

Dr. Forsythe:	Yes, it is.
Dr. Stengler:	Okay.
Dr. Forsythe:	And they're rushing a lot of these targeted agents out before they even know what all the toxicities are. You know, like Avastin, when it came out—or Bevacizumab, when it came out it was only prolonging life three months, Mark, and it cost $8,000 for a single bag every two to three weeks.
Dr. Stengler:	But the media reports were, "This is a breakthrough!"
Dr. Forsythe:	It was—it was a miracle drug! I mean, three months—really? $8,000 a bag—maybe I'll just go on that cruise instead, you know. It didn't make sense.
	But when you have—when you have the genes telling me what to do—because I always tell patients, Mark, "If I give you the wrong drug, I'm actually hurting you. I'm speeding up your demise." I don't like to say that to patients, but I said, "It's the truth." And you've seen patients, and I have many— in fact, I had a financial advisor recently that had neck cancer presenting just with a mass in his periclavicular area that was talked into going to UCLA, almost came to our treatment, but his—they gave him the million-dollar sell at UCLA. He died during the first cycle of chemotherapy at 60—age 60.
Dr. Stengler:	Yeah—so with your treatment, people come in, and then you're doing the testing.
Dr. Forsythe:	Yes.
Dr. Stengler:	Tell us about that and then take us through the treatments.
Dr. Forsythe:	So the testing basically is something—we take the blood. We're looking for circulating tumor cells, CTCs—has many names: it has genomic testing, DNA testing, gene testing, chemosensitivity testing, liquid biopsy, precision medicine, tailor-made medicine, the list goes on.
	There's about ten different names, Mark. And basically they're all true, but we prefer "chemosensitivity testing," because that's—it's like bacterial testing. If you had a bronchitis or a sinusitis, I would be culturing your sputum or your drainage to see what antibiotics work for you.

Dr. Stengler: But your—now your testing is unique though in that you're testing chemotherapy agents, you're testing natural agents.

Dr. Forsythe: Right, when the blood gets two degrees, it's good for first of all—when it leaves your arm mark it's good for 96 hours. Even if it arrived in Greece at midnight, they start working on it. Now, they are able to extract the cancer cells from the blood, put them into media in incubators and grow a plate of Mark's cancer. Your cancer is on that plate. And I'm a pathologist by training, but this is way above my pay scale.

This is very high-tech technology—laboratory technology. So once they have the cancer grown on the plate, then they tear it apart looking for your DNA, and your DNA is gonna tell them those four things: what drugs are best, target cells are best, and the supplements, which none of the American labs do, and what hormone, for hormone-driven tumors, are available for, and that would mean mainly blockers for your prostate cancer, let's say.

So all those four things are like handing you a blueprint or roadmap, as I said, that you hadn't had before. So you know I can guarantee you that what I'm giving you is all gonna work to a degree. Now, the drugs that come up, we never find a drug greater than 83 percent effective. That's the limit. And it will get better with time, but that's what we have to deal with now. That's the state-of-the-art now.

No perfect drug out there, in other words, Mark. But if we get two 80s, and then we have all the supplements—there may be 20 that come up for you—that combination, that calculus is determined by the University of Utah Math Department that we presented this idea to, to be over 95 percent effective in putting you in a good remission.

Dr. Stengler: So the synergistic effect, obviously.

Dr. Forsythe: The synergistic effect of all that ammunition going on the target. Now, I tell patients, "You know when the Seals team went after Osama Bin Laden, they not only had their helicopter gun ships and their rocket grenades, their stun grenades, their M-15s, their .45 pistols, everything with them, and if they failed a cruise missile ship was waiting

	offshore, and they were all gonna be gone, because they weren't gonna come back with that building still there. You know what I mean?
Dr. Stengler:	Yeah.
Dr. Forsythe:	So they—luckily they got him.
Dr. Stengler:	So—and you've been doing this for how many years now? And how many patients approximately do you think you've treated?
Dr. Forsythe:	I'm not a young man, Mark. I have to tell you that. I'm sorry. I've been doing in Reno for 44 years, but before that I was a pathologist.
Dr. Stengler:	And how many patients do you think you estimate you've treated?
Dr. Forsythe:	Several hundred thousand.
Dr. Stengler:	Wow, that's amazing. So in medicine, often our biggest advancements discoveries have been with mavericks. You know, I think of like just one classic example, Louis Pasteur in the 1860s showing what we call the Law of Biogenesis: life comes from life. You don't get life from nonlife, which at that time was very controversial, and people thought that could happen, so he disproved that. And he was ridiculed and obviously proven to be true. Now, let's take your situation. You'd be considered a maverick in oncology, I presume.
	(A) Would you agree with that? And (B) tell us maybe about a recent incident you had just trying to get the information out to a local hospital trying to help more people.
Dr. Forsythe:	This is a true story and happened recently. I went to the major hospital here in Northern Nevada to present my data to IS, and I said, "All I wanna do is tell your staff what I do." I was—been on the staff for over 40 years, not a blemish on my record, the head of many committees, no malpractice actions, no disciplinary action of any kind. So I showed them all my work with 1,250 patients. I showed them my survival rates.
	They looked at me, and they said, "This is amazing you did all this as a single person. It's hard for us to believe you

really did all this." But they said, "You know, our cancer institute is the engine that drives this hospital financially. Why would we wanna change anything we do?"

I said, "I got it. I do get it. Thank you." So so much for letting me know that. Hasta la vista! I left and basically it hit the newspapers because it was too good to let go. And they did publish it in the local newspapers that this is how—they weren't interested in improved survivals. They weren't interested in less toxicity. They weren't interested in the fact that it could be used safer on children's cancers. None of that. It was just that, "Leave us alone. We're making lots of money doing what we're doing. We don't wanna change."

Dr. Stengler: Sad.

Dr. Forsythe: Yep, pretty sad.

Dr. Stengler: Very sad.

Dr. Forsythe: Pretty cynical, and I tell this story because it is true.

Dr. Stengler: Well, you know what? This has been phenomenal information for our viewers. And I wanna thank you for just the tens of thousands of people you've helped, educating doctors around the country, like myself, so we can help people more effectively.

You know, you're the only one who's done it to this degree so far, and it's been a game-changer in helping people with integrative oncology. So thank you so much.

Dr. Forsythe: Thank you, Mark. It's been a pleasure.

Dr. Stengler: And what's the best website for our viewers out there to get more information, get help from you, get your books?

Dr. Forsythe: Well, we use info@DrForsythe.com, or EForsythe@SBC-Global.net.

Dr. Stengler: We'll put down a screen in DrForsythe.com. And again, thank you so much.

Dr. Forsythe: Thank you.

6 PROVEN WAYS TO BEAT CANCER

— DR. PATRICK QUILLIN —

Dr. Stengler: Well, hi, everyone. Glad to you have you back. I have a special interview today with Dr. Patrick Quillin, who I found out we're almost neighbors here in the San Diego area. And Dr. Quillin is highly experienced, highly trained in the field of nutrition and cancer. Uh, he's been around the world educating the public, educating doctors and professionals, and so it's great to have you with us today.

Dr. Quillin: It's a pleasure. Thank you for sharing your viewers.

Dr. Stengler: Now you've written many books on the subject.

Dr. Quillin: True.

Dr. Stengler: Perhaps the most well-known is this *Beating Cancer with Nutrition*, which I have had for years, excellent. Now it's sold, what, over half a million copies?

Dr. Quillin: Very, very true. Yes.

Dr. Stengler: Excellent, excellent. You've got some other ones. You've got, well, many, but here's another one, *The Wisdom and Healing Power of Whole Foods*, another great book. And for the professionals out there who are watching, we have a nice textbook on the subject, *Adjuvant Nutrition in Cancer Treatment*. So all great books to, uh, check out.

So, Dr. Quillin, maybe tell us about your background. Um,

especially when you started, nutrition and cancer, that really was pioneering work. It wasn't very common back when you got into this field.

Dr. Quillin: Uh, anyway, to make it very brief about my background, uh, um, as a child I was always interested in, "What makes it tick? What goes on inside here?" And as a child, uh, not out of maliciousness, but I just cut open a worm one rainy day. "What's inside here?" And I tried to do it delicately. The patient didn't survive, but I looked and learned a little bit about what's inside.

And, you know, doing—cutting up animals in our biology class was interesting. I took apart four watches four years in a row, much to my parents' dismay, trying to figure out, "What's in here? What makes it tick?"

And from that, uh, you know, I went into pre-medicine at Notre Dame, and from that moved into nutrition and earned my bachelor's, master's, and doctorate degrees in nutrition, a registered dietician, a certified nutrition specialist with the American College of Nutrition, um, fellow of the American College of Nutrition.

So all those degrees, for whatever they're worth. Taught college for eight years. Uh, worked at Scripps Clinic and La Costa Spa. Uh, was a grant reviewer for the National Institutes of Health Office of Alternative Medicine.

And then getting into the nitty-gritty of what did I do in nutrition and cancer, 1989 I joined Cancer Treatment Centers of America as their vice president of nutrition. And we—it was a team effort—put together a, uh, a great program, which was pioneering. Uh, in those days it was mind-blowing. Today it's still pioneering.

But it was using adjuvant, or helpful, nutrition as part of comprehensive cancer treatment. And up until then, 1989, people thought, "Well, it's nutrition or medicine." No, the two of them work well together. As a matter of fact, they— uh, synergism.

And so Dr. Stengler, I think of—they're rough numbers. One point six million Americans will be newly diagnosed with cancer this year. There are about 12 million cancer patients who are either in treatment or watchful waiting today. And most of them, I'm thinking 99 percent, feel like you have to choose one or the another: "Nutrition or my oncologist, who says chemo, radiation, and surgery are my only options."

In fact, if you use those medical oncology principles with an aggressive nutrition program, everybody becomes more of a hero. And so too many patients are like a child in a child-custody battle. The father and mother are arguing over and criticizing each other. Let's work together.

Dr. Stengler: Right.

Dr. Quillin: And so 1989 we said nutrition should be an integral component as part of comprehensive cancer treatment. It is not sufficient, but it is essential. That said, uh, we had—we organized three international symposia. These were Category 1 CME, continuing medical education, seminars in which we brought in the best and brightest around the world. Uh, we had, uh, 35 or 40 speakers at three different conferences. We had 400 to 500 attendees, most MDs and Ph.Ds.

And the soundbites were this. Number one, a well-nourished cancer patient can better manage the disease and the therapies. And that we can talk about in great length, but essentially if the patient is well nourished with food and supplements, they can better tolerate chemo and radiation and make it more of a selective toxin. There's the real rub. There's no doubt that chemo can kill cancer cells, and it sometimes kills the patient.

Dr. Stengler: Right.

Dr. Quillin: And radiation kills everything in its path, including the patient. What if you could make 'em more of a selective, uh, therapy, more of a, uh, a rifle rather than a hand grenade? And that's what nutrition does.

So, uh, over the course of three symposia, a textbook, my book, I think the, the, the groundswell movement, and the public is clamoring for it, is that, "I want my oncologist, my naturopath, my—all of my professionals working together. I don't want 'em arguing, and I want a team effort to show me how I can use nutrition to support my body," because here's the second soundbite.

And you learned this more than any of us in naturopathic medical college. A healthy human body is self-regulating and self-repairing.

Dr. Stengler: Mm-hmm.

Dr. Quillin: And this is so basic and obvious, you say, "Well, duh." But in fact, that's the essence of health, medicine, and healing, that if we're healthy—and the six major vectors that I have put together is nutrition; attitude; toxins; microbiome, the, uh, organisms in the gut; uh, energy alignment; and exercise.

Dr. Stengler: Mm-hmm.

Dr. Quillin: Those six major lifestyle factors create our body and make it healthy so that—the good news/bad news. Work done at the National Institutes of Health National Cancer Institute have found that the average adult gets six bouts of cancer in a lifetime. But only one-third of them will die from cancer, and today it's almost half will end up in a cancer institute, 42 percent.

So what about the other? They got cancer, but they beat it. Uh, what, what did they do? The body recognizes and destroys cancer. We have the immune system. We have DNA repair. We have collagen encapsulation. We have apoptosis and dozens of mechanisms in the body that know how to deal with cancer, recognize and destroy it, without a great deal of damage, collateral damage, as the oncologist will speak of.

Nutrition is an important part of that. It's not the only thing, as I said. It's one of six vectors, and we can go back through any of those as you would like.

Dr. Stengler: Okay, that's great. So as you said, you really were one of the pioneers in the field of integrative oncology, bringing especially the nutritional aspect in. Tell us about the mindset when you first started—I, I would presume you had a lot of resistance in the medical community—and how you've seen that change over the years, and how we need it to change a whole lot more.

Dr. Stengler:	Well, I give a lot of respect to oncologists. There's 10,000 board-certified oncologists in the United States, and then multiply that throughout the developed world. And they've got four years of college, four years of medical school, and four years of residency. And they're bright people, and they want to help people.

Unfortunately, their paradigm is in the complete opposite direction of nutrition.

Their thought is, "If I can give higher doses and longer cycles of an extremely toxic substance," and they'll tell the patient, "After you've had your IV of chemo, make sure that when you urinate, flush twice because the chemo that's left in your urine is so concentrated, it will kill all the microbes in the sewer system downstream."

If you spill chemo on a carpet, as I have seen in hospitals, you have to rope off the area because it's now an EPA—it's an Environmental Protection Agency toxic waste cleanup site. That's their therapy.

And so they're trained in, "How do we kill cancer with maximum sublethal chemotherapy?"

And then you and I come along and say, "And what if we nourish the patient at the same time?"

Dr. Stengler:	Right.
Dr. Quillin:	And that's the opposite of their paradigm. So it took a little rattling of cages. It took, uh, some education to bring some of them on board, and admittedly it's a minority. Of those 10,000, I'm guessing 90 percent of them are still oblivious or perhaps hostile towards nutrition in cancer.

And this is where this is a, um, a grassroots movement. The patients are driving this, not the FDA, not the AMA, not the ADA, none of those groups. The patients know enough, uh, through education, through programs like yours, through the Internet that they, they go to their oncologist and say, "What should I do with nutrition?"

The oncologist says, "Eat whatever you want." And hopefully they find another oncologist.

Dr. Stengler:	And that's a common theme I've seen with patients and the patients we've been interviewing for this series. So, yes.
Dr. Quillin:	So, uh, there is a dramatic, uh, education process that's going on in this country, and we're educating each other because, uh, I have found that, you know, among the many medical therapies, perhaps the most useful of all is pain management. Nutrition can only do so much. When you have a patient with stage VI bone cancer and the cancer is like a glass splint in their spine, you need some, uh, pain management, opioids probably.
Dr. Stengler:	Right.
Dr. Quillin:	Uh, and I'm a nutritionist, and I tell my patients, "Make sure you work with your pain management specialist." So I'm not against medicine. I'm involved in this integrative approach, and that's where we're gonna get the best outcome. For instance, there have been a number of studies that have looked at what happens if you take a patient who takes routine oncology, and then we're gonna compare that to routine oncology plus nutrition?
Dr. Stengler:	Mm-hmm.
Dr. Quillin:	Uh, there was a study done by Jaakkola and colleagues out of Europe in which they looked at, uh, uh, SEER data, Surveillance, Epidemiology, End Result, which means, "All right, we've had a couple hundred thousand patients with non-small cell lung cancer who have gone before you, and we have data gathered together.
	And here's the statistics, and here's the, uh, mean, median, and mode. And we're gonna take that and compare—we're gonna take our group, and we're gonna give them routine oncology plus nutrition, a decent diet and some decent supplements. Nothing extravagant, nothing exotic."
	And what they found is in routine oncology with lung cancer, you would expect one percent survival at 30 months. Two-and-a-half years later, one percent are still alive. In this group, six years later 44 percent were still alive. And what the oncologists noted was, uh, those patients who began integrative nutrition therapy earlier survived longer.

Dr. Stengler:	Mm-hmm.
Dr. Quillin:	Uh, what they said is there was no untoward effects in using nutrients along with chemo and radiation. So, um, there have been some brilliant docs, um, Charles Simone, a good friend, Chuck Simone. Got two children who are brilliant doctors.
	And they have written a, um, a review of the world's literature, and they looked at hundreds of studies with human cancer patients given nutrition and chemo and radiation and found no studies showing any neg—negative side effects.
	So the oncologist says—in their, their simplistic way of looking at things, they say, "All right, chemo is a pro-oxidant. Radiation is a pro-oxidant.
	Let's call it a minus one. And you come in with an antioxidant. Let's call it a plus one. And a minus one and a plus one equals zero, right?"
Dr. Stengler:	It neutralizes, right.
Dr. Quillin:	Right, that's their theory. However, cancer cells are very different than healthy cells. They are glycolytic, meaning they are obligate glucose metabolizers. They use a lot more sugar. They give off lactic acid as a byproduct of that obligate glucose metabolizer.
	And then they also—because they're anaerobic, they don't need antioxidants, the exception being vitamin C, and we'll come back to that, 'cause it becomes—now it becomes a selective anticancer agent because of the vitamin C.
	Anyway, you load up a patient with healthy doses of antioxidants, the healthy cells absorb those antioxidants. The cancer cells don't. And then you go in with pro-oxidative therapies, chemo and radiation, and now you're killing more cancer cells than healthy cells. Now the collateral damage is down significantly.
	So, uh, my theme is I'm not telling you either/or. I'm saying that when you find an oncologist who is intelligent enough to incorporate nutrition as part of their program, what I find fascinating, Dr. Stengler, is these oncologists, the few who will say, "All right, whatever you're doing, keep doing it.

Because you've—he's got a wait, waiting room with, uh 12 patients in there. Most of them look like death warmed over except one patient, who is following a good nutrition program.

And the oncologist says, "Just don't tell me. Just whatever you're doing, keep doing it." But they don't want to spread the good word because it's against—it's not a standard of care.

Dr. Stengler: Right.

Dr. Quillin: In oncology, if an oncologist gives nutrients, it's just not part of their practice, even though there's hundreds of studies to support it. So there are many reasons to incorporate nutrition as part of comprehensive cancer treatment, and we'll get to that.

Dr. Stengler: Yeah, that's great, and that seems to be one of the biggest problems, the myth that there is no science—there is not good research behind nutrition and cancer therapy. I mean, if you poll your average oncologist, they, they will tell you they're not aware of much good research.

Dr. Quillin: Yeah.

Dr. Stengler: Of course you've done a great job over the years letting the public and the health professionals know about this research. Uh, so it's really a myth. There's so much research now, it's just indisputable.

Dr. Quillin: Uh, I mentioned Dr. Charles Simone did a review article, hundreds of studies. Uh, Dr. Keith Block, another MD, did another review article, and he felt he was even more selective. So he said, "Well, if you criticize Simone's review, I'm gonna be even more selective."

And he reviewed the data, and it's beyond argument that nutrition improves outcome in cancer treatment. And so we're not talking about divorcing your oncologist. We're talking about augmenting, synergism, and making chemo more of a selective toxin.

Um, I have worked with so many patients over the 30 years, and so many of them have become the exception to the rule: someone who survives mesothelioma, someone who survives multiple myeloma. I'll give you an example.

Dr. Stengler:	Yes.
Dr. Quillin:	Um, the four big cancers are lung, colon, breast and prostate. So of the 200 different types of cancers that have been, uh, assessed and categorized by the oncologist, those are the four that comprise 75 percent of all cancers in America. Multiple myeloma is relatively rare, but it's also relatively lethal.
Dr. Stengler:	Mm-hmm.
Dr. Quillin:	Uh, it's a cancer of the bone marrow, myeloma, uh, and the body gives off abnormal cells from the bone marrow. Um, there was a—um, Michael Gearin-Tosh, uh, who was a professor at Oxford who was diagnosed with multiple myeloma, he was told by his oncologist, "Get your affairs in order. With my treatment, you might have a year."

He said, "That's not good enough." And so he did data gathering, fact gathering, and among the things he included, my book and some other good products. He didn't do any routine oncology, and he lived not six months, but 11 years.

Um, two patients that I worked with with multiple myeloma, one of them went through the whole routine. His oncologist said, "If you use any of this nutrition therapy, I won't treat you." And he died 18 months later. Awful story.

Parallel, and then we segue into the, the happy ending to this, another patient that I worked with where his oncologist said, "Do whatever you want. I'm your oncologist. Whatever you're doing outside of this office is up to you." And so we worked aggressively with food and supplements, and, uh, he lived 14 years, not 18 months.

So, uh, we don't talk about living forever. We don't talk about curing cancer. We talk about improving quality and quantity of life and chances for a complete remission.

And another study, um, Abram Hoffer, MD-Ph.D., worked with, uh, Linus Pauling, twice Nobel laureate. Could have had two more Nobel prizes. Uh, I, I got to meet the man, He was brilliant.

Dr. Stengler:	He gave a recommendation for your book in the past, yeah.

Dr. Quillin:	He did, yeah. Linus Pauling, brilliant guy. So Pauling and Hoffer did a study in which they basically took hundreds of cancer patients who came to Hoffer's office, and, uh, he would call them every month. "How are you doing?"
	"Fine."
	"What are you doing?" Well, some of them used Hoffer's nutrition as part of their cancer treatment, and some chose not to, possibly because of the scare tactics from their oncologist.
	So over the course of 12 years he followed these hundreds of patients, uh, and what he found out is the patients who used just medicine lived an average of six months. The patients who used nutrition and medicine lived an average of six years.
Dr. Stengler:	Absolutely. And, you know, it came out recently even in the, uh, conventional cancer institutions that 25 percent of all cancers could be prevented with proper diet. Now I think in certain instances the number could be much higher than that.
Dr. Quillin:	Yeah.
Dr. Stengler:	But it's finally being acknowledged. So, well, as you can all see, Dr. Quillin is just an encyclopedia of information. We could go on for hours, and that's why we're gonna have different modules with him. So look for the other topics and modules we're gonna talk about. And again, Dr. Quillin, thank you so much for this, uh, *[unintelligible]* piece.
	[Crosstalk]
Dr. Quillin:	A pleasure. Thank you for sharing your viewers.
Dr. Stengler:	Thank you.

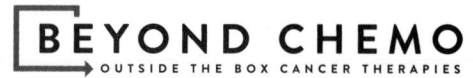

EPISODE 2: CANCER DETOX

Understanding the Root Cause
of Cancer—and How to Create
an Environment Where Cancer
Simply Can't Survive

HOW I USED NUTRITION TO CURE MY MOTHER'S BREAST CANCER

— DR. JOSH AXE —

Dr. Stengler: I'm here with Dr. Josh Axe and if any of you have been on the internet you probably are familiar with Dr. Axe. He's been a sensation in terms of natural health and getting great information out there on the internet. Ah, Dr. Axe is a certified doctor of natural medicine, a doctor of chiropractic, as well as a clinical nutritionist and he has a passion to help people get healthy by using food as medicine, which makes a lot of sense to me.

In 2008 he started Functional Metal, Medical Center in Nashville, Tennessee, which grew to become one of the world's most renowned clinics in that field.

Ah, Dr. Axe found one of the most visited natural health websites I told you about at draxe.com, which has a, astounding 15 million monthly visitors where the main topics include nutrition, natural medicine, fitness, healthy recipes, home remedies, and trending health news.

He's been a physician for many professional athletes. He traveled to the 2012 Games in London to work with USA athletes. And he's written several bestselling book, books, including *Eat Dirt: Why Leaky Gut Might be the Root Cause of Your Health Problems and Five Surprising Steps to Cure It, The Real Food Diet Cookbook, and Essential Oils: Ancient Medicine.* So millions of people have read these books and a couple of them tie into our topic today where we're talking about the connection between gut health and good immunity, helping people fight cancer, prevent cancer and then this very increasingly popular topic of essential oils

So Dr. Axe thank you so much for joining our program.

Dr. Axe: Hey Dr. Mark thanks for having me.

Dr. Stengler: So tell the viewers a bit more about your background. Like I said a lot of people are familiar with you, but you've got a unique background in terms of athletics and nutrition and how things have kind of just exploded in, in this field for you, so yeah tell us a bit more about yourself.

Dr. Axe: Yeah so I, ah, I started a practice here in Nashville, ah, a little over ten years ago and for me you know I really got into the natural medicine field through a health crisis in my own family. In fact, ah, you know some people know this, a lot of people don't, but, ah, when my mom, when I was in junior high my mom was diagnosed with breast cancer and that was really a shocking to myself and my family at the time, because my mom was my gym teacher at school, she was a swim instructor. So she was just really fit and everyone thought healthy, but she got that cancer diagnosis and our family lived in what I call the medical model at the time and she went through rounds and rounds of chemotherapy. She had a mastectomy. And I can still remember to this day seeing my mom's hair fall out, just remembering her on the edge of, of death.

And just saying to myself as a kid, "Man I never want to see anyone have to go through that again." And you know praise God she was diagnosed as being cancer free and healthy, but really for the next ten years after she went through chemo she seemed sicker than ever. She got put on multiple medications, antidepressant drugs, um, was diagnosed with thyroid issues, digestive issues, chronic fatigue syndrome.

And she was just sick and tired all the time.

One of the biggest things I remember about my mom growing up is that she had to take a nap every day.

And so this went on for ten years and then ten years later I'm, ah, I'm in a nutrition school, chiropractic school, and I get a call from my mom.

"Um, I have got bad news," in tears, she said, "I've just been diagnosed with cancer again." And she said, "Um, what do I do?"

And I'd been really blessed at the time to have been learning a lot of natural treatments and also being surrounded by doctors who were in the natural health field and getting counseling by them. I spent hours reading.

In fact one of the books I'll even mention was I think, I think even at the time, not then or soon after I had, there was a book that I think you, ah, co-wrote with, ah, Jim Balch, ah, possibly that you know we, we used some of those things as a guide in there.

I had a—we read a book by Jordon Ruben called *The Makers Diet* and we just started reading a lot of books and reading and we started realizing, just believing that at first we wanted to take care of her all naturally.

So with my mom she started juicing vegetables every single day. Started eating wild caught salmon, blueberries, we started supplementing with turmeric and reishi mushroom and a number of other supplements and really reducing those stress levels. And we did that natural health protocol for about four months. Went back to the oncologists and their exact words were, they, they called us after doing a PET scan, a CT scan a few days later and they said, "Ah, this is highly unusual. We haven't really seen this before, but the tumors have shrunk by more than half." They said, "You know come back in nine months." Went back nine months later, they'd shrunk again.

And at this point it's been, ah, it's been another 13 years since then and my mom is in the best shape of her life. In fact she's 65, her and my dad retired from Ohio down to Florida and just doing great.

The reason I share that with everybody is to say that's really why I practice even the way I practice. You know I know when my mom was sick she was like a deer in the headlights. There was so much information out there that that I really needed to put something together for her that was a compact and simple that she could actually do to change her health. But you know for, for me, ah, that's why I started draxe.com and some of these other things, but that's, that's probably the biggest part of my background.

And I tell my patients, I tell my patient Dr. Mark and I know you feel the way about patients you've taken care of, but I tell them that I'll take care of them like I would own family, because I know what it's like to have a family member who you know is, ah, you know confronted with a life-threatening crisis.

Dr. Stengler: Wow, that's, that's great information. So it sounds like you already were *[inhales]* very much interested in the field of chiropractic and natural medicine and probably into athletics yourself and then with what happened with your mom that, ah, you saw such good results with nutrition and holistic healing methods that your confidence must have just skyrocketed and it just took off from there.

Is that accurate?

Dr. Axe: It really did, very accurate.

Dr. Stengler: So in this series we're talking about many different aspects of helping people prevent and treat cancer with integrative therapies. Um, you really have great information on the connection between gut health and the immune system and so that's just so critical in knowing that 70 percent of our immune system *[inhales]* uh, originates in the gut. And so you've written many good articles on this and videos which people have access too.

Why don't you tell our viewers about the connection between a healthy gut, the digestive system, a healthy immune system and of course that's going to indirectly or directly tie into *[inhales]* ah, cancer as well.

Dr. Axe: Yeah absolutely. You know there, there are so many aspects of our health that are interconnected and the gut and the immune system is definitely one of the with maybe the strongest connection. And when you look at there's something I, I talk about in my book *Eat Dirt* and in this book we really go through how you treat things like—autoimmune disease and digestive diseases and even brain issues by directly treating the gut.

And your gut you have a lining in your gut that acts as a net. It's essentially your, your intestinal barrier and it's the barrier between your bloodstream and your intestines. And what can happen over time is a lot of times whether it's emotional stress and cortisol levels, ah, you know inflammatory foods. We have inflammation in that gut lining, imagine a fire there on that net. What starts to happen is these tiny holes in like the fishing net of your gut lining start to get bigger and bigger, bigger over time to where now things are leaking through into the bloodstream that should never get in there.

So think about this. I mean you're really, your lining should be allowing things like vitamins and nutrients and sugar and things into the bloodstream, but now things like gluten, casein, bad bacteria, toxins are getting into the bloodstream and your body says, "Whoa, this is a problem," sets off an inflammatory or an immune reaction over time. And if that continues to be, ah, continues all over time it can also start to cause things like autoimmune disease where your body attacks its own protein cells and tissues.

And so really what we want to do in treating a number of conditions is the first thing we want to do is we want to reduce that gut inflammation and start giving the body nutrients and things that really sooth that gut lining. Because what happens is most people's immune systems are overreacting, ah, over time as well due to like chronic inflammation that can happen in the body. So when that happens and I'll give you an example of this and this is something I love about some of the books I've read of yours Dr. Mark, because I've followed you for a long time.

Dr. Stengler: Well we've got a lot of common, you know athletics and I think we have the same spiritual background and so yeah it's interesting.

Dr. Axe:	Yeah my, in fact my mom, I mean every, you know of all the books and updated editions you know I, I know some of the things you've put out over the years, she has a lot of your books.

But you know getting into that like if, if I have a patient come in with Hashimoto's thyroiditis today, we know today for if you're watching this it's you know it's autoimmune form of hypothyroidism, that's simplifying, but that's essentially what it can be. A lot of doctors today Dr. Mark you and I see this you know the doctors wills say, "Oh here's some Synthroid or even maybe a natural doctor will say, "Why hey here's some Armour" or "here's some you know a few vitamins and minerals." But we know that Hashimoto's thyroiditis and autoimmune disease a big part of that starts in the gut. So if a patient truly wants to heal we've gotta heal the gut. We need to support the thyroid, we probably need to support adrenals, I mean there's a lot of things that go into play there, with you know really getting to the root cause of disease.

Dr. Stengler: Oh absolutely and with any chronic condition inflammation is always play a role. Now in terms of cancer *[inhales]* when you have this inflammatory, ah, condition going on, which certainly with a lot of people it originates in the gut, ah, it creates cellular changes, abnormal cellular metabolism, abnormal cell division in cancer. So it's critical that we cut that inflammation off so we can get normal cell division, healthy cells and that's where that connection with the gut comes in.

Maybe talk a bit more about, ah, types of foods you recommend people incorporate and then we'll get into some supplements and/or other techniques you recommend.

Dr. Axe: Yeah you know when we're talking about both cancer and autoimmune disease you want to follow an anti-inflammatory diet and you also want to give your body specific nutrients that are going to protect, regenerate, and rebuild within your body.

So talking about protection first antioxidants are really important. You know when my mom was sick and she's and having a number of these conditions from thyroid issues to cancer you know we started loading up on things like, acai, acai berry powder, goji berry powder, she was eating blueberries. We were doing a lot of those antioxidants, green leafy vegetables, so we were loading up on those antioxidant rich foods.

Ah, the next thing we started doing in terms of regeneration is consuming foods that really, um, in Chinese medicine or Ayurveda were known to lower stress levels and support tissue regeneration and so turmeric is one of those. Now a lot of people recognize turmeric for its compound for cumin, but it contains another unique compound called "tumerone," which has been shown, shown in studies to support stem cell production, so your body creating its own new and healthy tissue, so turmeric is one of those herbs that's fantastic at that.

Another one is reishi mushroom. We know in Chinese medicine reishi and cordyceps and maitake mushroom these were prized for their immune boosting abilities. So these are really supporting your own cells in one, killing off bad cells, but also helping your body support your body in new collagen production and creating new and healthy tissues; so reishi is great. And then other foods that help with regeneration beets, nitric oxide really important, ah, is important for improving circulation in the body as well.

And, and so those were some of things we did. And then we also did a number of foods that support rebuilding. Um, you know and things like collagen rich foods. My mom did a little bit of chicken broth every day. She did salmon with like the skin on it. We know the skin actually of the salmon is one of the most collagen rich foods in the world. And then even things like seaweed.

And so you know her daily diet I'll give you an example of what it looked like. She would wake-up in the morning and she would have a glass of herbal tea. You know it would be something like milk thistle and astragalus, but she would have that tea in the morning.

Then she would do some juices. You know she would do a juice blend of beets and carrots, but then lots of greens, ginger, turmeric, ah, spinach, lemon, celery. You know she would drink that juice down. And then for lunch she would have something like a super-food salad or a big bowl of chicken broth soup. If she did a salad she'd have a little bit of salmon on there, lots of veggies. Maybe she would have blueberries during the day and again a little bit of, ah, you know and then more vegetables and more vegetable juice. And so that was really a big part of her diet.

Now I'll, I'll just, I want to say one difference between if somebody has cancer versus somebody who has autoimmune disease if somebody has cancer I think they can go a little bit more raw in their diet. If somebody has autoimmune disease or inflammatory bowel disease they tend to have what's called a little bit dampness in Chinese medicine, so they really want to do less cold foods, even less juices and more warming things like warm bone broth soup. But, um, overall you know, um, as food is medicine it's lots of herbs, lots of—and I want to say this with herbs, when and this is something again I know that you've written about in your books, but when you look about at the United States today we consume probably less herbs per capita than anywhere.

I mean if you go to a market in Asia or the Middle East it smells like herbs, it smells like—but even someone's home it smells like that. You come into America today go in a grocery store it smells like nothing or maybe bleach, right?

Dr. Stengler: Right, right. *[Laughs]*

Dr. Axe: So we are getting almost none of these.

There's a, a book called *The Okinawa Diet* and they talked about our herb and antioxidant intake in the US compared to Japan is one-eighth. I mean it is that far off. So loading up on the herbs too is, is, is, ah, recommended.

Dr. Stengler: Well I don't think it's any coincidence you look at foods, you look at herbs our body has been designed in my opinion to interact with these natural compounds and so if we can tap into that our, our body is going to work better, our immune system will work better as well.

Um, why don't you tell the viewers about prebiotics as foods and/or supplements and probiotics? I, I know you've written a lot and done videos on that important topic as well.

Dr. Axe: Yeah I think the most important thing for people to understand is that I think a lot of times we look at labels and something says you know, "A hundred billion CFU, ah, probiotics," or this many prebiotics, the most important thing though it's those numbers when you're taking a supplement they can be semi-important.

The most important thing is we want to change your body's environment.

Dr. Stengler: Right.

Dr. Axe: You know I and I talk about this as I talk a lot about eastern medicine, but you think about if somebody has a dark, damp basement, like, in, in Tennessee here we have flooding years ago and I know in Florida recently where my parents were a lot of people were having mold issues. You know mold likes a, a damp environment. Well if your body is very, ah, damp it's hard, it causes certain bacteria or certain types of microbes to flourish like yeast and Candida and funguses.

So we want to do a few things as we cause the right type of bacteria to grow in your body. One, you know you do want to take some probiotics. You know you want to change your internal environment and you want to take what I would call "food-based and then soy-based probiotics." Food based you know, um, *[smacks lips]* you know, you know things like Bifidobacterium and, ah, Lactobacillus acidophilus, some of these other bacteria that you're going to get in you know kefir and sauerkraut, Lactobacillus plantarum, some of those species of probiotics.

I also think there's value in getting some of the probiotics that are our ancient, ancient ancestors would have gotten such as lack, you know such, such as some of the bacillus species, you know things like that, um, that are found in our soil today. So I think getting multiple types of probiotics predominately from your food, from fermented vegetables and things like that should be the first place.

Along with that prebiotic foods can great. I'm a fan of tiger nuts can be a very good prebiotic-rich food. Ah, plantains or, or bananas are a good, ah, chicory root. You know there are a number of good sources there of, um, *[smacks lips]* of, ah, and we see inulin a lot, in, in a lot of these prebiotic supplements. So prebiotics can be good as well.

The other thing I'll say though is along with those two things that all of us should be doing we want to change the environment of your gut also by consuming more bitter foods. It's known in Chinese medicine that bitter foods dry up dampness. In fact when you look at all the ancient remedy—

I mean if you've ever had you know it's funny like all of our alcohol today if somebody goes to a you know, ah, goes to a high-end, ah, you know, um, bar somewhere and they're serving cocktails you know a lot of those things were originally developed by monks or, ah, or, ah, or doctors as medicines so they had a little bit of alcohol in them. Well a marketer came along at some point and was like, "Let's back off on the herbs and up this alcohol and then people will drink it for pleasure."

But I mean traditionally people did a lot of herbs and that would help dry up this dampness in the body. So some bitter foods are things like arugula, watercress, ah, black cumin, um, artichokes. You know and then herbs like milk thistle and dandelion greens. I mean these are really bitter. So in addition to the prebiotics and the probiotics I think getting more bitter and warming foods.

You know warming foods like ginger and cinnamon. Do the blend of all those things to, together and then getting rid of the excess sugar.

All those things I think help with, with you know supporting a healthy microbiome.

Dr. Stengler: Oh excellent. Well that's so important. I know as, as doctors we, we test our patients and have for years and the vast majority of them have digestive issues, ah, they have increased intestinal permeability, which we have very good tests to you know find that out now. They got yeast overgrowth in the gut. They've got the malabsorption, ah, the bacteria balance is off. So I mean virtually everyone has some issue with that because of the standard American diet and other factors too, drinking chlorinated water, stress, pharmaceutical medications, steroids, and things like that, so it's just like you said foundational.

If you want to have a healthy immune system you've got to get that gut in order. And of course as you found out with your mother and studies have shown this, um, chemotherapy, radiation, other conventional treatments do cause gut damage, the increased intestinal permeability or leaky gut.

And so if your, if you've been dealing with cancer in the past or you currently are even more important you've got to work on that gut health.

Dr. Axe: Oh yeah. I mean when my mom was sick the first thing we did was really focus on healing her chronic constipation. We had her start doing magnesium. We had her, we drove out in the country and got this goat's milk kefir she started doing every day. Um, having her doing carrot juice, cod liver oil and we started doing all these things. We bought a mini-trampoline, one of those Rebounders, had her start jumping on that every day, doing acupuncture, all of these things to support that.

Dr. Stengler: Excellent. Now your mom obviously had the mindset where she wanted to get better. I mean my patients that come in with cancer and unfortunately we're seeing more and more every year, um, *[smacks lips]* you know I tell them, "Look diet is critical." The other doctors we've interviewed in a series if you currently have cancer or have a history of it it's not something you can just address lightly. We don't want to stress people out, but it's just critical. We find the people get the best results have to address their diet and it sounds like your mother had that mindset.

Dr. Axe: Yeah it's so important. You know I think the biggest thing I see when people are diagnosed with a chronic health issue is that there's a lot of fear. There's a lot of fear especially when they get into that conventional medical system and that's what doctors are trained to do in order to force them to do their treatments is instill more fear in them.

So for with my mom you know I think it helped her that we just laid out a very, very specific game plan from what she should do from when she woke up until went to bed.

And I do think taking care of those stress levels are really, really important. There's no doubt that emotional stress will cause disease.

And I'll say this as well, when I get in—I'll try and just keep this to a minute or two, [chuckles] but a lot of people don't realize how emotions cause disease in specific organs in the body. And within TCM it's called "The five elements of traditional Chinese medicine." They knew that certain emotions cause disease in specific organs. In fact if somebody experiences the emotion of fear it causes disease of the kidneys, adrenals, and reproductive organs, and bladder.

Think about how true this is. If you have a child that gets really scared they'll wet themselves. It causes them to lose or causes dysfunction on that lower area of the body of their bladder and kidneys. And but think about it a lot of people go through fear throughout their life, it causes disease there. So if somebody is struggling with cancer of the ovaries or uterus or prostate fear is an emotion that they have to combat through, through you know through you know spiritually, mentally they have to reduce that, um, that negative emotion that they're experiencing.

If somebody experiences anger, anger causes toxicity of the liver and gallbladder. Why do we call somebody an "angry drunk"? If you drink too much alcohol it causes liver toxicity makes you angry, you have a lot of anger causes disease of the liver and gallbladder, causes issues there.

And the same goes—think about if somebody studying real hard for a test or gets really stressed out well the emotion of worry causes disease in the stomach, the pancreas, and the spleen and then we can go on and on. If somebody has the emotion of grief or sadness or depression causes disease of the lungs and the colon. Um, and if somebody has disease of the, ah, of too high cortisol levels, fight-or-flight response causes disease of the heart and the central nervous system.

So these are things that people knew in Chinese medicine.

When people to see these ancient doctors they would treat their body with supplements and herbs and foods like we talk about, but also there was this understanding that we are body, mind, and spirit. And if we have a patient that comes in you know to do Hippocrates, Maimonides or another ancient practitioner you know they would have said, "You know what you're really dealing with a lot of fear in your life hey let's work on that as well."

And I know that not all doctors are trained in that, but I think it's important for just if, if you're a person watching this and you have thyroid disease or cancer or autoimmune disease it's really important that you follow the stuff that Dr. Mark teaches you every week on the program with nutrition and diet, but also that you really are proactive about healing yourself spiritually and emotionally as well.

Dr. Stengler: Well that's great information. I mean that's the way God has designed us, we're not just a material body. As you mentioned we've got a mind, we've got a spirit and so if you just address the physical will it help? Sure it will, but if you negate the other factors it's, it's, it can very problematic, you won't get the best results. And for some people *[inhales]* that's where the main focus needs to be.

So that's what we appreciate about holistic doctors like yourself looking at the totality and it's one of the weaknesses of conventional medicine. Conventional medicine has good aspects too, but it's just so narrowly targeted on the physical, it limits the results. So thank you for your insights on that.

[Inhales] So this has been excellent information the connection between gut health and emotion health and immune system for all you people out there with cancer. *[Inhales]* And of course Dr. Axe is just a very reputable resource in this area.

And so Dr. Axe thank you so much for your time today.

Dr. Axe: Awesome. Hey thanks for having me Dr. Mark.

UNLOCKING YOUR SUPERHERO GENE

— DOUG KAUFMANN —

Dr. Stengler: I have Doug Kaufmann, a friend of mine who's an expert in the relationship between fungal problems and cancer. So you know, in cancer today, as we've mentioned, there's many different causes or initiations of why cancer can occur. But probably the most underrated would be the link between fungal problems and cancer, and so that's why we have Doug here today, and Doug, thank you so much for being on.

Kaufmann: I'm honored to be invited. Thank you so much. It's fascinating, this whole word, fungus. Everything was bacteria, you know, now, fungus is becoming big, and when we look at the role of fungus in cancer, we know that, um, tobacco cigarette companies dip their tobacco in sugar, roll it tight, and yeast and sugar get together, and that might be why so many lung cancers ensue when we, uh, the fermentation process with cigarettes.

Alcohol, antibiotics, both fungal metabolites, are now inducing a dozen different kinds of cancer, the scientific literature is saying. So, we know, Mark, that there's a fungal component to some cancers, and very often, it requires looking at the patient's lifestyle.

Dr. Stengler: Absolutely. Now, you've been a pioneer in this category. You've really brought this to light, and you've been speaking to hundreds, thousands of medical doctors in the last number of years, educating them on this such important relationship between cancer and this organism. But Doug, you have a very interesting story—

So, if you would, can you maybe take us back, why you became so interested in the fungal connection to disease, and of course, you know, we're sitting here in your studio, such a generous person here. Your studio here in the Dallas area. You have one of the most watched television shows in America, in terms of health, and you've dedicated your life to helping people enhance their health, uh, in many different ways, but with a specialty in the fungal connection to disease. So can you take us through all these years, and what's been going on?

Kaufmann: Yeah, so, um, it's great to have you here, also.

Um, fascinatingly, so I'm in college, I get drafted. Uh, this is in 1968. Uh, ended up not wanting to go to Vietnam, because we could watch that on TV, you know, I didn't want to be in one of those body bags or helicopters.

So, uh, I enlisted in the Navy right away, and they made a bunch of us corpsmen, hospital corpsmen, and we thought, "Well, what's a hospital corpsman? Somebody that's an orderly in a hospital."

So, for a few months, they train you, then you go through specialized training for—we did for a couple of years. And you basically come out like a nurse, and you have a medical pack on your back, and then you're assigned to the Marine. I was with the Seventh Marines out in Vietnam, 20 years old.

Came home at 21 years old, and uh, came home sick. My skin was bleeding, hair was falling out, horrible stomach problems, horrible jungle rot on my skin, and so forth. And um, all the king's horses and all the king's men couldn't—I mean, I went to doctors, and "Here, take this cortisone," you know, uh, simple answers that we still get today.

Well, I—Dr. Everett Hughes, my boss at USC Medical School once said to me, "You know, you were overseas, could you have gotten into a parasite?" I said, "Aha!" So

I went over to get—we didn't have Google searches then, we had library cards—

Dr. Stengler: Right.

Kaufmann: So I get a library card, I go over, and I pull an old 1953, '54 book off the shelf, that says, "Parasitology," and you know the way God works, right? It falls open to, like, chapter 11, and it says, "Fungus," and I'm thinking—

Dr. Stengler: Oh, really?

Kaufmann: "Wait a minute, yeast and fungus. I got yeast growing all over my body, jungle rot. Could that have gotten inside my body?" And low and behold, the, the paragraph I, you know, if we had cell phones then, I would have taken a picture of the whole, uh, the whole, uh, chapter.

Basically, it said, "Yeast can parasitize man. Once on board, they must eat." My diet—remember, I'm 21 years old living in LA, so my diet is beer, and Oreo cookies, and Mexican food.

Dr. Stengler: Right.

Kaufmann: You know, and so I'm feeding this stuff, and I'm getting sicker, and sicker, and sicker. So, through all of that, I learned that it wasn't a tapeworm. It was a little tiny organism called a fungus. Thinking, Mark, I was the only guy in America that had this problem. So, I could fix myself by changing my diet. And back then, a change of diet meant go off Coors and on Budweiser, you know—

Dr. Stengler: Wow.

Kaufmann: That, that's just the way my, my 21 year old brain worked. Didn't get better for a long time until I finally decided I'm gonna go for this, 'cause I'm getting sicker, and I'm bleeding all over—

And I went for it, and I enjoyed weeks of feeling like the old Doug Kaufmann, the personality came back. And then it would take a few years longer for me to realize the impact of this fungus on other people, the fact that it can cause cancer is mind-boggling, 'cause there's a whole lot of sick people out there, who have no idea that if they're smokers, and they're drinkers, and they're eating a lot of peanuts, and a lot of corn, a lot of wheat, these foods commonly have mycotoxins in them, um, that might be causing, might be the, what we call the ideology or the cause of their—

Dr. Stengler: Yeah, tell the viewers a bit more about what a mycotoxin is. A lot of people have heard the term, but they don't—

Kaufmann: Yeah.

Dr. Stengler: Really quite understand what it's, what it's referring to.

Kaufmann: So, I put up a, a presentation graphic that said, "Myco," means fungus. Mycotoxin, poison made by fungus. Mycotoxicoses, any condition induced or caused by a mycotoxin. We have—

If you can imagine the, the gravity of this situation, there are thought to be 1.5 million to 2 million fung-fungal species. Today, we've discovered about 70 to 75,000 of them. We've classified them. Of those, we now know that 300 to 400 are pathogenic to man—

Dr. Stengler: Disease-causing, yep—

Kaufmann: Disease-causing, they can get on board, and cause disease. But there, that means there's 2 million species we haven't classified or identified yet. Of those, we have about 1,000 poisons made by these 300 species of fungi that can cause disease in man. One of them, called aflatoxin, and this is commonly made by aspergillus mold, that grows on our corn supply. Look at any agricultural report, there's a problem. Aflatoxin is impregnating our wheat, our corn, our peanuts, and we're eating it.

This is a known human carcinogen. It induces, it causes human liver cancer, amen.

They're now studying it for inducing other animals, which— or other diseases, other cancers in animals. Uh, other than just liver cancer.

Dr. Stengler: Well, I'm not seeing any signs in the supermarkets—

Kaufmann: Yeah.

Dr. Stengler:	With cancer warnings from these aflatoxins. But interesting. Have an interesting quote here. "The American Cancer Society defines fungal mycotoxins as mutagenic carcinogens." So, the American Cancer Society admits these things are strongly cancer-causing.
Kaufmann:	Yeah.
Dr. Stengler:	So—
Kaufmann:	And look at the date on that, by the way.
Dr. Stengler:	1995.
Kaufmann:	Yeah, a long time ago.
Dr. Stengler:	By the way, people, I got this from Doug's, uh, Powerpoint presentation, used with doctors, thank you very much.
Kaufmann:	Yeah, yeah.
Dr. Stengler:	But you know, also good data. Um, most are immune-suppressing, these mycotoxins. And here's one thing I learnt from you, I never realized, um, you know, all the biochemistry we took, and, and stuff, in medical school. Mycotoxins are heat-stable. They cannot be destroyed in boiling water, roasting, or even autoclaving—

In other words, we always, people always think, you know, I've cooked my food, it kills the bacteria, and all these bad bugs, and so, it'll take care of these mycotoxins Mr. Kaufmann's talking about. I mean, that is a big deal. |
Kaufmann:	It's a huge deal, if you think, if you boil your rice, sure, the fungus or bacteria on the rice will be boiled off. But if that fungus has deposited these poisons into that rice kernel, you can boil it, and boil it in autoclave, and you're going to eat it. That's big. Imagine, think about a colonoscopy. A reused metal tube that you can't autoclave off, you know, you—this has some pretty—you remember the TB tying test—
Dr. Stengler:	Yep, yep, used to do it, yep.
Kaufmann:	Used to heat up the, you know, so you're getting whatever that little boy in front of you had injected, if has mold you're maybe getting some of that. It has huge implications, and I don't mean to scare anyone.

Dr. Stengler:	Well, we did learn in medicine that aflatoxin, they always focus on peanuts, but it's a lot more foods than that—
Kaufmann:	Right.
Dr. Stengler:	As, as you've said, um, is one of the most carcinogenic, poisonous substances known to man.
Kaufmann:	Mm-hmm. And that's not ochratoxin, that's not any of these other toxins, deoxynivalenol, um, big names that are poisons, literally, and, and by the way, how do we induce cancer? Let's say you want to study a new pill. A pharmaceutical company can't give this pill to cancer patients, that's inhumane.
	So, we give it to mice, but all of these bunnies or mice have to have cancer, and they don't. How do you give 200 bunnies or mice cancer? Good question. You inject them with aflatoxin, made by aspergillus mold, and in a year, they all have cancer. We didn't inject 'em with cancer, we injected them with mold, and they end up with cancer. Do you think oncologists are missing a step here?
Dr. Stengler:	Well, we have this, uh, quote, from uh, the medical journal, *Medical Hypothesis*—
	It says, "Cancer is a hybrid," and I want you to comment on this. "It is due to a plant, candida spores derive from an asomisidi, or a sac strain of fungus," 1996. Tell the viewers more of what that means, in your hypothesis, which seems to blend in what they've described more than a decade ago, and how this ties into cancer.
Kaufmann:	So, these fungi, to kid or hide from the immune system, gather in a white rubbery sac, where they can reproduce. So, you're in the shower, taking a shower in the morning, you wash under your arm. Ooh, a little knot, that kinda hurts, no big deal. If you're a guy, you're not going to a doctor. Now, a woman would probably go to a doctor right away.
	A man gets in the shower four months later, ooh, it's a little bit bigger. A year later, wow, that's a mass growing under my arm. That will more than likely be scanned, uh,

MRI'd, uh, tested, and called cancer, right? Lymph cancer, lymphoma, or something.

But these fungi, it's so difficult to differentiate between an asomycota, a sac fungus, and a cancer tumor, no cancer center does it. You have to understand the laboratory. When, when you send a tumor in, and breast, origin is breast, and you wanna test it for cancer, that's what lab techs do, folks, they're putting cancer stains on it to see if it turns the color, so they can call the doctor, and say, "No laboratory tests for fungi."

And before I die, I would like to see that done. Every tumor gets a differential diagnosis. One is sent off, and they grow out different fungi, and the other is sent to cancer centers. And I think what you'd find is probably the convergence of two, in many cases, gosh it's showing positive fungus, and positive cancer.

Dr. Stengler: So, uh, these mycotoxins, I mean, they're directly carcinogenic, cancer-causing. Of course, they have other effects. They suppress the immune system—

Uh, they damage cell DNA, um, cause other imbalances in the body. For example, like insulin resistance, and things like that, which can connect the cancer, too—now, you brought up something I wasn't aware of, which I thought was quite brilliant. And that was the research on the P53 gene.

Kaufmann: Wow.

Dr. Stengler: You know, people are always hearing more about this P53 gene, 'cause you know, they're trying to develop drugs for it, and all these c- types of things. Now, this is a gene which normally would help protect against abnormal, uh, cell division, uh, in cancer. Uh, when it becomes damaged, mutated, so to speak, um, you have a problem, you're at high risk for cancer.

So, tell us about the research, actually shows the connection—

Kaufmann: Right.

Dr. Stengler: From mycotoxin to damaging this gene, 'cause something has to damage it. It's—normally, you're not born with it that way.

Kaufmann:	No, no, we all have P53 genes. These are called, uh, tumor suppressor genes. So, if you have a tumor, these genes suppress it from happening. We all, they say, get cancer from time to time, but the P53, and think of Superman, red S—
	On his chest, right? Um, the Superman gene comes in and defeats that cancer. What they're finding in over 50 percent of cancers now, damaged P53 genes. That's kind of exciting. Here's what's really exciting, that aflatoxin, those mycotoxins, fungal poisons, are what damages our superman gene.
	So, all a doctor would look at and say, "Yeah, that's gotta be cancer, look at his immune system is down. Right, he's finding himself eating a lot of cereal, and corn, and wheat, and man, he eats peanut butter every day. And he's—I've had him on antibiotics for a year, and he drinks a lot of alcohol. Something damaged his P53 gene. Well, that must mean he has cancer. What damaged the P53 gene?"
	One of the things we know that does is a mycotoxin. It's huge.
Dr. Stengler:	Well, now, for the health professionals out there, thinking, "Well, this is your guy's theory. We really don't know that."
	We've got the documentation. So from the proceedings of the National Academy of Science—
Kaufmann:	Huge—
Dr. Stengler:	Can't get more—
Kaufmann:	Right—
Dr. Stengler:	Mainstream than that. Here's what they say: "The mycotoxin, for example, one of 'em, aflatoxin B1, made by aspergillus fungus, is known to cause P53 mutations." This is not theory, this is fact.
Kaufmann:	And what I had to do, I was speaking to oncologists, "Oncologists, you're right." They're extremely scientific. They care. They really want to help those patients get better. If you don't know fungus, I don't think you know cancer thoroughly. Because if the P53 were any gene in your body can be mutated by fungus, why aren't we asking our patient about alcohol?

Alco—look, the—alcohol brewer's yeast is the fungus and the mycotoxin it makes, we call ethanol, or alcohol. Penicillium is the mold. The poison it makes is cold penicillin. There's thousands of penicillin-derived drugs.

Now, I'm not saying that your child taking a penicillin, PENVK or something like that, is going to end up with cancer. It's a poison, and it has to be. It has to poison bacteria in tiny doses. I've never worried about a round of antibiotics, especially if you chase it with a good probiotic.

Dr. Stengler: Right.

Kaufmann: I worry for the patient who's on antibiotics 'cause they're chronically immunosuppressed and they chronically get upper respiratory infections, 'cause I think we now have proper science that says longterm antibiotic use, uh, can induce, or a significant increase in five different lung, breast, prostate, colorectal, and uh, non-Hodgkins lymphoma, all induced by excessive antibiotics. We have to be careful.

Dr. Stengler: You know, in our book, we talk about kind of a newer theory, although it's been around, actually for quite a while, newer in terms of what people have been exposed to. But it's like the mitochondria theory of cancer. Um, it's basically saying that in this energy-producing warehouse of our cells, and we can actually talk about—

Just the cell in general, the machinery in the cell. You know, there's abnormal processes going on, and how the cell's creating energy, cancer cells use energy differently than normal cells. I don't wanna focus on that, but I always like to go a step before that, because right now I'm asking—oh, we're focusing on, there's damaged machinery in the cell, and so, let's try and figure out some ways to, you know, help people with cancer.

But we gotta go a step before that, and look at the triggers for that, and that's where the mycotoxins can come in, because what's causing the cell DNA damage, what's causing the mitochondria to be damaged so it's not producing energy properly.

Um, why don't you talk to the viewers a bit about that?

Kaufmann:	So, the new hypotheses is that it's not, uh, a genetic disease. It's a mitochondrial disease, and like Dr. Stengler said, a mitochondria is the powerhouse of our cells. Here's the important take-home message, and I've said this now for two years since the theory of mitochondria came up. The identical poison that can poison your pifty—uh, P53, your two—superman—gene can poison the mitochondria. I have a doctor friend in St. Louis who is going to speak on mitochondria. Everything's mitochondria all of the sudden. And so, I pulled her five or six off PubMed, five or six reports that said mycotoxins damage the mitochondria of the cell. It's not brain surgery, I mean, that's simple.
	I know science is saying, "Okay, it's not genetic. Only one to five percent of all cancer is genetic. Let's look at something else." Guess what? The same poison, fungal poison, that kills the mitochondria, will mutate the genes in the body.
Dr. Stengler:	Right. Well, now, let's get to the practical level. I mean, you've devoted decades to helping people with things they can incorporate themselves, and with doctors, of course, too.
	Um, you've got a show, Know the Cause, again, one of the most watched shows in, in America on, on health. Um, you've written several books on the fungal connection. You have the book, The Germ that Causes Cancer, exactly what we're talking about. And you wrote that book how long ago?
Kaufmann:	2001, I believe, we wrote that book. I mean, long time ago.
Dr. Stengler:	Way ahead of the curve, way ahead of the curve there. You probably just [unintelligible] find some of the theories and stuff since then, but that's great. Um, so with the viewers, in your books, maybe take my viewers through how you practically help people. Let's talk about the diet, you know, the basic things they need to do to treat this fungal problem, help their immune system, help with normal cell division, and then supplements, and then, then some of the more important medications, if you would.

Kaufmann:	Okay. So the first thing I learned many years ago, um, was that these fungi can get on board and parasitize humans. The second thing I learned was they need food. Once on board, if they don't eat, uh, they'll die, and they're not gonna die. They wanna go to your grave with you, they wanna go home to their relatives six feet in the dirt.
	And so, these guys are fairly persistent. So, in a human fungal cell relationship, another published from the scientific literature, guess which cell, a human cell, a fungal cell, when fungi get on board, which one becomes dominant? The fungal cell. You no longer eat chocolate, because it's sweet, and you kinda like it. You have to.
	You no longer go back to breads, which you've been away from for a long period of time, because you kinda think bread tastes good. You have to. The pasta you let go 'cause you didn't eat carbs, now you're craving, and you can't get enough of it.
	So, fungi must have grains, a grain-free diet 45 years ago when I got involved in this was called quackery.
Dr. Stengler:	Right.
Kaufmann:	You gotta have grains, you gotta have the vitamin E, you've got—
Dr. Stengler:	Probably lose your license if you recommended that.
Kaufmann:	Exactly, um, but that's what I was finding. If I stayed off sandwiches and things like that, I felt great. Um, so there is a diet that starves fungi, disallows fungi to spew their poisons in your body. In order to have a serious disease like this and look at fungus as a causative factor, or a causal relationship between fungus and this disease, you must consider two things: killing it and starving it.
	There are great drugs, diflucan, lamisil, sporanox, you know, older generation drugs like nizerol—
	That kill fungus in the blood stream. Most doctors who really understand the science of this understand that there are nutrients, you know, that have supplements that do just as good. Vitamin D3, cholecalciferol, resveratrol, but

you know, curcumin, they're very, very good, powerful antifungal supplements.

So, now you're starting to kill it, right? It's gonna resist, it's gonna fight you, and you're gonna feel horrible when you start to fight fungus. It's gonna win for a period of time, especially if you simultaneously starve it. Fungus hates your salad, hates your steak, hates your salmon. All it wants is sugar, carbohydrates. Wheat, when you chew, we masticate, mix enzymes, then we swallow. It now becomes glucose, no longer wheat. It's sugar. Fungus loves that, so you have to put together a diet that will starve fungus, and simultaneously just put your gloves on—

And start batting it. In worst case scenarios, like advanced disease, diabetes, heart disease, corona—uh, cardiovascular, uh, disease, cancers. If fungus caused it, it needs to be defeated, and it may take a few months to a few years, but generally, the patient will begin to notice tumor markers getting better, maybe the P53, putting its superman power back in.

And so, there's good news, how they feel, their laboratory test results, uh, begin getting better. So, it gives the oncologist, the clinician, and the patient a clue that I'm on the right track now.

Dr. Stengler:	And in a way, we like to see those die-off effects to some degree, because we know the mycotoxins, the fungus, is a releasing toxic metabolites when it dies.
Kaufmann:	Yep.
Dr. Stengler:	Maybe talk a bit about that.
Kaufmann:	You can't withdraw from something unless you're first addicted, right? Stop coffee for the weekend, oh, the headache, I gotta get my coffee, right? You're addicted to coffee, a lot of us are.

Um, once you stop feeding these little guys, they're no longer friend. They become foe. And they team up. Remember, they're growing in cysts in your body, uh, that, uh, has—may or may not be called cancer, right? Because doctors aren't aware of ascomycetes, or mycetomas. These are lumps that fungus grow in, and there's science in the case of mycetomas, that they can mimic cancer, but your doctor didn't learn about a mycetoma in medical school.

Walk into your oncologist, and say, "Can you define this word for me? Mycetoma?" "No, I have no idea what that is." Maybe that's what I have. So, you really—you have to go into this venture as the driver. You've gotta help your oncologist. You can send that biopsy off. It's in Paraffin now, at the hospital that did the biopsy.

You can take a piece of it, and send it to a laboratory who will do fungal and mycotoxin DNA testing, and tell you, "Uh-oh, we found poisons, fungal poisons—

"In that tumor." Maybe it's cancer, maybe it's the fungal poisons that have caused the lump.

Dr. Stengler: And of course, there's research now showing that what they had found unexpectedly, not you and I, but they have found that certain antifungal drugs, they're concerned now to have a good promise as cancer drugs.

Kaufmann: One of the—

Dr. Stengler: That's just a coincidence, I guess.

Kaufmann: Right.

In 1997, a medical journal reported that the drug, nizoral, helped reverse prostate disease in men. Nizoral only kills fungus. You see where I'm going with that. Nizoral helps men with prostate disease. But the most exciting one was the toenail fungus drug, called itrochonizal, or sporanox, to you and me. Sporanox has crossed, or jumped the shark, to cross the street. It's now an accepted cancer drug.

It's inhibiting angiogenesis, which means it's preventing cancer from metastasizing through their body. Why shouldn't every cancer patient in America be on sporanox? 'Cause the doctors don't know this yet. But the FDA has approved the toenail fungus drug for cancer. Gee, what must cause cancer if the drug that kills fungus is helping cancer patients?

Dr. Stengler:	So, it sounds like with your approach, and again, you *[unintelligible]* with tens and tens of thousands of people over the years. Uh, we've got the diet approach. In my book, I call it the "Kaufmann diet."
Kaufmann:	Thank you.
Dr. Stengler:	After a certain person. Um, antifungals, natural, and/or pharmaceutical, right? Helping with detoxification. Um, and, and then, changing the terrain of the gut, where really a load of these toxins can get into you by using good bacteria, and again, changing the diet. Uh, getting out of an environment, which is loaded with, with fungi, and-and mycotoxins.
	Would that be a summary, would you say, of, of your overall approach?
Kaufmann:	Sure. The, the one thing lacking in my humble opinion—
Dr. Stengler:	Okay.
Kaufmann:	Would be sweating—
Dr. Stengler:	Mm-hmm.
Kaufmann:	Far infrared sauna.
Dr. Stengler:	Mm-hmm.
Kaufmann:	Getting outside, even though you got a big lump here. Sweat, get outside, work out, it's amazing, folks, how you can—this is where Dr. Stengler—eh, this has been the core of his business for a quarter of a century. Detoxifying the body, these fungi are toxic, right? In your body. You need to detox. Very often sweating helps with that. Um, so yeah, that would be a good summary. The probiotics are so important, you know, because what happens here can grow a lump here.
Dr. Stengler:	Well, Doug, in ending, if you could, because you got millions of viewers with your television show, um, you're on the internet extensively, uh, you've talked to so many doctors, and, and people around the country, around the world, actually. Maybe just give the viewers a sense of what kind of feedback are you getting? When you're talking to

people and incorporating—

The kind of protocol you're talking about, this antifungal protocol, what feedback are you getting from your viewers, 'cause I know they e-mail and they write you, to the doctors you work with, which is an increasing amount now. Just in general, what is the feedback that you get, may-maybe give a few case examples—

Kaufmann: Uh-huh.

Dr. Stengler: If you want.

Kaufmann: Yeah, I was, uh, asked a couple of years ago to speak to oncologists. These are integrative oncologists, those who say there's gotta be something more than just chemo and radiation, so they began looking at diet, IV, vitamin C, good group of doctors. I spoke out in San Diego a few years ago to them.

I was nervous. For the first time, I was presenting not to television folks, not to radio or internet folks, not to the lay public, like I do a lot, but to real doctors, who could impact their patients' lives. You wouldn't have believed it. After I got done, doctors—

A line of doctors, and the questions they had changed my heart. I was angry at oncologists, I really was. I had friends, loved ones, uh, who had gone through and lost the battle. And I was very, very angry at oncologists. What I saw was the most humbled group of men and women from other countries, and here from the US, and they stood in line, some of 'em half an hour, 45 minutes, to tell me stories of how their, their cervical cancer patients had a 20 year history of vaginal yeast, and cervical yeast.

I mean, stories like this, that I just couldn't believe, or that most of their cancer patients they thought thrush was a secondary problem. But now they remember—when they first saw that breast cancer patient, and they looked in her mouth, she had thrush growing in there, so was it the yeast that came first or the breast cancer came first? The stories—I got on my cell phone and called my wife—and I was emoting, it was unbelievable.

Then I spoke again to groups of doctors, bigger groups of doctors, uh, to the point where you know one of the organizations I spoke to in Orlando, 2.1 million people watched it on the internet. Look, all I'm trying to do is plant seeds. When did that cancer start? Oh my gosh, it's when I moved into that old apartment, my wife and I love old architecture, and it did smell mildewy, it did smell moldy.

Or you know what? I've been on antibiotics for two years, and then my doctor felt my prostate, and said, "Man, you have cancer." I'll give him, there was a nodule on there. I won't give him it was cancer. So, if you can just look, assess that disease, when did it start, what were the parameters, what was happening in your life, Dad died, huge stress in your life, into a lot of mold. You've been drinking for 14 years, and it finally caught up with you, 'cause alcohol and cancer intermingle.

So, that's where I come in all of this, is going back to when it began, which your oncologist won't do with you.

And figuring out why that lump began growing.

Dr. Stengler: Well, you know, doc, in medicine, uh, the biggest changes in medicine have come through what we call mavericks, people who are thought to be kooky and crazy. But the biggest advancements in medicine, whether it be the MRI, the discoveries by Louis Pasteur, have come through mavericks. And that is the category you're in.

And just in ending, there's no doubt in your mind, from what you're seeing in medicine today, this revolution is underway, in terms of the fungal link to cancer.

Kaufmann: You cannot be hearing what I'm hearing from physicians, many of them. Not one, many of them. You cannot get the e-mails I get on "You saved my life six years ago with this antifungal program. I had cancer," and not believe in anything else. That there is a fungal component to cancer, I guarantee you, maybe it's not fully understood today, but why withhold treatment, if it might work for you today?

Dr. Stengler: Right. And then you have all the non-toxic options, too. Dietary changes and supplements—

Kaufmann:	You got it, simple stuff.
Dr. Stengler:	And all that. So, Doug, well, thank you not just for the information you gave the viewers, but really, I mean, it's only people like you and I who realize this took a tremendous amount of effort, and pain, too, to carry the truth for all these years, and finally get to the point where it's been accepted. I mean, people don't understand what's involved, you know, in the kind of fields we're in. So, *[unintelligible]*.
Kaufmann:	It's really exciting, isn't it?
Dr. Stengler:	Yeah, so I want to thank you for that.
Kaufmann:	Thank you.
Dr. Stengler:	Okay. Well, there you go, everyone. This is phenomenal information, cutting edge, and I know it's gonna help you and your loved ones.

THE IMPORTANCE OF DETOX

— DR. MICHAEL MURRAY —

Dr. Stengler: Well hi, everyone. Great to be with you again and I have the well-known Dr. Murray here!

Uh, Dr. Murray's one of the world's leading authorities on natural medicine. Published over 30 books featuring natural approaches to health. He's a graduate and former faculty member and serves on the board of regents of Bastyr University in Seattle, Washington.

He's also the Chief Science Officer at Enzymedica. And, you know, for the past thirty-five years Dr. Murray has been compiling a massive database of original, scientific studies from the medical literature, which helps all of us, including us doctors.

He has collected over 65,000 articles from the scientific literature providing evidence for the effectiveness of the things we're talking about: Diets, vitamins and minerals, herbs, other natural treatments, uh, to help prevent and treat disease.

And so he's constantly expanding this database and you can see all of this on his website, drmurray.com. You know, Michael, one of your quotes I really like and you've used for a long time.

Basically paraphrasing. It's a myth that there isn't scientific validation of these natural therapies we calmly talk about. Why don't you expand on that a bit?

Dr. Murray: Yeah, well, I think, uh, most doctors have their head in the sand and, and say, "Well, there's no evidence to support the role of diet and attitude, uh, lifestyle modifications and the proper use of dietary supplements that in the promotion of health and the treatment of disease.

And the fact of the matter is, is that we can build a stronger scientific case, the greater scientific validation, from the use of the natural approaches that we can for many of the drugs that are involved *[unintelligible]*.

In fact, I think that, uh, when medical historians look back in the last 100 years or so, yes there's been some major advances in medicine and, yes, they're, they're at certain times when, uh, pharmaceutical agents are very important.

But for the most part, uh, many of these drugs end up, uh, doing more harm than good and especially those that are just biochemical Band-Aids that don't offer any therapeutic benefits other than relief of symptoms and the—

Dr. Stengler: Mm.

Dr. Murray: And we know, as naturopathic physicians, the best medicine is the one that addresses the root cause of an illness, not one that suppresses the symptoms and, uh, we're going to have better medicines, uh, in the future and I believe that food is the medicine of the future.

Dr. Stengler: Right. You know, in a series we're talking about integrative cancer therapies to prevent and help people going through their cancer treatments.

Dr. Murray: Mm-hmm.

Dr. Stengler: Um, I've been studying, like, the laws of science and laws of logic, lately on my free time. *[laughs]* And there—they—there's this one law called the law of rationality, which, basically, says, you know, from the, um, evidence you draw a conclusion. So I'm still amazed.

Patient after patient comes in my office, seeing their oncologist, and they're told, you know, diet has no effect on their outcome. There's been no studies on supplements and, of course, you've documented these things in your many books, um, but it's not rational.

Dr. Murray:	It's not rational it's, uh, it, you know, doctors are like most of us. I mean, we're not up on something, we're down on it and, uh, what I found in, uh, dealing with doctors we probably just found the same thing, uh, they're even more skeptical than the average person.
	But, uh, many doctors are, uh, open minded enough to at least look at the literature when you share it with them and they may say something like, "Geez, I had—I had no idea that there was this amount of research on this approach." And, uh, both of the doctors I think are good doctors and, and, uh, there, there's hope.
Dr. Stengler:	Yeah.
Dr. Murray:	Others, others won't even look at it and they just dismiss it all the way, but, uh, I, I do think there's, there's a—a strong basis for, um, many of the things that we're talking about, uh, especially for after, um, treatment care, uh, and just makes sense. So if, if, if you—if you developed the cancer and you know that most cancers are related to diet, lifestyles and attitude and environmental factors, doesn't it make sense to address those, so you don't get another bout?
	You know, and to say otherwise, uh, that it doesn't have an, uh, an affect is just, just, uh, is just not rational.
Dr. Stengler:	Yeah. You—they, yeah. Irrational is a proper term, I think. You know, in this series, um, I was excited that you're going to talk about detoxification and use of enzymes, because as you know, in, in the medical world detoxification—the term is out there, but it's not really implemented in conventional medicine.
	Now as naturopathic doctors and holistic medical doctors. Detoxification is critical both preventing diseases, treating diseases, and especially with cancer.
	So I think, you know, there's more than 80,000 man-made chemicals in your environment.
Dr. Murray:	Mm-hmm.
Dr. Stengler:	And of course, uh, modern oncology is recognizing more and more how these environmental influences certainly can be a, a trigger for many different types of cancer.

Maybe just explain the basics of what, you know, we're talking about with detoxification and the basic pathways in the body and then we'll get into some more detail, if that's okay.

Dr. Murray: Yeah I, I think that, uh, the greatest threat, uh, to human health right now is not too much sugar, or not even the right types of fats. I think it's, uh, this ever increasing load of the toxic chemicals that are exposed to and the, the research is, uh, overwhelming. Uh, these, you know, pesticides, herbicides, flame retardants, solvents, uh, uh, heavy metals and industrial waste products.

Uh, these are major causes not only of cancer, but, uh, of other chronic degenerative diseases.

Uh, heart disease, uh, diabetes, obesity, uh, thyroid issues, so these are, uh, really serious chemicals and, and, uh, there's a lot of factors that have come into play in helping our body get rid of these compounds. Uh, obviously [laughs] the first [unintelligible] is to try and stay away from them as best we can, but that's, that's really difficult.

You know, I mean, it's kind of a, uh, I don't, I don't want to open up too big of a bag of worms, but, um, you know, the problem with some of the organic foods is, uh, let's, let's, let's take a look at, at how they're produced and, um, if you're using organic fertilizer some of those organic fertilizers are really high in, in heavy metals and, and other toxins and then you, you measure them in the organic food not so good.

So I think we want to—we want to promote, uh, sensible, organic farming.

Uh, you—what I've been amazed at this, if I'm getting off on a tangent—

Dr. Stengler: Sorry.

Dr. Murray: [laughs] Uh, overnight, almost overnight, it seemed like, uh, we had organic food available, produce and, and, and meats available in, in major supermarkets and drug stores where before they were always kind little niche, uh, place in your, in your grocery store, or health foods store, so what's really happened is that, um, the dirty little secret is that, uh, the—organic doesn't necessarily mean pesticide free. And, um, you really gotta—you, you've gotta really, uh, do a better job at cleaning up our food supply.

Our food supply is polluted and we are at the top of the food chain, so humans accumulate those toxins and, uh, so as we get older, it—uh, especially.

If we're not focusing on getting rid of those things, oh my god. They're, they're just going to, they're just going to wreak havoc and, and lead to, uh, not only cancer, but Alzheimer's and, and, uh, increased risk for, you know, obesity and diabetes and all these other chronic disease.

And so detox, okay, so learning how to detoxify is really important and I'm going to, I'm going to talk a little bit about diet, um, but I want to start off by—uh, I wrote a book on cancer and—many years ago and in doing the research on, on that book I came across a really interesting study.

A study looked at, uh, a person's, uh, ability to detoxify cancer causing compounds based upon their level of optimism.

Dr. Stengler: Hmm, wow.

Dr. Murray: *[unintelligible]* a pessimist, or had a positive mental attitude. They used a, a standard questionnaire to quantity a persons, uh, level of optimism and what—what they found was is the people that were, uh, negative, uh, were pessimistic, uh, they had an impaired ability to get rid of these cancer causing compounds.

Dr. Stengler: Mm.

Dr. Murray: On the flip side people that were optimistic, had a positive mental attitude, they were much more efficient at, uh, at, at getting rid of these toxic compounds. So, uh, we're influenced by, uh, not only what we eat, uh, but also what we think and what we feel and there's no question that, uh, those, uh, areas, uh, can play a huge role in reducing our risk for, for cancer and other product degenerative diseases.

Dr. Stengler: Yeah, that's, that's very interesting. You know, being in the industry you've looked at a lot of research, a lot of analysis. I have some, uh, friends of mine who own some, uh, production companies for supplements and herbs and things like that and they tell me, "You just be amazed if you saw, saw these herbal compounds that come in, especially from other countries, and they bacteria and the heavy metals and the pesticides."

They say we—50 percent of stuff we've got to turn back. Um, I know you've looked into this in detail so people, you know, they buy their teas and all of that and it's, it's—people are just bombarded, like you said.

Dr. Murray: Yeah and, uh, you know our, our bodies and—are really, uh, you know, resilient and can, can do a lot. Uh, the, uh, these manmade chemicals in particular; they're very sticky substances, uh, they're very difficult for the body to get rid of, so we really have to, to, uh, do all that we can to stay away from them and then, uh, you know, fortunately there are mechanisms, uh, in, uh, supporting our detoxification instead of some that we can take advantage of, uh, through diet and proper supplementation.

And I think it's really important the—not only in prevention of cancer, uh, but also in helping people recover, uh, and, uh, I just don't—I don't get it, because these, uh, conventional oncologists—they see the, the devastating effects of their, their treatments and, yet they're into rebuilding and they're not helping people recover and, and, uh—

Dr. Stengler: Yeah I haven't met an oncologist yet who, um, had a post-treatment detoxification protocol.

Dr. Murray: That's great.

Dr. Stengler: Yeah.

Dr. Murray: Yeah, it can really make a big difference, uh, cause, uh, let's face it those are pretty toxic chemicals that people are ingesting and, you know, having, uh, injected into them and, uh, if they're not going to get rid of those compounds, uh, they're, they're, they're health's going to suffer.

Dr. Stengler: Well, maybe for the viewers just on a basic level, uh, of course there's just many different categories of toxins and you mentioned a bunch of them. On a basic level how do you explain to the viewers how it increases the risk of cancer? You talk about damage to DNA, um, changing the environment of the cells. How would you explain it to the viewers?

I mean why, why do these chemicals, uh, these toxins—how do they contribute to the formation of cancer?

Dr. Murray: Well, uh, it's really interesting, Mark.

Um, the conventional theory is that a toxin, uh, damages the DNA in our cells and that leads to, uh, a mutation and, and, and cancer formation. Uh, and, you know, some of the common toxins that can do that will, uh, ultraviolet radiation, uh, uh, you know, toxic chemicals in, in, uh, cigarette smoke. The, uh, uh toxic chemicals in our food. Uh, you know, we ingest these compounds, we're exposed to them, and we—and they're, they're kind of like, uh, uh, uh, bullets in a, in a gun.

You want to get rid of, of as many of those bullets and kind of empty your chambers as you, you possibly can, uh, the—I think, I think there's, there's challenges to that, to that theory. Uh, and I don't know if any of your guests have talked about the mitochondrial theory of it.

Dr. Stengler: Mm-hmm.

Dr. Murray: So one of the—has anyone talked about that?

Dr. Stengler: Yeah we have a bit, but go ahead and review it, because you were at different segments there, so review it a bit, yeah.

Dr. Murray: Yeah, so what they, what they've done is they've taken, uh, cancer cells and they, uh, and, and normal cells and they have, uh, swapped DNA so they put the normal cell DNA and the cancer cell and the cancer cell DNA in the normal cell.

Now, uh, the thought was is that the cancer cell would become normal, because the DNA could become normal and vice-versa.

Dr. Stengler: Then what they found out was, is that the cancer cell was still cancerous even though the DNA was fine and, uh, likewise the normal cell was still normal.

So the outcome was that they think that, uh, mitochondrial damage and mitochondria are the energy producing, uh, components of our, of our cells and they have some DNA as well.

So for some cancer maybe a high percentage, uh, it's not the human, or somatic DNA, that's damaged and forms mutation and that leads to the cancer's growth. It's more the mitochondrial, uh, DNA that's, that's damaged.

And, and, uh, there's support for that and it, it's kind of, it, it's kind of, uh, uh, a big issue. *[laughs]* Because all of chemotherapy agents are directed towards, uh, the human DNA and they—that may be why we don't see as good of results, theoretically, as we should, uh, by, you know, killing, killing cancer cells. Because it's not the human DNA it's the, the, the mitochondrial DNA.

Dr. Stengler: Yeah, you hear a lot about, uh, treating the DNA in oncology and by big medical centers, but when you really look at the data it, it's quite disappointing at this point.

I mean, it's not the breakthrough people had thought. I mean, you look at some drugs and, and you know, they, they're proclaimed as a breakthrough and you look at the literature and they extend lifespan, like, two months, and things like that.

Dr. Murray: Yeah, if it was for $100,000, or $200,000 and it's, it's, it's interesting. Uh, you know, there was a big break in the, in the '30s and '40s away from biological therapies into more toxic therapies, like chemo therapy. But there's a resurrection of those, uh, biological therapies and I think we're going to be looking at cancer a lot differently, uh, in, in the very near future. And, uh, there's—you know, we're—we have breakthroughs that are occurring, uh, rapidly in science.

Science reflects the desire to understand our environment and, you know, I just wrote a book, uh, called The Magic of Food.

Dr. Stengler: Hmm.

Dr. Murray: What, what I tried to get across in this book, uh, Mark is that the greatest technology in the world is nothing that man has created. It's nature.

Dr. Stengler:	Mm.
Dr. Murray:	And the way in which we commune with nature on a daily basis is through the food that we eat.
	And we're just scratching the surface in understanding how that food affects our bodies and, and our cells. I, I wanted to call it the magic of food, because, uh, Sir Arthur Clarke, who wrote 2001: A Space Odyssey, said that any sufficiently advanced technology is indistinguishable from magic.
Dr. Stengler:	Huh.
Dr. Murray:	I just told you that the greatest technology in the world is nature and food represents that technology.
Dr. Stengler:	Mm-hmm.
Dr. Murray:	And the way it works in our body is, is magical. You know, I, I, I don't know how, I don't know how my phone works. Uh, to me it's magic. Right?
Dr. Stengler:	*[laughs]*
Dr. Murray:	But I'm sure something that could explain, you know, very, uh, in detail fashion how that phone really works. Uh, and, uh, my book kind of shares with people some information on how food works and, um—
Dr. Stengler:	Well that will be interesting. When's that book coming out?
Dr. Murray:	It, it, it's out.
Dr. Stengler:	It's out now? Okay, good.
Dr. Murray:	Yeah it's out. Yeah, The Magic of Food and people get to drmurray.com. There's a magicoffood.com. If they go to magicoffood.com they can download the practice in the first chapter for free and, and get a taste of it, but, uh, I have no doubt that the, um, um, that the, the future in, in both prevention and treatment of cancer is going to be food first and, and I can't wait for that.
	I hope I—I, I think I'll see it in my life.
Dr. Stengler:	Yeah. Well, that kind of brings up the topic of epigenetics. Not to get too technical with people, but that ties into the food. You want to just touch on that a bit? Um...

Dr. Murray:	Well, yeah. The, the human genome project is this, uh, this idea that we were Going to solve all these, uh, issues of health, uh, and develop new drugs and treatments based upon understanding our DNA, uh, and the sequence of our genetic code.
	Uh, what the scientists have found out is, is that our DNA is a lot like a computer hardware and while that's important, you want to have healthy hardware.
	If the hardware is fried, the computer's fried.
Dr. Stengler:	Yeah.
Dr. Murray:	If the DNA is damaged, if you have a true genetic defect, you got problems. Uh, it's hard to overcome. Uh, but what they found was, is that what is more important to the computers, the software, and what's more important to our DNA is the, uh, epigenetic factors, factors that influence the expression of our genes and those things are attitudes, emotions, experiences, diet, lifestyle, and the environment.
	And so to a very large extent those are things that we can control.
	Interestingly enough identical twins, when they're born, they expressed their DNA almost identical, but by the time they're 50 they only expressed 3 percent of their genetic code in common.
Dr. Stengler:	Mm, hmm.
Dr. Murray:	So they're, they're really not, uh, that, uh, identical anymore. And also, keep in mind, that you have the microbiome—to take into consideration where you have a much greater, uh, diversity of DNA, than you do even in, in your, in your body cells.
	So, um, there's a lot of factors that go into, uh, how we can influence the expression of our genes. Um, and that kind of explains why, uh, some people could have a very high risk of developing breast cancer, or prostate cancer, and yet never develop it.

And, on the flip side, like, some people who have, you know, really shouldn't have, uh, breast or prostate cancer from a genetic standpoint they develop it.

If, if they're just, uh, these factors that, uh, influence the expression of genes and the damage to genes that are not related to the DNA itself.

Dr. Stengler: Yeah, that's good information. Well, maybe take us through some things you typically recommend to people. You do it all lectures and talk to people and patients.

Take us through some of the things you find—uh, beneficial in terms of detoxification for those viewers trying to, you know, do their best to prevent cancer, maybe have been through cancer treatments. What are some of the things you think are real workable, safe and, and effective for them?

Dr. Murray: Well, first let me tell people what not to do.

Dr. Stengler: Mm-hmm.

Dr. Murray: Um, one of the worst things that people could do right now, I think, is to go on an unsupported, uh, water fast, or even a juice fast.

Uh, you need food to help detoxify, uh, I just think one of the problems with a water fast is that these toxins that we're most concerned about, they reside in fat cells.

And, uh, if you're, uh, loosing, uh, or breaking down fat too rapidly you're, you're releasing these compounds and they get mobilized and our, our brain is like a magnet. Uh, cause our brain is like a magnet. Uh, cause our brain should be the largest collection of fat in our body.

For most people it's not, it's your—around your belly, but, uh, so—you know, it—when people are going through a, a juice or a water fast often they, they experience flulike symptoms, dizziness, headaches, uh, cloudy thinking, uh, uh, severe fatigue, joint pain, uh, skin eruptions, and people tell them, "Hey, that's all good! You're, you're, you're having a, a cleansing, uh, process. It's a, it's a healing crisis." And, um, I don't think of it like that. I think it's a crisis. I think its auto-intoxication, meaning they're poisoning their body, because they're releasing all of these toxins that were stored.

Uh, I don't think you should have just sort of the, uh, a reaction. Uh, and, and there are ways to prevent that.

Detoxification is something that we have to pay attention to on a daily basis, so I do recommend a cleanse as I developed one for Enzymedica that I really like, obviously.

Dr. Stengler: Yeah.

Dr. Murray: It's the, uh, a 10 day cleanse and people who go to Enzymatica.com and, and, uh, and learn about it.

That's in the purify line. But, uh, you know, my point is, is that I think you have to eat, uh, good food and eat clean while you're, you know, detoxifying and my goal with that program was to teach people, uh, how to eat and help them feel better quickly, 10 days, uh, I want them to feel better. I don't want them to feel worse, uh, like some of these cleanses.

I want them to feel better, so they understand the connection between how they eat and how they feel. Uh, there's so many things that you have to be cognizant of to, uh, eat clean these days, um, and I'm a little concerned about some of the, the recent dietary fad and, uh, they may be helpful for some aspects of our physiology.

I mean, people are always focused on weight, right?

Dr. Stengler: Right.

Dr. Murray: It's such a big issue so we see, you know, diets like, uh, the, the keto diets, like, did right now, and paleo, um, the, the problem is, is that any sort of animal-based, focused diet—and I'm not saying you should be a strict vegan, but if you're just, uh, you're just you're just eating meat—I just had a, uh, uh, uh, a friend of mine on Instagram just posted his, his diet pyramid and it was, it was, a diet pyramid like all the rest of that you had, it just had pictures of steak, uh, bacon and eggs. That was it.

Dr. Stengler: Oh, wow.

Dr. Murray:	We—that, that was your *[unintelligible]*. I guess, those were his three food groups that he was focusing on and, um, the problem is, is that, um, we, we think about talks and being, uh, really a problem of in produce and there are bigger problem in, in animal foods.
	Uh, meats and, and, uh, and dairy product and that is because, uh, the animals, uh, concentrate those products just like we do.
Dr. Stengler:	Right.
Dr. Murray:	I think it, you, you—we, we always focus on eating organic produce, but the bigger, uh, message should be, uh, you know, eating organic, uh, uh, meat and dairy. Uh, so I'm a little concerned about, you know, people that are out there really, uh, eating a meat center diet.
	Because, um, I just think that they're going to increase their, their load. So I, I like to recommend a diet high in plant foods. You don't have to be a strict vegan, um, you, you know. Uh, uh, I, I was a strict, uh, vegetarian for, uh, six years in my 20s and in—it just didn't, didn't agree with it. You know, you know.
Dr. Stengler:	Yeah.
Dr. Murray:	Uh, you know, but I, I think it does agree for many people and for many people that, that's the best diet for them and we kind of just got to try different things and see what we're, um, I, I think, uh, you know, we all have our, our philosophies on, on what, what people should eat, but there's no question that most people recommend, you know, having to focus on vegetables—good oils and, uh, uh legumes and other, uh, plant foods. Nuts and seeds, et cetera.
	So, uh, those are really important in helping to detoxify as well, uh, so, um, you know, learning how to eat in a way that supports detoxification involves eating more high fiber, high water content food, lots of greens, lots of colors. Uh, one of the concepts that I got at *[unintelligible]* the, uh, The Magic of Food is if you look—if you look globally at, um, blue zones, or, uh, places where people live a long and healthy life.

You can start seeing certain dietary patterns. Now the foods maybe different, you know, and, and, uh, and Italy, uh, Mediterranean, southern Mediterranean, you know, maybe it's red wine and in, in Japan maybe it's green tea.

Dr. Stengler: Right.

Dr. Murray: But, similar compounds, flavonoids, you know, uh, so I, I believe that, uh, one thing that, that you see is—in healthy people is that we eat a high content of, uh, flavonoid rich food, colorful food. Because flavonoids are plant pigments that had been referred to as, uh, nature's biological response modifiers.

That's a big, long, uh, description, but what it means is that these compounds modify our response to the environment. This is noted by their anti-cancer, anti-oxidant, anti-inflammatory, anti-viral affect, so, uh, we, we have to take advantage of those compounds, um—[sound of phone ringing] I'm sorry about that.

Dr. Stengler: That's alright.

Dr. Murray: Uh, so, uh, you know, one of the, the principals that I, I recommend is eating a rainbow diet; five servings of, uh, of, uh, vegetables a day. A serving is defined as one-half cup cooked, or one-cup uncooked vegetable, uh, uh, uh, a day. Five, uh, servings, uh, and French fries and potato chips don't count.

Dr. Stengler: Yeah.

Dr. Murray: And, and, uh, you know, we [unintelligible] the color, try and get a variety of different colors. Two servings of fruit, uh, handful of nuts, uh, nuts are very healthful, just make sure they're not covered in yogurt, or, uh, or chocolate. You know, just focus on, on good, high quality nuts and see—as well as things like avocados, uh, olive oil, uh, cold-water fish, uh, fish oil supplements.

Those are all really good sources of, of oils. So very important to support our bodies nutrition and detoxification, uh, from a foundational aspect first and then we can look at this, the various supplements.

Uh, uh, most of the supplements that people think of for detoxification enhancement involved, uh, enhancing the liver function. But, detoxification occurs in, in just about every cell in the body.

Dr. Stengler: Right.

Dr. Murray: Our liver is critical, uh, and, and it—certainly the major organ is detoxification, but this process is occurring in every cell and so we have to, to kind of, uh, you know—treat, treat the whole body and some of the things that, that I think are quite helpful and things that help boost Glutathione. Uh, Glutathione is a, uh, a pre-amino acid peptide that is really important as an intra-cellular anti-oxidant and it's very important in, in, in getting rid of what are called "Persistent organic [unintelligible]." So pesticides, herbicides, flame retardants, et cetera.

These compounds are hard to get rid of and, uh, Glutathione is very valuable to our cells and so what happens when we're exposed to one of these compounds then, uh, it defeats our Glutathione spores and that makes our cells more susceptible to damage. So things that lower Glutathione levels, like cigarette smoking, or taking Tylenol.

Tylenol is one of the worst drugs ever invented, uh, 50 million people take it on a day—on a weekly basis, rather. And it—what they don't realize is that it's, it's really poisoning themselves and making them more susceptible to, uh, to damage. And that can include increased risk for cancer, uh, Alzheimer's disease, early aging.

So, um, you know, that's where people really need to be looking to, uh, natural approaches to treat many of these common issues that they're taking drugs, like, uh, Tylenol, or proton pump inhibitors.

There's a long list of drugs that, that really are quite damaging, because they interfered with some basic physiology and, again, medical storage; they're going to look back and they're going to think, "What the heck were they thinking? These drugs are poisoning, uh, people."

Dr. Stengler:	Well, you wrote a whole book on that. Now what was the title of that book, again? I have it in my library.
Dr. Murray:	What—yeah, yeah. What the Drug Companies Won't Tell You and the Doctor Doesn't Know.
	And, uh, it's, and I look at every class of drug there, their, their problems. Uh, because their, their mechanisms are—
Dr. Stengler:	Unnatural, yeah.
Dr. Murray:	Not—yeah, they don't address the underlying cause, or they're blocking enzyme systems, uh, they're, uh, interfering with normal physiology. They're producing, uh, some significant, uh, uh, side effects.
	So there, there's a better way to approach these issues.
Dr. Stengler:	Now what other supplements do you, in general, uh, recommend for people to take a look at in terms of detoxification?
Dr. Murray:	Well, you know, herbal medicine; I know that's a love of yours as well as me. And, uh, you know, Milk Thistle Extract is, is one that, uh, most people are familiar with.
	I like to use a special form of milk thistle called, uh, Silybin Phytosome Siliphos. This—in this form the milk thistle components have been bound to the phosphatidylcholine and that increases the absorption and utilization and when you do that with an herbal substance, generally you get better results and that's what the clinical studies have shown.
	Other things that can be quite helpful in supporting, uh, liver health is artichoke extract. Uh, um, you know, in the N-acetyl-cysteine uh, I didn't mention that when you look at nutritional compounds that boost, uh, Glutathione. Those are some of the, the, the key ones that I recommend.
Dr. Stengler:	Oh, yeah, that's great. And, uh, water. Do you have a general water intake, uh, recommendation? I know it depends on the body size and the environment you're in and all of that. Do you have some basic parameters you'd like to recommend?

Dr. Murray:	Um, you know, when I lived in Seattle I didn't worry too much about the drinking enough water. It seemed like I just had to step outside and take a deep breath and have it *[unintelligible]*.
Dr. Stengler:	Yeah.
Dr. Murray:	But I live in, uh, Arizona now and, uh, what I learned about water consumption is that—and then, and in the, in the, in the desert here is you've got to be drinking enough water during the waking hours so that you're, urinating every two, to two-and-a-half hours if you um, if you're not doing that you're, you're dehydrating.
Dr. Stengler:	Mm.
Dr. Murray:	Uh, so you, you really have to—it, it does depend upon your locale and I found that as a good a rule of thumb, uh, uh is in the winter months now, but, uh, in, um, in general in the, in the summer, uh, I make a concoction, uh, of, of it, it, it—it may not sound good to people, but, uh, I, I know it's really good for me, so I do it.
	I, uh, I, I, I juice, uh, two lemons. I, uh, juice a big chunk of ginger and I put in, uh, mineral water, uh, make a gallon and, and I, and I drink that gallon every day.
Dr. Stengler:	Right and then you know you meet your quota there. Yeah.
Dr. Murray:	Yeah. Yeah, so, uh, and the, the lemon juice and ginger are great for anti-cancer, anti-inflammatory affects, so it's, it's, you know, I'm, I'm adding a little bit to the water to make it more interesting and, uh, provide more motivation for me to drink it.
	But, yeah, we, we have to be well hydrated, or our body just doesn't function properly. And, um, that's a big issue for a lot of people.
Dr. Stengler:	Yeah, that's great. Maybe let's just a little bit on enzyme therapy. You're one of the world's experts and just understanding how enzymes work and using nutritional enzymes. Uh, people are interested in enzymes. Lot of people know you can help them for digestion.

Dr. Murray:	Yeah.

Dr. Stengler: Uh, but they're—they have many other uses, maybe take the viewers through that; how they can be helpful for people to enhance their immune system, detoxification, energy, all that kind of stuff.

Dr. Murray: Yeah it—enzymes are really interesting. I think, uh, you know, if people had heard me talk first in the last thirty or forty years I've always said that the enzymes are, are underutilized and they're probably the most valuable natural products in health food stores and available to physicians.

And there's so many great benefits to, uh, you know, therapeutic enzymes as well as digestive enzymes. Just to, to— tell people what enzymes are.

Dr. Stengler: Mm-hm.

Dr. Murray: When we're talking about supplemental enzymes we're, basically, talking about molecules that can, can break down other molecules.

Uh, enzymes can either build new molecules or break them down, so digestive enzymes, for example, break down food components and, and so, uh, the digestive enzymes can be fantastic for, for helping, uh, improve digestion, especially in helping with, you know, gas, bloating, indigestion, occasional heartburn, uh, leaky gut. All of these, these sort of things.

But when we're looking at, uh, kind of systemic effects, like, producing a, uh, a benefit in cancer patients, uh, enzymes that we're, uh, looking to, uh, behave a little bit differently than, um—

It's, it's, it's really interesting, because what happens with these enzymes that we take, uh, orally, these digestive enzymes, is they do get into the blood stream.

Now when they're in the blood stream it would be counterproductive if these things were breaking down our proteins, fats and carbohydrates. So, uh, we have, uh, factors that block the activity of those enzymes.

So what they found when, uh, certain, uh, enzymes is that by taking them in supplemental form in patients who have cancer it increases the production of uh, like, a protease inhibitor.

So, you know, proteases is your protein digesting enzymes, so, uh, the explanation is some people do—the, the way enzymes work in cancer is that oh the, uh, you take the protease that get in your blood and they go in there and they, they, they go there and they digest the cancer.

Dr. Stengler: Right.

Dr. Murray: No. That's not what's happening. Uh, what's happening is that the enzymes that get into the, the body and get into the blood stream and the body responds by increasing the amount of protease inhibitors.

Now this is important, because what a cancer utilizes to grow is that it secretes proteases and other enzymes that break down the surrounding tissue, so that it can grow.

Dr. Stengler: Mm.

Dr. Murray: So what happens when we take these enzymes orally and they get into the blood system; they actually increase the level of inhibitors of these growth, uh, producing enzymes that the cancer cell produces.

And that's why we, we see if we look at the natural products that have been studied in, in clinical studies in patients with, with, uh, with cancer; the ones that have—were done with these, uh, enzyme preparations are, are really quite, uh, um, significant. They show significant, uh, improvements in survival rates and, and effects.

Uh, so, um, I think they're, they're underutilized, uh, uh. It, it, you know, uh, and I know that it baffles me.

And in our book, uh, I, uh, you know, we, we rated them, uh as, uh, the number one, uh, natural approaches to helping people with, with existing cancer based upon the fact that they had such good, uh, research behind them.

Dr. Stengler: Wow.

Dr. Murray:	Yeah. I, I think, I think, uh, they're underutilized and I think what's great about them, Mark, is that they help all these other natural therapies work, work better, too. In other words curcumin, or berberine or some of these other, uh, anticancer compounds from, from plants.
Dr. Stengler:	Mm-hmm. So probably some of the history of cancer, or being treated for cancer now, it would make a lot of logical sense to take enzymes to help break food down, get better nutritional value, less toxins, better immunity, because of it and then take, like you said, the protease enzymes between meals more for, like, a direct anticancer effect. Would you say that'd be true? Or...?
Dr. Murray:	Mm-hmm. Very well said, yes.
Dr. Stengler:	And enzymes really have improved over the last—I mean, enzymes compared to—I started medicine 21 years ago.
	I mean they're... they're just superior now.
Dr. Murray:	Yeah it's, uh, it's fun. Uh, you know, and two science officers were in Enzymedica and, uh, we, we have, uh, a product called Digest Gold, which, uh, it's the best-selling digestive enzyme supplement in North America and, uh, the reason is, is that there's a lot of the proprietary technology in there and, um, in the past, uh, the enzyme therapies primarily used animal-based enzymes; Pancreatin.
Dr. Stengler:	Right.
Dr. Murray:	Uh, the problem with, uh, our own digestive enzyme as well as those from, from pigs is that, uh, these enzymes, like proteases, have a very narrow pH range. Of the digestive enzyme supplements that are available right now they're generally produced from microbial sources and concentrated and these enzymes are not only stronger—but if you mix them properly they are active at more, uh, sites on a protein and they have a broader range of pH activity, so they're able to digest food much more efficiently. They're quicker and they're stronger than our own digestive enzymes and certainly, uh, far superior to, uh, the enzyme that we used, uh, 30 years ago.

Dr. Stengler:	Yeah, that's great. Well, it's good for the viewers. A lot of people have heard about enzymes, are not exactly sure how to use them. Lot of people do use them for digestive issues, but, like you said, people can take that way beyond that, especially people battling cancer. Um...
Dr. Murray:	Yeah. You know, enzyme therapy is great for inflammation, it's been shown to be helpful in osteoarthritis, in rheumatoid arthritis. Any, any person with an auto-immune disease: multiple sclerosis, lupus, the anchylosing spondylitis, rheumatoid arthritis and, uh, they should be taking, um, these, uh, protease, uh, enzyme formulas.
	Uh, anyone that's dealing with a viral infection, uh, there's some great anti-viral effects.
	And there's just a whole cascade of benefits. So when, when you, when you take these, these enzymes that, uh, would occur and, uh, they're, they're useful in so many, uh, different things.
	You know, a lot of thing mucus that, you know, it breaks down the mucus. If you have a sports injury; swelling, pain, you know, these enzymes could be really helpful.
Dr. Stengler:	Well, nice things with enzymes: someone new to, let's say, natural medicine. I mean, you use enzymes with them; and you had a very high likelihood they're going to notice benefit and their confidence in natural medicine goes up pretty quickly.
Dr. Murray:	Absolutely.
Dr. Stengler:	Yeah. Well, Michael, you've shared great information. Anything you want to just say in summary? I know we've covered a lot of areas, I guess, um, you know then I assume with the work you do, you help people to become educated and be more proactive, so they can have a better life. Uh, they can have better outcomes. But how would you summarize your thoughts on this topic?
Dr. Murray:	Well, uh...
	You know, Mark. We, we share a lot and, uh, we're mutual admirers of each other's *[unintelligible]* and we're very

supportive of each other and, uh, you're doing a fantastic, uh, service here and I, I'm just thankful to have any opportunity to, to be part of this program.

And I encourage people to, to, uh, you know, uh, watch and view and learn as much as they can, uh, from all these wonderful experts that, that you've, you've brought together and, most importantly, uh, listen to you.

Dr. Stengler: Oh. Well, hey, we really appreciate it. I mean, we're thrilled to have you on the series, so thank you again.

Dr. Murray: Okay, thank you, Mark.

Dr. Stengler: Thank you.

THE TOXIC EFFECT

— DR. PAUL ANDERSON —

Dr. Stengler: Hi, everyone.

Today, we have an expert in integrative oncology, Dr. Paul Anderson. You know, Dr. Anderson, one of the things that concerns me, and I, I see with some patients, they come into my clinic, uh, for a totally unrelated condition, you know, they're coming in for a certain condition, and in talking to 'em, going through their history, "Oh, yeah, I had cancer five, six years ago, but you know, it's been five years, so I'm you know, it's, it's cured."

And in, in my mind, I'm always thinking, "Wow, I'm concerned, because I know what the relapse rate is with cancer." Uh, maybe speak to that a bit, why it's just, there's no, there are so many people out there with a history of cancer, they feel—

You know, optimistic, which is good, but we know this relapse rate is so high—

Dr. Anderson: Right.

Dr. Stengler: Speak to that, if you would.

Dr. Anderson: Yeah, I think that's, that's very, very critical, and it, um, I think that the, a couple of things are very important to consider. One, one of them is, uh, I'm sure you and I probably do the same thing, which is you're, you're careful how you talk about that, because you know, hu-human nature, and you can think of this with any major disease, is, well, it's gone, they said it's gone. It's been five years, it shouldn't come back, right?

You, you don't wanna rain on their parade, you know, and make—uh, but on the other hand, the other thing that I see human nature do is, you know, a-absence doesn't make the heart grow fonder for cancer, absence makes you forget. And so, if you look, and you see, and wow, you're really living a lifestyle that's fairly pro-cancer, you know, and you've already survived it once, um, how many people do we see that ten years later, maybe they have a different—

Cancer that, you know, whatever. So, I think that the, um, the—it's sort of, a, a, a double-sided balance. One is saying that's great, I'm so glad that you're five years clear of that.

Dr. Stengler: Yeah.

Dr. Anderson: But we need to be proactive and we need to, you know, clean things up as much as we can, and, and you know, what I always tell my people who, now we get them, a lot of times, will come in actively, whether, whether it's after that conversation, 'cause they came in for some other reason and you found out they have cancer. Or they come in and say, "I don't want to get breast cancer again. Can you help me with any of this?"

Um, either way, the best thing to do is to kinda break it back down, and say, "Look, here's, you know, whether it was genomically triggered, or a stem cell issue, or metabolic, or all three, uh, here's the biggest triggers, so why don't we just make sure you don't still have a bunch of toxins around in you. Why don't we make sure—

"There's not some infections kinda hanging out that, that don't give you symptoms anymore." Or, uh, "Let's, let's take a good look at your dietary intake, and you know, your stress levels, and all that." And, and that makes a lot more sense to them, 'cause it's not like you're saying, "Well, you know, oh you had cancer, it's probably gonna come back."

You're saying, "Let's just be proactive, and be as healthy—

Dr. Stengler:	Yeah.
Dr. Anderson:	"As we can be."
Dr. Stengler:	So, there are a lot of things people can do in terms of prevention, if you have cancer, even more important, you get focused on these things, and then take care of 'em.
Dr. Anderson:	Mm-hmm. And I think that's the, you know, w-whether it is a preventive aspect or it's during cancer, the other thing that we see a lot now, which I-I really think probably you and I see more now than we did 10 or 20 years ago, is the person who comes in and says, "You know, I had this stage one or the stage two cancer, and they did standard treatment, and they say it's all gone. I don't want it to come back. And I asked them what to do, and they said, 'Well, we—you know, live a healthy life, and go on, and—
Dr. Stengler:	Right.
Dr. Anderson:	"Call us when you get cancer again."
Dr. Stengler:	Right.
Dr. Anderson:	Uh, so we see that a lot, and so, really, in those cases, we focus heavily on all of these trigger areas, we try and detoxify their home, uh, we, we often do detoxifying therapies with the person. We do check them for, uh, chronic kinda latent infections that are not so symptomatic, and of interest in, in our practice, especially with people who, you know, say you get an early stage prostate—
	Or breast cancer, or somebody catches a colon cancer really early, and it's, you know, no evidence of disease after treatment, we commonly find latent infections in that population. We commonly find they've been exposed to toxins that they, they forget they work somewhere, and got exposed or whatever—
Dr. Stengler:	Right.
Dr. Anderson:	And as you were mentioning, hormonal shifts, you know, because our, you know, we all have stress. There's no way to be alive and not have stress, uh, but it, it tends to be more the way we deal with it. And so, we see a lot in these

folks is just the, the treatments they've undergone are very stressful, and it's—

Dr. Stengler: Right.

Dr. Anderson: You know, so we spend a lot of time kinda getting that system back under control, and balanced, and trying to do that. Um, so whether it's what we would call primary prevention of I'm—I've got a one in three chance of developing cancer I don't want to, or active treatment, I've got cancer, don't know what to do, or secondary prevention, which is well, they've got the cancer, and it's out, and I don't ever want it to come back.

Really, it all comes back to the same things.

Dr. Stengler: Right.

Dr. Anderson: It's these triggers. It's just where you prioritize them as you're treating.

Dr. Stengler: Right, exactly. For, for example, someone was in a workplace near exposed to some, uh, serious toxin, some carcinogenic toxin, and we know that was a, an exposure and maybe run lab tests, we see it is. We gotta focus on that, and still address the diet, and the stress, and all that, but that may be a priority for a period of time.

Dr. Stengler: And I find all the patients and the health professionals are very impressed with the tools we have to really look into these things. Taking the history is one thing, but for a lot of things we're talking about, we have great testing, uh, scientific tests we can do to identify these problems, and the degree they're a problem, and then hone in on 'em, more in the more important root causes, maybe just speak to, uh, the viewers a bit about that, the kind of, um, you know, we got blood tests, we got urine tests, we've got all sorts of tests to look into infections, uh, look into different toxins.

Maybe talk a bit about some of these tests, just some of the common ones we've used to look for root factors—

To help people more proactively.

Dr. Anderson:	Right. And I think that's, uh, that is a huge benefit that has a, im, improved over the last 10, 15 years is just the technology we have available. Um, it's not that long ago that, that most of the infections that were related to cancer, the tests were so unspecific that you could, you might know, or you might not, right? Or there might be a history.
	Uh, kinda the same with toxic testing and other things of that nature. And like anything, because it's, it's almost never one thing that did it, you know, unless, I mean, somebody could have an overwhelming exposure to a, a drug or a toxin or something—
Dr. Stengler:	Right.
Dr. Anderson:	But then you know—
Dr. Stengler:	Right.
Dr. Anderson:	But most of the time, it's a little bit of everything, so, um, the things that I've been most, uh, benefited by, I think, clinically, are in the area of chronic infections, we, we now have lab tests. They're not perfect, but they're, they're 100 times better than they were—
	Ten, 15 years ago, as far as identifying, uh, you know, and, and this is something I think that's good to be clear about. People think, "Well, infection. Shouldn't I have, you know, a fever or pneumonia, or something like that?" Most of the ones that create cancer are a little more stealthy.
Dr. Stengler:	Yeah.
Dr. Anderson:	You know, they're, they, they've been with us so long we don't get symptoms anymore. So, we have much better ways of looking in there, and, and what we usually will tell people is, "Look, if you haven't been checked for the more likely causes, we can do panels that will look into that, and if they're not there, great, we don't have to worry about it, but don't not check for it."
	You know, because I've had many people, where they had two or three things that are treatable, but they just didn't have any symptoms from it, right?
Dr. Stengler:	Yeah.

Dr. Anderson:	So, there's, there's that. Then, within the toxin world, there's two things, I think, that have become very incredibly helpful. One is the sensitivity of testing for things, such as certain, um, carcinogenic, you know, metals, or chemicals, or whatever, is—
	You know, is, is really light years ahead of, of what we had when we were in school for example—
Dr. Stengler:	Things like arsenic, mercury, lead—
Dr. Anderson:	Yeah, oh, and, and now, um, even better, uh, for some of the chemical toxins—
Dr. Stengler:	Oh, yes.
Dr. Anderson:	Like the persistent organic, uh—
Dr. Stengler:	Right.
Dr. Anderson:	Ch-chemicals, and all of that. Um, but the other thing that has been a benefit is you might have been able to test for it before, but it was very hard to infer, is that small, medium, or large, as far—like, is that a good number or a bad number, or whatever?
	The, um, government has been tracking, uh, large, meaning, you know, tens of thousands of people, over time, and uh, so they now have standard norms for what healthy people are supposed to have, as we all get exposed to toxins. I mean, you can't—
Dr. Stengler:	Yeah.
Dr. Anderson:	You can't live a non-toxic life.
Dr. Stengler:	Right.
Dr. Anderson:	But they have norms for tens—literally, tens and tens of thousands of people, so big numbers, which equal good statistical significance.
	And so, you can look, and with, depending on what it is, either a blood test or maybe a urine test, etcetera, you can match that against the healthy normals, and actually have a, a gradient of, you know, the small, medium, and large, and percents.

And so, if we see somebody that's all, you know, off the chart, above that, and they've been exposed to whatever, say a metal or a pesticide or something, that we know is carcinogenic, um, we know that now, uh, there's things we can do to depurate and detox that person—

Dr. Stengler: Right.

Dr. Anderson: Which we talk a lot about in the book. And um, and so, I think that the—not only the ability to test, but now the ability to have data that's really reliable, to say, "That is a lot, that—you shouldn't have that much." You know, which 20 years ago, didn't even exist. You know, they've been—

Dr. Stengler: Yeah.

Dr. Anderson: Actively collect—for this reason. So, I think having the data, having the specificity, and now the tools to actually do something about it is very, very important.

Um, and, and then there's other things that relate to—certainly, we can ask people what they're eating, we can ask them about all sorts of things, and we can tell them to change their diet or something. But there's, um, markers now that we can look at in the blood that actually show, you know, is your, is your diet having an inflammatory effect or, or some other thing.

But if we've narrowed it down, and the diet's the last thing, and they're still really inflamed, then that's probably time to step back and say, "Maybe this diet isn't the right one for you." You know?

Dr. Stengler: Right.

Dr. Anderson: So I think that the testing is, when, when you combine it with what we've always done clinically in asking, looking, you know, taking the whole case, um, the testing and also kinda the, the norming of the data that we have now is so much better and allows us better window—

Dr. Stengler: Yeah, that's great. Well, just for the viewers, just some examples of tests we may run, depending on what's going on with the person, we may do stool tests, look for intestinal infections, how you're breaking food down, as Dr. Anderson has said in previous modules—

Seventy percent of your immune system, approximately, originates in the gut. Look at things like heavy metals with urine and blood tests, mercury, cadmium, um, arsenic, uh, a variety of different carcinogens. Different, uh, chemicals, like pesticides, or benzenes, other chemicals you got from the workplace or the environment.

Again, blood and urine tests, you can test for these things. Nutritional deficiencies, so much research on vitamin D related to the immune system and the risk of certain cancers we talk about in the book. Um, and the list goes on and on. Inflammation markers, I always like to run a big panel of inflammation markers, because, and maybe you could speak to this just for a minute, uh, chronic inflammation, you know, it's related to all chronic diseases, you know—

Dr. Anderson: Yeah.

Dr. Stengler: Including cancer. Maybe talk just a little bit about that.

Dr. Anderson: Yeah. I think that, uh, and I was alluding a little bit to it with just general sort of lab tests, and we think—

Dr. Stengler: Yeah—

Dr. Anderson: You know, sometimes, we think of lab tests, there's kinda two ways that they can be used, many of them. One of the ways is sort of a blunt measurement, as in—

You went to the emergency room and you got this big problem they're trying to sort out, and if you got one or two of these that are way, way out of whack, uh, well, you know, maybe your liver's shutting down, or your kidneys are shutting down. That's one way to look at them.

But there's a lot of inflammatory markers, like the C-reactive protein or lactate dehydrogenase or alkaline phosphatase, or all—a lot of these others that, that might in previous times, have only been looked at in, say, an emergency situation, or the ICU, or just generally making sure you're not gonna die tomorrow, you know?

Dr. Stengler:	Yeah.
Dr. Anderson:	Uh, we can now use those and many, many others that have been developed since then to see if the, the, the is—our, our friend Nasha Winters, calls it the train, you know, inside of the person—
Dr. Stengler:	Yes.
Dr. Anderson:	Is more inflamed, or less inflamed, etcetera. And the reason inflammation becomes such a problem is, is that really, if you look at any, any of the three major theories of cancer—
	As a trigger, inflammation is non-specific across all three of them. Inflammation doesn't help anything.
Dr. Stengler:	Yeah.
Dr. Anderson:	So, one thing it does is it requires your body to expend energy to shut it off, and if you're expending energy to shut inflammation off, that's the same biochemistry that is normally keeping cancer cells from growing. So, you're diverting your troops, you know, elsewhere.
	Uh, but the other thing is is that inflammation generally creates the kind of chemistry that if you had a couple of cancer cells, either metabolically stimulated, genetically stimulated, you know, or otherwise, uh, inflammatory, uh, chemistry around them tends to feed them. And, and that's really where that, that comes in.
	And it's probably where the crossover with toxins cause inflammation, infections cause inflammation, bad diet, bad gut causes inflam—so you know—
Dr. Stengler:	High blood sugar levels, high insulin—
Dr. Anderson:	Tons of things.
Dr. Stengler:	It's all sorts of things, that's right. Being overweight, so—
Dr. Anderson:	Sure.
Dr. Stengler:	Well, this has been great information. I wanna encourage the viewers, you know, seek out doctor—doctors, like Dr. Anderson who can help you look for the triggers, the initiating factors of cancer, um, whether you have had a his-

tory of cancer, whether there's a family history of cancer. I mean, the statistics are just so high that 40 percent of people will develop some type of cancer in their lifetime, and that number continues to increase.

So, why wait until you have cancer? Be proactive. Now, if you've had treatments in the past, chemotherapy, radiation, things like that, I mean, those are toxins, which served a purpose, but they are toxins your body's been exposed to. And so, doctors like ourselves can help the, the cells, the body to recover, to a certain degree from those treatments, and we talk about that in our book, *Outside the Box Cancer Therapies.*

Dr. Anderson: Thank you.

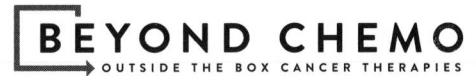

EPISODE 3: CANCER'S KRYPTONITE

Watch as the World's Best Oncologists Reveal Their Top Cancer-Killing Secrets (Including One that's 35 TIMES More Effective than Chemo)

BOOSTING YOUR IMMUNITY THROUGH IV THERAPIES

— DR. PAUL ANDERSON —

Dr. Stengler: Well, welcome back to *Outside the Box Cancer Therapies*. I'm here again with Dr. Paul Anderson, an expert in integrative oncology, and we have a very important topic today, one that we help a lot of patients with, as do other integrative doctors around the country, and that's the concept of injection therapies. Also can be in the category of intravenous therapies.

And so, Dr. Anderson actually teaches doctors around the country how to do these therapies safely and effectively. He's also written extensively on the tremendous amount of research behind them and how they help the immune system, how they can help to fight cancer, how they can help patients who have fatigue problems, uh, and other side effects, undergoing conventional cancer therapies.

So, Dr. Anderson, welcome back again.

Dr. Anderson: Thank you.

Dr. Stengler: So, this whole concept of injection therapies, intravenous therapies, people kinda have a basic idea, if they've been in a hospital, what we're talking about. But give an overview of what it is—

Dr. Anderson: Sure.

Dr. Stengler:	And we're gonna get into some of the specific therapies—
Dr. Anderson:	Yeah.
	And, uh, I think probably one of the—it's, it's different now. I think originally when we started doing it years ago, um, the most common question we would get would be, well, can't I just take like that vitamin by mouth, and not have to worry about the needle?
	Uh, which i, is true, you can take many things by mouth. Um, so the first thing I think is the theory behind why one would even do this, because sometimes, what we hear from our colleagues at the hospital or out in primary care, where they really don't do this sort of therapy, is wow, you know, the, the only IVs I've ever seen have been, you know, hydration in the ER, or uh—
Dr. Stengler:	Mm-hmm.
Dr. Anderson:	You know, someone gets low potassium, and they have to replete it or—
Dr. Stengler:	Yeah.
Dr. Anderson:	Antibiotic.
Dr. Stengler:	Yeah.
Dr. Anderson:	So, why are you giving a patient an IV of anything? You know, that, that's sort of the, the idea, and a lot of patients will feel like, wow, I—that, that seems intense. Well, the first thing about it is it bypasses your digestive system, and—
	As we've talked about, the digestive system is probably one of the first systems to kinda go down or go dysfunctional when you start to get sick, of, of any kind of illness, but especially in cancer, in any chronic illness, and especially during cancer therapies in the digestive system is, is very, uh, low functional, okay.
	So, you can be taking a lot of things early, and they may be w-working a little bit, but not, not very well. So, in intravenous therapies, the idea is of course to go around the digestive system, put it right in where the cells can take up

all the nutrients or whatever you're putting in. And, and it's quite frankly, why if you have a very bad infection you go to a hospital, they don't give you antibiotics in a pill form. Usually, they give it to you in an IV so it gets to the infection—

Dr. Stengler: Right.

Dr. Anderson: Faster.

Dr. Stengler: Right.

Dr. Anderson: So, what we've done over the last few decades, really, is, uh, kinda springboard off the work of some early pioneers in—

The IV nutrient therapy world. Um, and we talk about a number of these doctors in, in the book, but uh, um, this idea goes back, really, to the 40s, and before. And it was really, in my mind, fairly intrepid physicians who were really going against the system, because there wasn't a lot of IV therapy done back then anyway.

Dr. Stengler: Right.

Dr. Anderson: And then they were doing nutrients, you know, uh, and actually having quite good success with it. So, what, what I feel that the—I consider myself in sort of the modern wave of IV nutrient and IV natural therapies, uh, work, is we, we worked off sort of those intermediate groups of people from the '40s to the '70s, who really tried what they could with the materials available, and developed some protocols that would say, gee, you know, turned out safe, and many of the patients got some benefit.

And what would happen, you know, if we had—

More available, more nutrients, or even maybe some, uh, you know, medicines that came from an herbal base, or medicines that came from some other chemistry, you know, base.

Dr. Stengler: Right.

Dr. Anderson: So, that's really been the purpose of the last 35 to 40 years of doing this type of IV therapy. So, technically, it's the same as if you've ever been or seen somebody getting an

IV. There's an IV catheter that's in a vein, and there's a tube, and a, and an IV bag. The difference is what's in the bag normally.

So, in the world of cancer therapy, um, whereas, let's say 15, 20 years ago, there might have been two, or three, or four type of therapies that we would've done. Uh, now, there are literally, uh, at least near, you know, in our clinic, near 100 different variations of things that can be done. Because technology's expanded—

Availability of things has expanded. But really, our knowledge has expanded.

Dr. Stengler: Right.

Dr. Anderson: So, so we have a number of categories, and I think the best way to do it would be to describe the categories, and maybe we can talk about specific items—

Dr. Stengler: Yeah, sure.

Dr. Anderson: Within it. So, one would be what I, what I would call restorative or quality of life IVs, so this would be, um, you, your, you're back home from surgery, you wanna heal up. You haven't been able to eat well, etcetera. We have a lot of nutrient therapy mixtures that would replace the amino acids and the vitamins and minerals and fluids, etcetera, that your body, you know, may just not have had enough of to heal up afterwards—

Dr. Stengler: Right.

Dr. Anderson: So it's a little boost.

Dr. Stengler: Right.

Dr. Anderson: The nice thing is—

Dr. Stengler: The hospital food just didn't supply enough—

Dr. Anderson: Yeah, the, the hospital food, or, or whatever IV they give you at the hospital, just wasn't quite enough, right? And, and there's actually—and I believe we, we speak about it in the book, but there's data that shows, um—

If you look at some of the more common, just, just surgical

procedures, such as orthopedic surgery, very common, up to, you know, 70 to 80 percent of people are malnourished, technically before they get surgery, so then you know, you've got surgery. It's, it's not going well. Kinda the same with cancer patients, right?

Dr. Stengler: Yeah.

Dr. Anderson: So, we do, we do a lot of that. Sometimes, if we have time to plan, we'll, we'll build them up with some before surgery, then stop in a reasonable time, let them have surgery, and then afterwards, at a reasonable time, restart.

Dr. Stengler: And that could be things like amino acids, which helps you make muscle and tissue, uh, vitamin C, immune system tissue healing, B vitamins for energy, magnesium for energy, detoxification, um, minerals, detoxification, tissue healing. So, things like that we're talking about.

Dr. Anderson: Yes. Yeah, very, very—uh, things that are already on the inside of you, just that you probably need a bit more of after whatever you know,—

Dr. Stengler: 'Cause the body doesn't heal by magic.

Dr. Anderson: Right.

Dr. Stengler: It requires these nutrients.

So, between the, the American diet, maybe the hospital food, being on medications, high stress, um, we can get these high levels of nutrients, in a safe manner still, sometimes I call it supraphysiological. Um, and we cite data in the book, for example, you can get up to 100 times the blood level with some of these nutrients, vs. taking them orally.

Dr. Anderson: Yes.

Dr. Stengler: So, we're forcing—not forcing, but we're, we're more aggressively supporting—

Dr. Anderson: Yeah.

Dr. Stengler: Tissue healing, if you will.

Dr. Anderson: Yes. And it's, and it's all—you know, I think something that's important to state is whether we're doing, you know, ten times or 100 times, or whatever, uh, the normal amount, one of the nice things of the last 30 or 40 years is there's been a lot of work done by people who preceded me and people of kind of our generation that really tried to map out the levels that were safe and that were effective, and you know, sometimes, you need a certain amount—

But you really don't need more, you know, or, or sometimes—

Dr. Stengler: Yeah.

Dr. Anderson: You, if, if you give too little, it's like why even bother. So, we have very safe parameters around which we can do it. And often, they're, they're quite different from what people would see in a hospital IV, so that's usually the first discussion that has to go on, is, well, we're doing this for a very specific reason.

And I think the other thing to, uh, kinda segue, 'cause it's very similar IV therapies, is the patient who needs, um, a boost of quality of life, say they didn't have surgery or anything, but just the process of their cancer and their cancer therapy has just worn them down—

Dr. Stengler: Right.

Dr. Anderson: And they're, um, you know, just, just not having, not only energy, but it's hard to focus, and think, etcetera. In many cases where the person will come in and they'll say, "Look, I—you know, I, my cancer, I understand, I know where it's at. You know, I, I, yeah, I'd like it to go away, but that's not a big deal.

"But what I would like is to be able to not have to sleep 20 hours a day, and I would like to be able to speak to my family, and all of these things." And we've had many, many cases like that, where we do similar things with amino acids, and vitamins, and minerals, and certain, you know, very—what I would call physiologically balanced, but as you say, kinda supraphysiologic dose.

And we do a few of those, and it just supplies, whether it's muscle, liver, brain, gut, whatever the tissue is that was the weakest. It supplies them with the substrate they need to work. And we've had people literally, um, in—you know, whether it was end-stage of life, or just they need to be kinda perked up after all the therapy, and they were gonna live a while longer.

We've had people go from, you know, very dysfunctional, and having to take a lot of medications, and, and really being kinda groggy or sleepy—

Dr. Stengler: Yeah.

Dr. Anderson: To being able to engage with family and be on lower amounts of pain medication, etcetera. So, so in that—

Realm, whether it's, uh, you know, to help you heal from something, or just to help you kinda get back some health, that's a huge area of, of the IV, IV *[unintelligible]*—

Dr. Stengler: Oh, yeah, and I see that consistently helping people.

Dr. Anderson: Yeah.

Dr. Stengler: You know, the fatigue and the brain fog, people who have been through chemotherapy and radiation, uh, weak community, getting sick easy, wow. I mean, I'd say the vast majority of people, we do these, uh, nutritional IVs with notice a significant improvement. They really do.

Now, Dr. Anderson, you know, when the patients come in my clinic, and now yours too, you know, we talked about different, uh, therapies. We have formed different modalities, and I talk to 'em about nutrition, I talk to 'em about detoxification, and I talked to them about herbal medicine, and things like that.

But I do tell 'em probably the closest thing we have to conventional medicine is some of our intravenous therapies. Now, not necessarily like in a, in a treatment where there's side effects, but in terms of potency, um, let's get into this big category, what we call oxidative—

Therapies. What that means in some of the more important treatments, and, and how they work, and a little more detail on that.

Dr. Anderson: Yeah, so those, uh, oxidative therapies are, to lump them into a big category, would be therapies that would actually create an oxygen reaction within the system, usually in the plasma or the extracellular space. And an oxygen reaction actually creates then a trigger for other chemistry that, uh, really calls the immune system to reactivate, reenergize, etcetera.

So, whereas, what we're just talking about being more palliative or recuperative therapies, where we're giving sort of a broad base of amino acids, vitamins, etcetera.

Oxidative therapies are, uh, a very targeted treatment, where you're trying to get the immune system to go and do something specifically, whether that's to focus on killing a pathogen, like a virus, or something, or, or whether it's—

Get—trying to get the chemistry around the cancer to stay involved in the fight with the cancer. Uh, etcetera. That's really the goal of most oxidative therapies. The one people have probably heard the most about is high dose vitamin C, and it's uh, been—it was popularized, uh, in Scotland before, and then, the line *[unintelligible]* popularized in the US.

And, and uh, if you've read the history of that, you know it kind of goes back and forth between oh, it's a good idea, it's a bad idea, and all that. Uh, and, and we've certainly seen that whole spectrum of things. Uh, but one of the things that was, uh, of interest was, in, in uh, the research that the National Institute of Health funded that we were involved in all those years ago, the very first thing that we did in the IV therapy service was high dose vitamin C, because that's the one thing everyone knew about—

Dr. Stengler: Right.

Dr. Anderson: And uh, even though, the, the, the structure of the research was not set up to be an IV research, eh—

They wanted something for IV, right?

Dr. Stengler: Yeah.

Dr. Anderson: And they'd said, "Well, we've heard about vitamin C, so why don't we test that out?" So, um, and we had been doing that for years before, so we kinda had a roadmap for that, and all. The idea with it is, because people say, "Well, wait a minute, I—you know, vitamin C, my doctor says an antioxidant, right? So, how could vitamin C be an oxidate pro-oxidant. That just seems not possible."

What happens is if you eat vitamin C in a food, or you take pills of vitamin C, or even if you get an IV, like we were talking about before with just a little bit of vitamin C.

Dr. Stengler: Yeah, low dose.

Dr. Anderson: It's a, it's an antioxidant. It goes to your cells, and it helps shut down oxidation. When you—and you can only do this through IV, an IV therapy, and it's been studied numerous times, but especially in the mid-2000s, a lot of landmark papers came out, and we referenced those in the book, showing that if you get the plasma levels up to a certain level, it goes from—

Being an antioxidant to an actual pro-oxidant. So, the goal with the IV therapy would be to get the plasma to those levels. Now, it's an incredibly safe modality, because if, if you do the right work up on people, and make sure that they don't have kidney troubles, and certain genetic problems, etcetera, which we test everybody for, but if, if you, if you rule out those people who may have a problem, uh, it is incredibly safe therapy.

And the thing that we see with it is it's, um, there, there was a lot of hope for a long time that maybe if we just got enough vitamin C in a cancer patient, you know, all the cancer cells would die and all that. We don't really see that, but what we do see is we see improved immunity, improved immune function.

We often see an extension of life over, uh, the you know, standard lifespan one might see—

With that type of cancer. And uh, we definitely see in most people quality of life improvement.

Dr. Stengler:	Yes.
Dr. Anderson:	Which is very important. And, and so, it's not a one—you know, kind of one trick therapy, but it's a very good base therapy, because it's, um, it, it does many, many things. And without getting too deeply into it, and having, having had to both defend and also explain it in research, because when you're working with other doctors, they wanna know, "I don't get this. Why are you doing it?" You know? You have to, you have to come up with not only research studies to back it up, but a good explanation for it.
Dr. Stengler:	Right.
Dr. Anderson:	So, without getting too deeply into that, what we, uh, noticed was the high dose vitamin C, probably the reason that people get both a quality of life benefit and, and an immune benefit is there's a time where the high dose is doing that oxidative type therapy. But then, that level starts to go down—
	And it doesn't just magically disappear. Your normal, healthy cells are sucking it up, because they love vitamin C. So, the kinda what you might call the leftover, or what we used to think was non-usable vitamin C, 'cause it wasn't a high dose, is actually helping the healthy cells stay healthy.
	So, you get kind of a double benefit that way.
Dr. Stengler:	Yeah.
Dr. Anderson:	So, that, that's the main one. Now, there's others, uh, that are common, but sometimes controversial, uh, ozone therapy, which is an oxygen, uh, instead of O2, it's O3, so it naturally drops off into oxygen, so it creates an oxidative burst. And that has a similar but, but quite different effect, really.
	Really, what that does is it delivers the oxygen in that oxidative, uh, cleaving, and burst that happens at the tissues. Instead of like with vitamin C, where you create peroxide, and there's this whole other cascade that goes on, it—
	It, it, it kinda short-circuits that system and just, it really goes and turns on all of the, uh, immune triggers that are, that you know, to say, "Okay, let's go after this." So, you see ozone

therapies used in, in infections a lot, and, and also in cancer.

And, and then the other one that's probably one of the most common oxidative therapies, uh, that is also sometimes con—you know, considered bad or good or whatever, but certainly been used for a long time, is the actual use of dilute hydrogen peroxide, which sounds really odd, you know, because you see it bubble, and that might be bad.

But it's—uh, a peroxide therapy for IV is a very specific thing, and it's made by a pharmacy—

Dr. Stengler: Right.

Dr. Anderson: So there's not the stuff that's—

Dr. Stengler: Right, right.

Dr. Anderson: You're, you know, you're cleaning your, your stuff with. Uh, so, so and the thing that, uh, is, is interesting in, in speaking with doctors about this, is they'll think, "Well, okay," they, they know if they're—especially if they're [*unintelligible*] oncology, they know that there's petri dish studies—

Where they'll take peroxide, and they'll put it with certain types of tumor cells, and peroxide will kill many tumor cells, right?

Dr. Stengler: And your immune system produces it naturally in small amounts.

Dr. Anderson: And your immune system uses it to help—

Dr. Stengler: So, people are surprised—

Dr. Anderson: All sorts of stuff—

Dr. Stengler: To find that out, yeah.

Dr. Anderson: It's, it's part of you, already—

Dr. Stengler: Yes.

Dr. Anderson: What the doctor will miss is the fact that, um, you're putting the peroxide in upstream, you know, whether it's through a vein here, or through a port, or whatever, it's going into your plasma. It becomes, uh, broken down immediately. So, then, there's sort of two arguments there.

One is, oh, well, the peroxide's not gonna get to the, uh, tumor, which, which is true. It's not.

And so, uh, therefore, it's, it's totally worthless. And the other is, well, I've certainly seen patients benefit from it. Well, what is the benefit? I-if it's broken down in the past, then what in the world's the benefit?

Well, it turns out that the benefit is actually, let's say, you know, you put it in my arm here, and by the time it's in the blood up here, it's broken down. The process of the breakdown of it is actually where the, the medical benefit happens, and that is, there is in breaking the peroxide down, there's a release of these chemicals that go downstream, and they don't get broken down, and they will float through your plasma, and they'll go, and they will turn immune activity on.

So, peroxide has multiple ways of going. Now, the way to get actual peroxide to a tumor tissue is actually, that's one of the things vitamin C does, that high dose. It actually delivers it at the tissue. If you're doing it dilute peroxide pharmaceutical version in the IV, you're delivering immune chemistry.

So, just, just different ways of the same thing—

Dr. Stengler: Yeah, yeah. Now, one of the treatments we use at my clinic would be a substance called artesunate, often used before the high dose vitamin C for more aggressive treatment.

And uh, I think you're to be credited with that. Aren't you really the one who helped bring it into the, into the, um, kinda the integrative oncology world a number of years back, or tell us about the history of that and what it is and how it works.

Dr. Anderson: I-I'm one of, I'm one of a group, yes.

Dr. Stengler: Okay.

Dr. Anderson: Yeah, it's uh, so, most of the group doesn't want anyone to know who they are, so, uh, so thank you—

Dr. Stengler: Oh, okay.

Dr. Anderson: For asking me on camera, though, that's good. But no, I write about it extensively, in the IV chapters—

So, there's nobody who's not gonna know. Um, it, it is, it is a part of the wormwood plant family. So, uh, and the wormwood plant is used for many, many things in, in plant botanical medicine, but um, in Asia, the uh, ar-arte-sunate, and then the oral version is called artemisinin, and we write about both in the book. Um, artesunate has been used for—

Decades, uh, for malaria, as a malarial treatment. It is relatively inexpensive to produce, there's a lot of malaria in Asia, and in, in certain other parts of the world, and uh, and, and what they found is there's different pieces of the wormwood plant, but the artesunate as far as an injectable is the safest.

And so, I often have doctors say, "Well, I've read about, you know, this other injectable, or this one," and, and, and I have, too, and I tell them not to use those, because they're, they're not nearly as safe as artesunate, and it works quite well.

So, so the next question comes, uh, how did anyone get from, uh, you know, malaria treatment or—and they use it for other infections, too—uh, to cancer. That, that seems like a leap right there, right?

Dr. Stengler: Yeah.

Dr. Anderson: Uh, so, I, I think that's where sort of, uh, uh, definitely a small group of us in North America, um, and uh, maybe a little bit bigger group in, uh, in Europe, and that actually some research—

Maybe a little more forward thinking research in Asia where they're very used to using it for malaria, all started to say, "Well, wait a minute. How did, how does it work to kill a, a pathogenic bug?" And, well, there's two things it does, which is—I, I really think artesunate in its injectable form, is actually a bit safer than the oral version, as we talk about in the book with the oral one, you have to rotate it, and do all these things, you know, and it's not, it's not that dangerous, but it's, you know, it's, it—you have to keep up with it—

Dr. Stengler:	Yeah.
Dr. Anderson:	And so, wormwood is a tricky plant to use. And in the injectable form, what we learned was the reason that it would go and kill something like malaria or some other type of infection is it would create a similar, but different oxidative burst to what we would see with, say, ozone or vitamin C. So, not quite the same, but similar.
	So, what, uh, and, and um, the, the part, partially, I'm credited for, because it was part of the research we did, so it was sort of legally protected to try it and use it, was, um, uh, we literally had a, a meeting, and uh, we would periodically have meetings, and we'd look and say, "Okay, of our stage four cancer patients in this category, who is living and who is doing better than the others? And are they doing anything different?"
	Because we were searching for any answers we could, right?
Dr. Stengler:	Yeah.
Dr. Anderson:	One of the things that we found in that early—and this was very early on—was there was a woman who had very advanced stage four breast cancer, gone all over the body, and um, she really should not have been alive, and she was. And we started to kinda look at her case, and the one difference—
	She had from the rest of the group was she had gone over to Germany, where uh, an oncologist was doing this combination therapy, using artesunate IV and then high dose vitamin C. And he says, "There's no reason that Dr. Anderson can't do that in the US," um, so he sent her home with the drug, and uh, with a very tiny piece of paper, writing out, uh, "This is how you do it." It's just not a terribly elaborate protocol, but uh, that, that was that.
	And, and we had a little bit of communication. And I thought, hmm, okay. 'Cause this, you know, I, I had thought about it, and read about it, but it, it was never really available in the US. So, uh, we started to do the therapy with her, and she continued to stay alive, but also was pretty functional, like considering the level of disease she had.

| Dr. Stengler: | Yeah. |
| Dr. Anderson: | Um, what really happened was that this oncologist had sent her home with so much— |

Of the artesunate that she could never use all of it, and I don't know if he did it on purpose or not, but um, we decided well, let's, let's, let's actually study a group of breast cancer patients using it.

And so, we were the first to actually do a, to track patients with and without artesunate and vitamin C. And we, we took a group of, uh, 40, and this is part of what was, uh, what was, um, reported at Society for Integrative Oncology, the year that Medscape wrote it up, which I think was good, because it was very good outcome.

Uh, but actually got the attention of people, and we, we took a group of 40 people who were all doing integrative cancer therapy, so it wasn't like, you know, some were just getting chemo, and some weren't. They were all getting the same thing, and we offered all 40. They all had stage four breast cancer.

| Dr. Stengler: | Yeah. |
| Dr. Anderson: | We said, all, some, or any combination of you— |

Can get this combo of, uh, artesunate, and then a vitamin—high dose vitamin C. Or you can just continue to do all the other integrative things that we're doing with, with no IV addition. And we just wanna track you over time.

| Dr. Stengler: | Yeah. |
| Dr. Anderson: | And so, what it was, it turned out to be a, a one-third, two-thirds. So, it was about, I believe 10 in the treatment group who were getting integrative oncology, plus the IV artesunate, vitamin C, and then, uh, 30 in the integrative oncology without the IV. |

And we track, we tracked them actually for five years, but the statisticians have the data on the three years. And there was a, a very significant, uh, statistically, uh, survival advantage in those who did the artesunate and the vitamin C over those who just did the integrative oncology.

Now, to, to be fair, those who did the integrative oncology without the IV still lived longer than if they wouldn't have done it.

Dr. Stengler: Okay.

Dr. Anderson: So, but—

Uh, to see the benefit on top of it was—

Dr. Stengler: Yeah, to *[unintelligible]*

Dr. Anderson: Quite remarkable. So, we then started to expand that out, and use it in, uh, people with prostate and other types of cancer, and since then, we've used it for many, many other things. Um, and uh, the um, then some of the, you know, technical things, such as getting it, because it's—you, because it, we are not considered to have malaria in North America. It's not really a big drug here, right?

So, it's had to be, uh, made specifically through, uh, an FDA cleared source, and we have availability, etcetera—

Dr. Stengler: Yeah.

Dr. Anderson: So, we, we at least now don't have to get it from Germany or some other place—

Dr. Stengler: Yeah.

Dr. Anderson: But, but that was, um, that was a very, um, I mean, it, it was one of those things that looked great on paper, but you know how that is.

Dr. Stengler: Yeah.

Dr. Anderson: Doesn't always work.

Dr. Stengler: Till you see it, you—

Dr. Anderson: The one thing I would say about ar—artesunate is, and this would be the whole wormwood family, but as an injectable—

What, what we discovered later was, was not a new discovery. It was just in reading the data deeper, trying to look for, this is doing more than just probably an oxidative treatment. It turns out that the doctors who do autoimmune disease have been researching artemis and then artesunate and wormwood for about a decade.

And so, they don't like oxidation in that end of medicine, usually. So, we started reading their research, and the reason that they believe that it works there is, in addition, totally separately from the oxidation, it has a immune modulating or an immune sort of calming effect.

So, one of our working theories was, especially with the breast cancer, these are metastatic breast cancers, so they've got in the bones and everywhere, is not only do you get that burst of oxidation that helps the vitamin C work, but way after the oxidation is gone, the chemistry of the—

Uh, artesunate is going to places where tumor cells may be hiding, or metastasizing, and not turning up or down their immunology, but actually leveling it out, which tends to slow them down. And so, that's something that we see with a lot of other therapies, but this was just sort of a— we, we believe a very fortunate bonus from—

Dr. Stengler: Yeah.

Dr. Anderson: You know, a, a—well, probably more than a two-for-one from that plant. But that, that's been a very, very big, uh, benefit, and it's used quite a bit in, uh, in, as I said, Germany and a lot of Europe in cancer—

Dr. Stengler: Yes.

Dr. Anderson: And they're, uh, experimenting in Asia with many different cancers [unintelligible] right now, so—

Dr. Stengler: Yeah, it's a great addition. Uh, another IV therapy, uh, you have a lot of experience with, poly MVA. Tell the viewers what that is, and of course, we do talk about in our book, *Outside the Box Cancer Therapies*, both orally and intravenously.

Dr. Anderson: Right.

Dr. Stengler: But, uh—Tell us about it.

Dr. Anderson: So, it's a, a, the poly part comes from it being a polymer, so in, instead of, uh, say, a ionic or crystal substance, like a mineral would be, or, uh, or an organic substance like a vitamin would be. It's a combination, really, and it's an, it's an unusual molecule that was developed specifically in looking for something that would weaken cancer cells, ma-many, many decades ago now.

Um, and it's actually been used, um, prior to in humans, it was used a lot in veterinary cancers, which is where we got a lot of the original data to show it actually did make differences in certain types of cancers in dogs and, you know, other animals, which is always helpful to see if, you know, there's something that goes on there.

And as you mentioned, it comes in an oral and an IV version. The reason that we started to use the IV version, because the oral version actually works quite well, and it's pretty easily absorbed.

Its, its structure, one of the reasons they designed the structure the way they did as a polymer was so it would absorb easily, so it, it is used orally quite a bit. In its IV form, uh, we use it, usually to synergize other therapies, and it's, it's a little like vitamin C in that it can be used as a restorative, so if someone has a neuropathy after chemotherapy, we might use a lower dose of it as a restorative with other IV therapies.

In moderate to higher doses, it actually can go and it takes advantage of something that we, uh, talked about in an earlier segment, which is the metabolism difference between a cancer cell and a normal cell.

So, a normal cell would take it up, use it, kinda like, uh, it uses vitamin C as more of an antioxidant supportive nutrient. Cancer cells have a part of them where if they were a normal cell—

Energy would be generated, and in the cancer cell, that's a real dysfunctional place, and it's, it's what allows a cancer cell, in part, to divide as fast as it does, and it's, you know, it's sort of a, it's a fast dividing but not terribly well-organized cell.

Dr. Stengler: Right.

Dr. Anderson:	Smart, but not well-organized. The poly MVA actually has an affinity for that part of the cell. So, like I said, it goes to the normal cell, it just helps it work better.
Dr. Stengler:	Right.
Dr. Anderson:	Goes to the cancer cell, it kinda turns on some processes, and this is something that when they, when they first were putting it together, they, we didn't even know exactly how that part of the cell worked, right? So, they kind of were guessing a little bit, and then as time has gone on, they researched it, and found, "Oh, it does this."
	So, in a cancer cell, it actually goes in, and it causes pieces of the energy creating mechanism in the cell to work at a, at a level that is, um, uh, unhealthy for the cancer cell. So, it makes, again, it's like we talked about—
	With the metabolic therapy you're doing, metabolic diet therapy, it makes the cancer cell in a weakened state.
Dr. Stengler:	Yeah.
Dr. Anderson:	And then that gives it more, uh, uh, more availability for immune function to come and get it, or, or just for the cell to, to, uh, have what we call an apoptotic effect, where the cell realizes it's not normal and actually kinda involutes and dies. And we've actually seen that in, uh, in cell line studies that we've, we've done with it.
	Um, so the reason that we, we use it as a couple things. Like I said, it can be on the restorative side, but on the treatment side, um, getting it to the tumor cell can be of great benefit in getting the cell to actually realize it's a tumor cell, and then your tumor cells, once they realize that they're actually a tumor cell, have a natural, uh, internal death, a thing we call apoptosis.
	Um, so, so that's one of the main reasons that we're using it a lot now, and—
	So people will say, "Well, if I can take it orally, do I have to do it IV," etcetera. Kinda the same as the other things in the beginning. We might do an IV just to kinda get, you know, more going in there.

Dr. Stengler:	Right.
Dr. Anderson:	And then we will maybe switch people to it, uh, as an oral. Um, just of note, because, because it's an unusual, you know, it's, it's a very unique molecule, and uh, there's a laboratory that, you know, owns a patent and all of those things, um, and so, over time, people have thought, "Well, you know, is it just a gimmick, or whatever?"

We actually cite in the book now, um, uh, even NASA has been using it in experiments on, uh, protecting, uh, astronauts from radiation, so doing a radiation protection, et-cetera. And it, and, uh, that's actually led us to e-expanding it from just a cancer treatment side or the restorative side to, uh, some post-radiation work with it, too. Um, so it's, it's something that's actually kind, kind of—

Like a lot of the things we've talked about. The longer they're around, if they keep working, somebody says, "There's gotta be a reason," and they study it deeper. |
Dr. Stengler:	Yeah.
Dr. Anderson:	That's something we see with poly MVA.
Dr. Stengler:	Yeah, it's very unique. Um, the last injection therapy, let's talk about mistletoe extract.
Dr. Anderson:	Mm-hmm.
Dr. Stengler:	Um, for our friends from Europe, uh—
Dr. Anderson:	Yeah.
Dr. Stengler:	Developed that over the years.
Dr. Anderson:	Yes.
Dr. Stengler:	But talk about that.
Dr. Anderson:	Yeah. Um, mistletoe, as, as we all know, is a plant, or most of us probably know as a plant, we think of it around the holidays, hanging up in the ceiling. Um, and mistletoe comes in a number of different, uh, forms, as a plant. So, it's essentially, uh, it's, it's a parasitic type plant that lives off of other plants.

So you usually find it, you know, trees or bushes, etcetera. And so, um, the, the Europeans, uh, probably are most credited with looking at it, and saying, "Well, that plant acts different than a lot of other plants, and that plant seems to be able to—

Take advantage of other plants," and it, so there's sort of bred this whole idea of, oh, well, maybe it would do something to disease cells. Um, and so, i-if you look at it in a—if it's—eh, if you were to take it, you know, mistletoe orally, it'd be quite toxic, right? So, that was, sort of, the first experiments, uh, where that was—many, many years ago.

Dr. Stengler: Yeah.

Dr. Anderson: Um, and then what they, what they realized was if you, um, kind of like the wormwood to artesunate idea of a purification of just one piece of it, if you take the piece that is probably the most potent, but purify it, and make it sterile, what they would do then is they would inject it, uh, just under the skin, into the fact under the skin, and they would find that they would get an immune response.

So, it was, it was not a, you know, not, um, a, you know, an allergic, bad response. It was just your immune system reacted to it.

Dr. Stengler: Yeah, you want a mild, inflammatory reaction to—

Dr. Anderson: Yeah, so it was—

Dr. Stengler: Activate the immune system, right.

Dr. Anderson: To say, "Hey, immune system, let's do something. We've got this, you know, cancer." So, they came up with a very elaborate, um, not only some of the different species of mistletoe, but also you start with a very, very, very low dilution of it, and see how the person responds, and *[unintelligible]*.

Dr. Stengler: Right.

Dr. Anderson: And nowadays, uh, there's—you can do it by that subcutaneous kind of injection, kind of like someone would do with, uh, insulin if they had diabetes. Uh, and then there's also an intravenous version. But really, the bottom line of it is, it is one of the most global, uh, immune stimulating injectables that, that are available.

So, just as we talked about ozone, peroxide, high dose of vitamin C, etcetera, downstream, they trigger these chemicals that start the immune system. You can kind of think of mistletoe as, um, a giant version of that. So, where the oxidative therapies may trigger little—

Sections, uh, mistletoe triggers bun—lots of sections.

Dr. Stengler: Yeah.

Dr. Anderson: You know, of, of this immune reaction. So, one of the things that we, we had talked to patients about is, you know, we, we want an immune response. We, we want a certain amount, but we want an immune response. So, if you get a fever, or if you get, you know, inflamed, or something, that's not always a bad thing, but we need to know, 'cause we—then we don't give you, you know, a higher dose, or something.

Dr. Stengler: Right.

Dr. Anderson: The other thing that, that mistletoe has been really excellent at, has been, um, really in two areas. One is in people, where they've had a therapy, sometimes certain chemo, certain antibiotics, other things, will shut down the, the bone marrow, and will quit making blood cells.

Mistletoe actually will often turn that system back on, and, which is something that vitamin C usually won't do, etcetera. So, we often will use mistletoe in a restorative or a rescue, uh, event.

The other thing is similar to high dose vitamin C in, in some cases where the patient obviously, the cancer is just too advanced, and it's not responding to anything. In many cases, um, the, the patient will have decreases in pain, improvement in mobility, eh, so, so as a quality of life measure, you know—but ideally, we like to use it in the person where the fight can still go on, and has a chance, you know, to win.

But mistletoe is, is probably one of the broadest, uh, immunologic stimulating, uh, medications, and if you look, you know, just, and there's different ways of, uh, assessing research, you know, around the world, and we only cite a few studies. But i-in the United States, there's, uh, trials going on right now, major, one major university in particular, using mistletoe with cancer, so it's, you know, kinda made it here.

And, and if you look at the US criteria for studies, there's o-over 100 easily of studies that they would say, "Yeah, those are valid studies that show that there's a benefit."

Dr. Stengler: Yep.

Dr. Anderson: If you look at the Europeans, uh, who've been studying it forever, um, and using it forever, you know, there's, there's hundreds and hundreds and hundreds of studies that are, that are available and out there. They're just, you know, um, they're, they're just categorized differently in the US than there.

So, it's probably one of the most studied alternative, integrative therapies is mistletoe, really.

Dr. Stengler: And it's used routinely by conventional oncologists in countries like Germany, Switzerland, for example. So, um, very common there, the oncologists.

Dr. Anderson: Yes. Yeah, and, and as I said, finally, kinda getting into some major university research here. I think simply because it's, it's been used so long in other countries, it—you know, there, why would we not look into that, and—

Dr. Stengler: Yeah.

Dr. Anderson: You know, one thing I always think about is all of the money—

Well, not all of the money, but a majority of the money in, in recent years as far as drug development and oncology has been focused on immunologic drugs, so either starting or stopping a process. Usually, starting or stopping one process. Mistletoe, uh, does a whole lot of that all at once, and so it would be, you know, it would fit right in with what we've been studying anyway.

Dr. Stengler:	Very unique in that way. Well, this has been great information from Dr. Anderson on the different injection therapies, the ones integrative doctors commonly are using across the United States, Europe, and uh, Asian countries, and so, just powerful, powerful anti-cancer treatments, treatments to help support, uh, those undergoing conventional treatments, offsetting the side effects, chemotherapy, radiation.
	And so, as always, great information, Dr. Anderson.
Dr. Anderson:	Thank you.
Dr. Stengler:	We really appreciate it.
Dr. Anderson:	Thank you.

THE SECRET TREATMENT THAT IS 35 TIMES MORE POWERFUL THAN CHEMO

— DR. JAMES FORSYTHE —

Dr. Stengler: Well hi everyone! I'm really excited today. I'm here in Reno, Nevada, with the most well-known integrative oncologist in America, probably the world. And we're gonna talk about his experience in treating tens and tens of thousands of patients with a variety of different types of cancers using integrative oncology, which this series is all about. So Dr. Forsythe, so great to have you

Dr. Forsythe: Thank you, Mark.

Dr. Stengler: Outstanding! And so we want to get into integrative cancer treatment with you today, of course, being you're the premier expert, in my opinion. But tell us a bit more about your background. I mean, you're a very interesting guy. You're a medical oncologist. You're Board Certified in Internal Medicine.

Dr. Forsythe: Yes.

Dr. Stengler: You're certified in Homeopathy. I mean, I don't know of anyone else has those types of credentials and, of course, decades and decades of experience.

Dr. Forsythe: So since the year 2000, I've done about four outcome-based studies. This is survival ship studies, Stage 4 cancers, adults only—that means over 16 years of age—all types of cancer—blood diseases, solid tumors and so on—all takers—in other words, anyone—and my first study was for Nature's Sunshine out of Utah, and I did the Paw Paw study, which is a product from the Paw Paw tree, indigenous to the southeastern United States. And that came out favorable, and it's being used worldwide now, as you probably know, Mark.

And then I was introduced at various meetings to Poly-MVA. I was seeing patients there who were saying, "You know, I've got—I've had multiple myeloma for five years, and I attribute it all to Poly-MVA," and things like that.

Dr. Stengler: Tell our viewers a bit more about what Poly-MVA is.

Dr. Forsythe: Poly-MVA was developed in '91 by the Merrill Garnett Laboratory in Long Island, associated with Stony Brook University. Merrill Garnett is the genius behind that. It's a type of energetic medicine. It's a product that is a nutrient, but it's also an energetic nutrient, and it causes cancer cells to undergo, in layman's terms, a mini-electrocution. Most cancer cells—in fact, all cancer cells, Mark, don't have the energy to get up and die.

They don't know how to die. They don't know how to go into apoptosis, which is programmed cell death. The Poly-MVA stimulates the energy in the cancer cell from anaerobic metabolism, gives them enough energy to actually force them into apoptosis. And that's obviously a simplification of what happens, but rather than get into the biochemistry.

Dr. Stengler: Yeah, yeah—so you had kind of read about this. You were intrigued by it, and then you, of course, had to see it for yourself and—

Dr. Forsythe: I did.

Dr. Stengler: —do further research. Is that right?

Dr. Forsythe: And then I went to the principals of the company, especially Al Sanchez, Sr., who is the local west coast distributor. In fact, he was the countrywide distributor of Poly-MVA. And I said, "We need to do a clinical study, because I think you have a product here that is really worthwhile, but you know there's no study to back it up." So he furnished the Poly, and I did—went about it to about 500—600 patients, and found that the survival rate was about 32 percent in 6 years.

Eventually, that came out to be the figure, and that was beating by 16 times the conventional results. So that looked very good. So during that study, unfortunately, I ran into a buzzsaw with the FDA. I was doing anti-aging medicine at the time with HGH, which only was used for adults with low-HGH levels. It was not due to enhance sports performance in professional sports, in college sports or high school sports. So it was strictly for anti-aging because thanks to the article that came out in the '90s by Redman—you may have heard—a professor from Wisconsin, who showed that older men getting HGH had many benefits. Their skin was better. Their bones were harder. Their sexual performance was better.

Their cognitive functions were better. And their exercise tolerance was better and so on—many other things; in fact, many things that we've learned since then that also show improvement with very little downsides to the HGH. And remember, we learned in medical school, as you know, Mark, that you can replace any hormone deficiency with a replacement hormone, and that's the standard. However, the FDA didn't see it that way. They—that was the only hormone you couldn't replace with impunity. They didn't like it, and probably because it was abused in athletics and so on.

Dr. Stengler:	Right.
Dr. Forsythe:	You know about Barry Bonds and so on.
Dr. Stengler:	Right.
Dr. Forsythe:	So anyway, we were using it, and of course the 84M was backing it completely, and it turned out maybe there were 20,000 to 30,000 doctors throughout the country using HGH, and they were flying under the radar basically because the FDA—it was illegal according to them.

In fact, the only legal way to use HGH was for traumatic brain injury, for short bowel syndrome, or for kids that were on HGH to make them taller and bigger in their growth and using it as they became adults. So those were a few of the only ways you could give HGH. It didn't seem right to me, frankly. It didn't seem right to anyone in the 84M establishment that was the case, because there are many benefits. And as we age, it is the major hormone of aging as you know, we reach our peak between 25 and 30, and from then on it's all downhill as far as our HGH is concerned. And does it cause cancer? Well, that's always been a question mark, but they're crossing curves, Mark. That means, as you age, HGH goes down, so they don't meet; they're inverse curves.

And also patients who have pituitary tumors that secrete lots of HGH don't die of cancer. They die of congestive heart failure. Or kids that have had a lot of HGH to make them taller never get cancer as adults—almost never, as far as we know and throughout the literature, they don't ever develop cancer. And they're still on HGH, most of them.

Dr. Stengler: So you're doing this Poly-MVA study, and the FDA started coming after you because of using HGH or growth hormone, which kind of erupted things, right? And I know you fought them on that. Tell the viewers about that.

Dr. Forsythe: Yeah, it was a nasty thing. It was—gave me a few gray hairs, to say the least. They came into both my clinic and home with three agencies: the FDA, the FBI and the ICE, Immigrations Customs Enforcement. We all know about ICE now.

Dr. Stengler: Even though you're a citizen of the U.S.

Dr. Forsythe: I'm a citizen. I never had a malpractice suit.

I was head of many hospital committees and chief—assistant chief of staff. I ran the cancer wards at all three hospitals, ran the VA program here in Reno. So I said, "What's going on here?" And so they came up our driveway one morning. My wife and I—our kids were all gone, all grown—and I said, "Who did you invite for breakfast?" Well, there were three dark SUVs coming up the driveway, and out poured about four to five people from each IV—from each SUV.

And by the time I got to the back door, Mark, they had the

door buster ready, they had their guns drawn, and they all had their block letters on their black sweaters. It was in February of '05. They pushed me back in the house on the floor with a gun to my head. My wife came running down the hall; she was hysterical. "What did my husband do? What did he do?"

"He used human growth hormone off label." Well, as you know as a doctor, Mark, we all use off-label drugs. Aspirin!

Dr. Stengler: We're allowed to do that, yeah.

Dr. Forsythe: Aspirin is an off-label drug if we use it for anticoagulation or heart disease rather than headaches. So it's crazy. And oncologists, of course, use off-label chemotherapy every day when they go to a second, third or fourth or fifth line chemo; it's always off-label because there are just no studies to back it up. Anyway, I went through a long period, about—it was from February of '05 to '07 when the trial was in actually October of '07. So about $1 million in legal fees. And then before the trial, they had the nerve to tell my lawyer, "Well, we think he knows a lot about HGH for adults.

"We want him to write our national protocol." I said, "Oh, my gosh! This is great. That probably means that the whole case is going away." Well, it wasn't quite that simple. They still wanted $150,000 in investigative fees, and they wanted me on probation for three to five years, and that would have been my license right there. So I said, "No, we'll go to trial, and we'll take our chances with the jury."

And after a—in October of '07, we went to trial, and I had a unanimous "not guilty" verdict. They had no—they had nothing on me that was gonna stick at all. And it actually allowed for a precedent to be set for other doctors in the country, and there are about 20,000 to 30,000 estimated that were flying under the radar using HGH for anti-aging purposes. So that was a kind of a feather in my hat, and after that I started writing books.

And I wrote—I've written 24 books since then.

Dr. Stengler: Yeah, we've got a couple here. We've got—I mean, like you said, many great books—but *The Forsythe Anti-Cancer*

Diet, which is excellent. We've got *Take Control of your Cancer: Integrating the Best of Alternative and Conventional Treatments*, like we're talking about today, and many other books people can get from your website and online.

So then you were able to get back on track with the treatments you were studying and proving in research, whether they worked or not?

Dr. Forsythe: Yes, I decided after the trial to go back and do the survivor studies because I felt that we still hadn't hit the jackpot yet in terms of the best system to treat patients using the combination of the best east-west medicine, or we call it "integrative medicine." I prefer the term "integrative oncology," Mark, because that really clearly states what we do.

And no doubt I was very much influenced by 2003 when the Human Genome Project was completed and we were able to tell then by circling tumor cells in our genes what is best in terms of the best drugs, the best targeted agents—the newer form of chemo—the best supplements—by that, I mean vitamins, minerals and herbal products and some prescription drugs even—and the best hormones for hormone-driven tumors.

That would be in a male, the prostate, testicular tumor; in the female, the breast, the ovaries, the uterus, cervix, sometimes the vagina or vulva. So that part is all good, because when you have that information, you're basically handing the patient a blueprint or roadmap to get better. And so we started doing that. We looked at around the world for the best genetic labs. So we found three throughout the world, believe it or not.

The ones in the United States weren't up to par, and they weren't fully developed yet, and they still aren't. So we looked at Korea—South Korea, that is: The Good Gene Lab. We used that for a while, and in a couple years it just didn't measure up, Mark. We felt there were problems with the reporting, the inconsistencies and reliability. So we went to Germany, the Biofocus Lab, and that was better, but still not quite what we wanted.

We ended up in Greece, even though their economy is a bit shaky, but they are the tops in terms of genetic technology. So when we take them—for instance, let's say you had prostate cancer—God forbid—and you came to me, and you had some bad experiences either through family members who'd had full-dose chemo or you're reading or whatever, Mark, you said, "I don't want any of this.

"And I really don't want hormone therapy and drop my testosterone level to zero and—

Dr. Stengler: Yeah—muscles and bones break down.

Dr. Forsythe: —my muscles flabby—

Dr. Stengler: Your memory and your energy and sexual function and all that.

Dr. Forsythe: You get osteoporosis, energy, sexual—all that—you said, "Not for me." And you heard about my low-dose insulin potentiated therapy, and you knew that I do genetic testing, so that's what I do for every patient. We currently have 1,250 patients at 7.5 years in our study seeing a survival rate, a prospective study, of 70 percent.

Dr. Stengler: And how does that compare in general to conventional research?

Dr. Forsythe: Thirty-five times greater.

Dr. Stengler: Thirty-five times greater!

Dr. Forsythe: So if we—if you take 600,000 deaths per year in cancer in the United States, conventional medicine can prolong their life 12,000 people out of 600,000 for greater than 5 years: only 12,000. If you take what we do, and it was used nationally, it would be over 400,000, Mark.

So that's quite a difference.

Dr. Stengler: Yeah, that's great.

Now, you're unique in that—and you and some other doctors around the country—you're unique—when you do use the chemo, which you do, you're using low dose. Why don't you go through that process, because that's very unique.

Dr. Forsythe: Yeah, we're doing the IPT, and I have altered the IPT. In-

	stead of shooting the insulin—
Dr. Stengler:	IPT for insulin potentiation therapy.
Dr. Forsythe:	Insulin potentiated therapy—basically, it's low-dose. It's—we add the insulin to the bottle right with the chemo rather than shoot it in, because in those cases they do have fairly high instance of severe hypoglycemia. When we do it in the bottle, it doesn't happen.
	We never run into that. The patients do well, and then at the end of the bottle, we bring their blood sugar back to normal.
Dr. Stengler:	So basically, for the viewers, you're giving the patient insulin simultaneously with the low dose chemo, so you can use much lower doses of chemo and drive it into the cells. What percent less chemo would you use compared to what a regular oncologist is using?
Dr. Forsythe:	Ten to fifteen percent dose on every drug.
Dr. Stengler:	And so obviously, the side effect potential drops way down.
Dr. Forsythe:	No hair loss, no rashes, no cytopenias. If you're a therapeutic virgin—I tell this to my women—if they come to me and they haven't had any prior radiation or chemo, they're a therapeutic virgin. Sometimes they don't like to hear that. They'll tell me, "Oh, I haven't been a virgin for years."
	But they're therapeutically naive, and that's good, Mark. That means that we have a lot to work with. Their immune system is intact. Their blood counts are intact. Their bone marrow is preserved. They don't have organ damage or neuropathies. They don't have hair loss.
	So they don't have all those toxicities.
Dr. Stengler:	And then—so you have the IPT, and then of course you're using all the other tools you talked about. Why don't you talk to us about some of the other IV therapies you use and—
Dr. Forsythe:	Well, what we do with the chemo is give it two days a week: Tuesday and Thursday usually. And in between that, we sandwich immune IVs of various types. High dose C, 50 to 75 grams, the L-Glutathione, 100 to 200 milligrams, the hydrogen peroxide infusion—because remem-

ber, cancer grows favorably in a hypoxic environment. That's how cancer grows. They don't like your body to be rich in oxygen. Then the Poly-MVA product from—as we mentioned, from Stony Brook University, which causes cancer cells to hurry up and die. And then the last one is the Myer's Cocktail with DMSO, which we call the Forsythe Immune Protocol.

Everything together really is called the Forsythe Immune Protocol because we're really combining immune therapy with low-dose chemo, and we're seeing very good results. Our patients leave the office not with a bag over their head. They're not bald. They're not sick and rundown. They're actually energized, Mark.

Dr. Stengler: Yeah, well, a lot of the nutrients you talked about in the IVs, not only are they anticancer, but they help with cellular energy in a healthy way and offset any other kinds of side effects a lot of people with cancer experience. So—and then, of course, to set it off you work with supplements and diet. Tell us about that.

Dr. Forsythe: Yeah, one other thing.

Dr. Stengler: Okay.

Dr. Forsythe: After three weeks of therapy, we do put them on the best oral medicine that comes up on the gene test. And for breast cancer, that could be Xeloda, which is a form of 5FU. It could be an alkylator or alkylators like Cytoxan, Alkeran, Chlorambucil—any of those—or VP16, which is etoposide.

Any of those would work if they're—again, they have to be close to the 80s—above the 80. And they take that in a half-dose—half the conventional dose, Mark, because they're getting all the supplements, too. You don't need to do the full dose, which makes it much easier on them.

And generally insurance will cover that. We do have a foundation that helps pay the bill. Otherwise, it's all cash, but sometimes insurance companies will cover the cost of the chemo, but not the alternative IVs.

Dr. Stengler: Good, and so then you're definitely integrating very spe-

	cific nutritional supplements and diet. Tell us a bit more about that.
Dr. Forsythe:	Well, we have our diet book, as you see. There is no one single diet for every patient. All the diets cause weight loss. They're all weight-loss diets. We have the Paleo, the Mediterranean, the South Beach Diet, the Zone Diet, the Gerson Diet, the Budwig Diet, the Atkin's Diet.
	All of them fit different people different ways, and we have to find out as much as we can to which one's gonna suit them. Sometimes we look at their blood type. That may be important. If they're meat eaters, then we wanna give them a diet like—O, if they're O-positive, they do well on the Atkin's, and Atkin's—the ketogenic—which is also called the ketogenic diet—works better for some people.
Dr. Stengler:	And what do you find with the nutritional supplements? How beneficial do you find those with your patients; just as part of the overall synergistic program?
Dr. Forsythe:	They are, and they very—they're on a lower scale of efficacy, Mark. They can go from as low as 5 percent effective to as high as 60 percent or more. Very rarely above 60, though. And if there are certain things of the supplements that can be given IV, like curcumin, artesunate, DCA—which military lingo would be "Delta Charlie Alpha" we call it, or it's dichloroacetate with Vitamin B1.
	We give them that as well.
Dr. Stengler:	And I wanna thank you for just the tens of thousands of people you've helped, educating doctors around the country, like myself, so we can help people more effectively.
	You know, you're the only one who's done it to this degree so far, and it's been a game-changer in helping people with integrative oncology. So thank you so much.
Dr. Forsythe:	Thank you, Mark. It's been a pleasure.

THE POWER OF OZONE

— DR. FRANK SHALLENBERGER —

Dr. Stengler:	Hi, everyone! Welcome back to Outside-the-Box Cancer Therapies. I'm here in Carson City, Nevada, with a very special guest, Dr. Frank Shallenberger, who is an expert in integrative medicine, very experienced also in integrative oncology, and we're here at his beautiful clinic. And Dr. Shallenberger, great to be with you.
Dr. Shallenberger:	It's nice to be with you, Mark.
Dr. Stengler:	And so we're talking about many different topics in terms of helping the viewers out there understand the different natural ways they can help themselves work with holistic doctors in terms of cancer therapy—integrative cancer therapy. And you're definitely one of the experts I'd say in the world in terms of oxidative therapies, especially ozone therapy. You mind telling the viewers what is oxidative therapy, and what's ozone therapy, and what's so unique and special about it?
Dr. Shallenberger:	Okay—well, oxidative therapy refers to, you know, I guess scientifically speaking, therapies that initiate the movement of electrons. Now, that's probably not telling your listeners very much, but technically speaking, that's what it is.
	But it's—we stay alive through this process of electron movement. We stay alive through the process

of oxidation. And when the oxidation decreases in efficiency, that's when we get vulnerable to getting sick, and particularly with cancer. Cancer is caused by a deficient state of oxidation. So if you're wanting to get through that—if you're wanting to get over cancer or even present cancer, you gotta make sure that your levels of oxidation are well balanced. And the fact is that you can have a situation they call oxidation stress where there's too much oxidation. That can happen say with toxicity.

Or you can certainly with chronic as you get older and you get a little out of shape and so forth and so on, you can have levels where you have deficient states of oxidation. So what we're doing with ozone therapy, which is a very powerful oxidant, ozone being oxygen itself.

Normally, oxygen is with two oxygen atoms. It's a strong oxidant that way. Ozone is three oxidant atoms, so it's 50 percent stronger in the sense of its capacity to oxidize. So that's where we got with ozone, directly rather than with just pure oxygen. But when you administer that to people, it has an effect similar to exercise—a little bit more powerful, but similar to exercise in that it just improves your oxidation efficiency, and things just work better.

Dr. Stengler:	And you've written on a subject, you have a couple books out on ozone therapy. Wanna give the names of those just for the viewers?
Dr. Shallenberger:	Okay, sure—yeah. So for laypeople, I've write something called *The Ozone Miracle*, which I wrote that to help people know how they can actually administer ozone to themselves or to members of their family at home and take care of a lot of problems. And then I wrote a book more for professionals called *The Principles and Applications of Ozone Therapy*.
Dr. Stengler:	And I know you've been president of a medical association for ozone.

Dr. Shallenberger:	Yes, I'm President of the American Academy of Ozone Therapy.
Dr. Stengler:	So a lot of people are surprised to find out ozone as a medical therapy has been around for quite a while. Tell us a bit about the history and—
Dr. Shallenberger:	It's got—that's one of the things that intrigued me so much—when I first learned about ozone, it was almost 40 years ago. But one of the things that intrigued me so much, Mark, was that there's such a rich history behind it. Ig goes—it literally goes back to the 1700s. But the clinical use of it goes back a good, solid hundred years. Luminaries no less than Richard von Siemens, the guy that invented the x-ray tubes and a bunch of other things. He's known as the Father of Electro-engineering. He was involved in ozone. He made one of the first ozone generators.

And Nikola Tesla, who I think everybody knows about. Tesla actually made the first ozone generator in the early 1900s, but that was strictly for medical use.

We have publications that came out of the Florida State Medical Association in the early 1900s about ozone therapy. We have studies coming out of the University of Chicago in the late 1800s. We've got studies all throughout the 20th century and culminating now in studies that I would say over the last 10 years probably had about 1,500—2,000 articles in the last 10 years published just on the medical use of ozone.

So it has a very rich history with a lot of important people going back a hundred years or so. And that's one of the things that is so attractive about it, and we know so much about it and how to use it and how it works.

Dr. Stengler:	Yeah—that's great. I've talked to doctors and patients from countries like Russia, Germany, talking about ozone where here people think it's a new

	things, they're like, "Oh, we've been using ozone medically for decades."
Dr. Shallenberger:	Exactly! Yeah, yeah—so part of the reason that we have this American Academy of Ozone Therapies is to kind of get that word out and teach doctors about it. Because it's still pretty unknown here in the United States.
Dr. Stengler:	Well, you've got a very interesting background. You got training in conventional medicine. I think you even worked in the Emergency Room for *[unintelligible]*, didn't you?
Dr. Shallenberger:	Yeah, that's right.
Dr. Stengler:	And so then you also are trained in holistic, nutrition and natural hormones and ozone therapy and injection therapies and vitamins and minerals and all these types of things.
	And so ozone, you just continue to be very impressed with it. It's hard to beat. Is that an accurate summary?
Dr. Shallenberger:	Over the years, you know, if I tried ten therapies, probably one or two of them really pan out to be great, and the other ones just fall by the roadside. Ozone is one of those things that you just don't wanna be without. Once you've got that thing, and you're using it with your patients, and you see the results—
	If you didn't have it, you would be—feel like you were at a loss.
Dr. Stengler:	Yeah, I agree. I've been using it more in recent years—
Dr. Shallenberger:	Good.
Dr. Stengler:	—because of people like you making it more well-known to doctors like myself and very impressed with it. Take the viewers through—say someone comes to your clinic, and maybe they've got cancer. Tell us how you integrate ozone therapy into their protocols, because I know, like any good doctor,

you don't just use one thing. It's a multifactorial approach when people have cancer. And how exactly do they get the ozone, because there's different ways here in your clinic you utilize it?

Dr. Shallenberger: And so—which is one of the other really fantastic things about ozone therapy is that there's so many applications. You rarely—well, I don't know if I will say "rarely," but it's unusual for you to find a patient that couldn't benefit in one way or another from one of the many ozone therapies. For one, it will take away pain. So if you've got a pain in your hip or a pain in your shoulder—and I don't care what's causing the pain. It could be osteoarthritis.

It could be any kind of cause of pain. It'll probably take that pain away. If you have a damaged joint— for example, many knee surgeries can be avoided simply by injecting ozone into the knee.

Dr. Stengler: Which you teach doctors how to do as well. Yeah.

Dr. Shallenberger: I teach them how to do that. And then you can give it systemically. We give it through the skin in the form of a sauna. We can give it intestinally in the form of a colonic. We can give it into the bloodstream. There are so many ways to administer this therapy. There's a technique where you can put it in sinuses. You can put it in ears. You can inject it in just about any place you wanna inject it. It's so safe!

There's just another part of the principle. None of us wants to do anything to hurt people, and this is one of those things. You could—unless you went out of your way it would be pretty much impossible to hurt anybody with ozone therapy.

And as you pointed out, integrated is really a great term to use with ozone therapy. And when I teach doctors how to use this, one of the first things I tell them is, "Listen, whatever you're doing, don't stop doing it. This is not necessarily a substitute for what you're doing. You just add this into what you're doing. If you're a cardiologist, do your thing, and add ozone in. If you're an oncologist, it doesn't matter what your specialty is—a homeopath, an acupuncturist. If you add this into what you're doing, it just amplifies the results."

Dr. Stengler: In your mind, what's happening inside their body that's so beneficial? Take them through the many benefits.

Dr. Shallenberger: Well, okay—so, for one, you're forming lipoperoxides. So these are lipids—they're fat-soluble molecules that have electron potential to them, shall we say.

And the point is that these lipoperoxides can last in your body for days. So if I were to treat you with an ozone therapy, the effects of that therapy will linger for days, maybe even weeks, depending on what sort of dose I gave you. So it goes on. If you just give a therapy once a week, that whole week you'll have this going on.

One of the things that it does is it modulates the immune system. A lot of why people get sick—and you could make a case for the primary reason people get sick across the board is some imbalance in their immune system. Ozone has an immune balancing effect to it. So if you have too much of the wrong thing, it'll decrease that. If you don't have enough of the right thing, it'll increase that. It just tends to be very immune system balancing. It stimulates the body to detoxify. It stimulates the circulation, stimulates the delivery of energy, stimulates metabolism.

One of the reasons that we all face when we start having a lot of birthdays is that we don't efficiently utilize oxygen. We don't efficiently process that oxygen into energy, because that's the only reason we're taking in oxygen is to get energy from it. And ozone will stimulate that, improve the way we deliver—the way we process oxygen. Some of the listeners might realize this in the sense of mitochondrial function; if they know that term, mitochondrial, it stimulates mitochondrial function.

All these principles that I've listed so far—it's amazing that one thing can do all of that, unless you just start to think and remember, "Oh, yeah, this is oxygen. It's not this—

Dr. Stengler: Fundamental *[unintelligible]*, yeah.

Dr. Shallenberger: It's—what is more fundamental—what do you really—what's the most important nutrient you need by far? It would be oxygen.

Dr. Stengler: So what—what was—what in your opinion is happening inside say that cancer cells or tumors when people get ozone treatments?

Medically, what do you think's going on there?

Dr. Shallenberger: Well, I guess the first thing I wanna say is that, with few exceptions, ozone is not actually a treatment for cancer. I don't want people to get that idea. There's a couple of exceptions to that, but that's not at all typical. What ozone is is it's something that can be used in combination with other therapies that are more anticancer. For example, and I'm thinking of the main conventional therapies like surgery, chemotherapy and radiation, ozone has two principal effects with this, and one is when given simultaneously to those therapies, it'll improve the outcome. The patients heal better.

If it's a surgery, they'll be out of the hospital in half the time. They'll have much lower chance of complications. They'll heal faster, etcetera, etcetera. If you give it in combination with radiation therapy or with chemotherapy, they'll—the efficacy of those treatments will improve, and the side effects will decrease.

Dr. Stengler: And it's because of all the things you said. It gives you healthier mitochondria producing energy inside the cell. Healthy cells will produce energy efficient-

	ly are not as hospitable to cancer growth. Immune system activation, controlling inflammation—
Dr. Shallenberger:	It exploits the difference between healthy cells and cancer cells. Ever since Warburg first brought this up back in the '30s, we know that cancer cells differ from healthy cells almost 100 percent of the time with the way that their mitochondria work or don't work.
Dr. Stengler:	Yeah, talk about that for just a minute, the Warburg Effect—for the layperson out there. How would you explain—how do you explain that to your patients?
Dr. Shallenberger:	Well, I guess one way to understand it is if you take healthy cells, and you deprive them of oxygen, they die.
	You take cancer cells, you deprive it of oxygen, they don't die. They don't seem to notice it, because they live in a space that doesn't use oxygen. They don't particularly like oxygen. And in fact, oxygen is harmful to them.
	It slows their growth. So it's a unique thing. You give a patient, who has, of course, most of the cells in his body are healthy cells. He's got a few bad cells—a few cancer cells. You saturate that patient's body in oxygen, and the cancer cells don't like it, and the healthy cells are happy. They like it. So it's differential.
Dr. Stengler:	Yeah—and like you said, you're using it and the rest of us use it as a therapy to potentiate the other therapies. By itself, we don't find it cures cancer. But it potentiates the other therapies that—and the synergistic effect, people get better outcomes and better quality of life.
	Energy, less side effects, less inflammation and pain and all that. Maybe just in ending, tell the viewers just how—well, some of the other therapies you integrate into your treatments for people who have cancer: you know, IPT, intravenous vitamin C.

I know—like I said, any good practitioner, you're using a multifactorial approach, of course, along with diet and supplements and exercise and stress reduction. But maybe give the viewers sort of what you've found to be just very important in terms of a comprehensive approach to get the best results.

Dr. Shallenberger: Yeah—everybody's so individual. The one thing is you definitely can't cookbook it. You can't have, "This is my protocol; you do it," type thing.

Dr. Stengler: Right.

Dr. Shallenberger: But certainly inflammation is in there, right. So you have to have some sort of therapies that are focused on the inflammatory process and decreasing the inflammatory process. In that regard, I find certain herbs—you know, curcumin, turmeric—

—frankincense, black cumin seed—so these have a nice anti-inflammatory potential. There's even some studies—you probably know these—that show the NSAIDs—NSAID medications, leaving aside their side effects, have a strong anticancer potential to them. And in cases like prostate cancer, it can almost be completely therapeutic there. So you wanna get something that hits the inflammatory cascade nicely.

Then you wanna get something that boosts up the antioxidant system, because these people normally with cancer are completely—if not completely, but very depleted in their antioxidant potential. Normally, that would be vitamin C and glutathione for me. One of the things that I discovered—well, I learned about—let me put it to you that way—about five years ago was melatonin and the incredible effect—

Dr. Stengler: There's a lot of studies on melatonin.

Dr. Shallenberger: —that high-dose melatonin has on cancer potential. So I love incorporating that in with my patients.

Dr. Stengler: And people are shocked to find out that it's a very powerful antioxidant: melatonin.

Dr. Shallenberger:	Mm-hmm—these most powerful in the central nervous system. Has a strong anticancer potential to it as well.
Dr. Stengler:	So you get patients who come in with a variety of different types of cancers. Probably like me, they've under—they're undergoing conventional treatment—chemotherapy, radiation, surgery—maybe they've had those treatments, and then you're integrating the kinds of things we're talking about. Would that be a typical kind of case for you?
Dr. Shallenberger:	Yeah, so I have two ways that patients can deal with me. One is I can administer the chemotherapy, and I use a low-dose form of chemotherapy with insulin, and then I'll of course integrate all these other aspects in there with that. Or some of my patients get conventional. They have their conventional oncologist, and simultaneous to while all that's going on, they'll see me to help detox them from the chemotherapy, improve the effects of the chemotherapy.
	But here's one of the things that really listeners need to know so much, and it's so aggravating to me and—with this whole idea of cancer recurrence is the conventional approach is typically, "Oh, okay, we finished our therapy. You can go now. We don't need to do anything else. You're either cured or whatever you are. You're in remission or whatever you are. We finished that therapy, and off you go." No proactive aspects to that. No discussion of diet. No—the cancer is gonna come back!
Dr. Stengler:	Not changing the environment.
Dr. Shallenberger:	Yeah, they can—yeah. So what I really want people to understand is no matter what form of therapy they've had for their cancer, if it is successful, if God was good and they're successful and they've got into remission or they can't find the cancer on the scan, the game is not over. You're on first base now. You've still gotta complete the whole circuit.
Dr. Stengler:	It's a lifelong—

Dr. Shallenberger:	Yeah, it's a lifelong deal. We gotta make sure it doesn't come back, because when it comes back, then it becomes, as you know, quite difficult.
Dr. Stengler:	That's true. So just in ending, you've practiced for 45 years. I think we know the answer, but would you say these nutritional therapies and integrative therapies we're talking about—ozone—just in general for patients' cancer, whatever treatments you're getting, it's a mild benefit, moderate or tremendous benefit? What would you say the range is and what you see in people?
Dr. Shallenberger:	I'd have to say it was critical. I'd have to say the benefit is really huge.
Dr. Stengler:	Well, there you have it, people, from an expert. Excellent information. Use it to your advantage. And again, thank you, Dr. Shallenberger, for your time.
Dr. Shallenberger:	Okay—thanks, Mark. Okay.

THE PROVEN STRATEGY THAT WEAKENS CANCER CELLS

— DR. PAUL ANDERSON —

Dr. Stengler: I'm Dr. Mark Stengler, here with Dr. Paul Anderson, co-author of *Outside the Box Cancer Therapies* book. And in this series, we're gonna talk about really the, the nuts and bolts of integrative cancer treatment, metabolic therapy. How can we best affect the cell machinery to help fight cancer, prevent it from replicating, uh, preventing abnormal changes in the cell?

And so, Dr. Anderson's the perfect person to talk about this topic, and it's—you know, it can be a very complex topic. I know you'll make it simple for the viewers. But first, let's start by talking about what do we mean by metabolic therapy?

Dr. Anderson: I think that's a great place to start. The idea goes back to something that we speak about in the book in the, um, theories of how cancer develops, and one of the theor—theories, is the metabolic theory. And so, that's a very simplified term for kind of a lot of chemistry—

But to get into it, a metabolic therapy's goal is to take advantage of the metabolic differences between a cancer cell and a normal cell. And one of the things that, um, is sort of, this is not a, really a disputed theory or idea, but like other things that we've spoken about, it's something that goes back a long, long way.

And so, if you think about things that, that were o-observationally, uh, you know, brought up through science, or with, you know, very, maybe rudimentary testing methods that may have been available in the teens and the 20s and the 30s, vs. now, it's not that the older idea was necessarily wrong. It's that we know more about it. We know about kinda the depths of how much activity goes on, etcetera.

So, the idea of a metabolic therapy is literally to say what's the difference between many cancer cells—

And our normal, healthy cells? And is there something or somethings that we can do that will make the cancer cell either weaker or a better target for the immune system, without harming our normal cells?

So, the majority of cancer cells, though, uh, have this ability, which makes them, um, neoplastic, or cancerous, to, uh, replicate without the normal triggers for, uh, cell replication that normal cells have.

Part of that is predicated on the fact that they operate their internal machinery in much more of a simplified manner, and the chemistry is quite a bit different than a normal cell. A normal cell not only has to follow—

Very proscribed triggers and signals to divide and replicate, etcetera, so it's done normally. But also, it has a lot of internal machinery that works, uh, at very many levels. Cancer cells, for the majority of them, replicate without those normal triggers, which was what makes them, you know, cancerous cells, and they also operate using, uh, very, very simplified chemistry inside to keep them going.

So, it'd be like having, you know, two cars that look the same on the outside, two different motor systems inside—

Dr. Stengler: Right.

Dr. Anderson: So, the idea and, um, it was popularized and, um, actually named after, uh, Dr. Warburg, who is a Nobel Laureate, uh, in the 1920s, and it was called the Warburg Effect, and that is actually when, uh, he described the difference between these two, sort of the engine systems of the two different, normal vs. cancerous cells.

And then what ensued from there with the metabolic theory of, uh, cancer was, well, what can we do to take advantage of these? That led to there could be dietary things that could take advantage of it. There could be things that change the chemistry, uh, and to go back to our car, you know, model, it might be that, uh, you, you know, you have the normal cell, uh, with the normal engine in it, and uh, it can run on, you know, a multitude of fuels, uh, and fuel varieties.

Whereas, the one with the, you know, the sort of fast replicating, but not too efficient engine takes only one fuel. So, if you take, and take advantage of that, and say, well, the normal cell can survive very well if we give it this sort of fuel system, the cancer cell can't, that was sort of the first idea, was could we change people's diet? Could we do particular things—

That will get in and adapt in a little bit later that might change it. Then what really ensued from there is that became an area of a lot of research up until the point when we started to look more at genetics and genomics, as far as a, a cancer therapy. And there's been in the last ten years, a huge resurgence as cancer as a metabolic disease, and treatments around that, etcetera.

And we started to say, well, if there's merit to this, then we should be able to start to change the metabolism of a patient and see something happen with their cancer, either it slows down, or the patient feels better, or maybe it, we get some regression. Something's gotta happen there, right?

Dr. Anderson: Yeah.

Dr. Stengler: So, what we did, uh, and then hence the term, combined, is we started to look at, well, are there ways, uh, beyond—

Dietary changes, which are very important, that we can also take advantage of this weakness that some cancer cells have? And so, we started to look at all manner of different ways into the problem. And through a, uh, uh a bit of our own experimentation and, and research with our, with our human patients, uh, we started to see some early responses.

One of the things that we started with was restricting, uh, the amount of sugar sources in the diet, making sure people had certainly enough calories, and enough nutrients, and all of that, but restricting the sugar sources.

And uh, you know, s—in, in the book, and in other, uh, parts of the film, we've talked about, you know, people, uh, oncologists get upset when you say, "Well, you know, sugar—

"Feeds cancer," 'cause it's—it's not that simple, right?

Dr. Stengler: Right.

Dr. Anderson: But in a sense, um, it—sugar is, it does not create a good environment for cancer. It actually creates a good environment for the cancer cells, but not, not for them, uh, dying.

So, it, it's sort of a how you deal with the word. So, the first thing that we worked on was well, can we get people good nutrition, um, a, a good enough variety, and yet restrict glucose sources, or, or sugar sources generally?

And so, and there's many, many ways to do that. There's a spectrum of, you know, you can do low carbohydrate type diet, um, you can do a ketogenic or a keto-adapted diet, there's are the more common ones nowadays. Um, and what a lot of people don't know is there's, there's versions of those that, uh, are done with vegetarian foods, like there's—there, there's a—because it works, and because it's being published so much, there are nutritionists working on ways to do this—

Dr. Stengler: Yeah.

Dr. Anderson: So, we started with the dietary interventions, and, and I really our initial dietary interventions were, were fairly straightforward. We put together, um, diet plans that included a lot of high fiber vegetables, so they got nutrients, but not a lot of sugar from it. Um, they, they had a certain portion of, uh, proteins, depending on what they were eating for proteins, a certain amount of fat, and some other things.

And, then, we also started to work with a combination of two metabolic, um, rea-really metabolic supplements/medications that took advantage of this weakness in the cancer cell, as well, because we knew with diet, I had actually previous to, to the research, I had had three patients in, in my career—

Who had done just ketogenic diet, and a sense of basic nutrition, with some stage two medium, medium sort of stage breast and other cancers. And it actually lived between 10 and 15 years with only diet as an intervention. That wasn't my idea. They just came in and said, "Hey, this is what I've been doing, and I just want you to monitor me."

You know, they, they weren't interested in—and we would do little bits of this and that, but basically, it was diet intervention, which got my attention, and, and of course, what you see is with any intervention, if you just do one, eventually, the cancer figures out a way around it.

So, we knew that we couldn't just do it with the diet, but then we had to figure out, well, what would work here, and this. Well, one of the differences in—that Warburg did point out that's, that is still true to this day—is that the cancer cells that we're talking about that fit this model, uh, they like glucose—

And they take it up rather rapidly, but they metabolize it down only part way. And so, they break it down, so our normal cells right now would take glucose, break it all the way down, and essentially, take it apart, and use it, put it in the mitochondria that make our energy, and uh, and, and produce a great amount of energy out of it.

Cancer cell doesn't really need that, because its job is just, just to get down and, and divide as quickly as it possibly can. It gets part way down, and then it stops, and there's, there's a lot of—and we go deeply into this in the book, but there's a lot of enzyme differences, and it basically stops with a little energy, and then it creates lactic acid.

Now, most people who have worked out or read about working out, or whatever, have heard of lactic acid as the stuff that makes you hurt after you work out and you're out of shape, right? Well, that's because you're doing the same thing—

You go out and run, and you've not run in years, your legs are gonna hurt, because they build up lactic acid, and it's because you ran out of oxygen, kay? Well, this is what your cancer cells are doing all the time.

So, one of the weaknesses is if you can stop that creation of lactic acid, that does a bunch of things, but to just simplify them, 'cause this—that's a very deep well of discussion, um, when you do make lactic acid and pump it out of a cancer cell, it's part of the recruitment process to get normal cells to possibly become cancer cells. It's also part of potentially what can create more cancer stem cells.

But the other thing that it does is it turns on an accessory feeding mechanism for the cancer cells, so it's a self-replicating process. So, shutting that off does many, many beneficial things. The other thing is, although not terribly efficiently, it forces the cancer cell—

To do more of like a normal, uh, oxidation reaction in the mitochondria, which the cancer cell doesn't really operate well with.

Dr. Stengler: Right.

Dr. Anderson: So, then comes, well, what would work? Is there anything natural, semi-natural, drug world, anything, that would shut that off? Well, there's a few agents that do that. One of 'em that we used, which, because it was available in the United States, uh, as a, a, as an orphan drug, was called DCA, it's like chloroacetate.

And it was literally designed originally for lactic acidosis, so it just blocks that step. So, there's that. We use that, but we knew that that wouldn't be enough, because the—this is a complex system, so the diet's important. The DCA became important, and one of the problems that DCA has is that, um, it-it's been used, as we've talked about with many other things, it's been used in Europe for a long time with cancer—

So, it's a lot of research. If you use too much, it can create side effects, obviously, because it, it is a metabolic manipulator. And, uh, we had stopped using it, uh, for that reason, is we would get a dose that was effective, but then the person would get side effects, and we, we don't want that.

So, we, um, came upon a, uh, another product that had been developed for cancer purposes that, uh, again, on paper, would appear to be supportive to protecting against the side effects of the DCA, but also, supportive to this, um, forcing the mitochondria of the cancer cell into a, a weakened position or a changed position.

Dr. Stengler: Yeah.

Dr. Anderson: Something it didn't like. And here's the really good thing. The normal cells for the most part were, were not bothered—

By these two things, as long as you didn't overdose with the DCA. So, what we did as a proof of concept was, uh, had a laboratory actually test the two together, and what—and, in cancer cells, in just a petri dish—

Dr. Stengler: Yeah.

Dr. Anderson: And, um, what we found was that you not only got synergy where more cells died if you used them together, but you could lower the dose of the DCA, which was the, the one that gave us the side effects. And so, it was on paper a bonus that we would cut off the side effects anyway, and we didn't need as much of the DCA.

And the poly MVA, the other, uh, product, would actually fo—kinda force the mitochondria into a weakened state. So, now we've got multiple pieces, you know, of the, the wheel turning here. So, we actually started in, uh, 2009 with a small group of patients.

And so, what we did is we put together, um, our best assessment of this, this is the diet we would use, this is the ratio of DCA and the poly MVA, um, and here's how we would do it, and we will only do it with people where no standard therapies or chemo surgery, radiation's not gonna work, or didn't work.

No natural therapy had worked, either, so we had already tried vitamin C and all these things that we've spoken about, and, and will—so, it was a small group, but there's, there's always people where they have aggressive cancers, and they're just not responding—

Dr. Stengler:	Yeah.
	So, um, I would present the idea to them, which seemed—originally, when they found out, especially the very first patient found out that no—no one had ever done this before, uh, that, that was a—he had a lot of questions about that, and uh, I said, "Well, but here's the thing, you know, not—your oncologist said, 'I can't do anything for you with the type of cancer you have.'"
	And he had a very aggressive, kinda large cancer, um, and we had tried all of—you know, all of the natural things we could try, and he was, he was a very good patient. He was really trying, and everything.
Dr. Stengler:	Yeah.
Dr. Anderson:	Um, and so, then, when I said, "You know, this, this is kinda the next step, and here's why," and I explained it to him, he went home, he did some reading. He says, "Well, okay, it looks like you can't hurt me with this, or maybe not too bad. I don't have other options."
	So, we started to do it, and, and work with him on it. And um, one thing I will say is he was, he was extremely—
	Extremely, uh, particular about the way he did things, which means that when we changed his diet, he really changed his diet, like, he did, did everything we said.
Dr. Stengler:	One hundred percent.
Dr. Anderson:	And he was, he was 100 percent on what we had him take and schedule. So, he was kinda the, a, a good first patient. And he was literally getting to the point where he was needing to go to a hospice. So, he was that bad.
	After about a month, he—we checked in, and he'd been doing the therapy, and the diet, and he, he wasn't, you know, remarkably better, but he said, you know, "I, I was pretty much unable to get off the couch, and I'm going for walks every day now." And he says, "Yeah, it tires me out, but I couldn't do that before."
	And part of the problem was one of the tumors was decreasing his lung capacity, so that wasn't so good. At about the

second—so about week 8, 9, 10, he went back to his oncologist, and they redid his imaging, and the oncologist said—

"You know, your tumor shrunk." And he says, "Oh, that's probably why I can breathe better." He says, "Yeah." So, and about that time, he was not getting tired from his walks, and he was, you know, kinda moving.

And then about, um, weeks, you know, 14, 15, 16, and he was the same therapy through the whole time. Uh, they got another, um, another X-ray of sort of that was you could see the tumor that easily. Um, and the oncologist said, "It shrunk some more." And it's shrunk, you know, this is not a—just some fluke. He says, "Something you're doing is doing this."

And, and he said, "I still—there, there's no chemo I can give you or anything, so don't stop doing whatever you're doing." And so, this, this got our attention, certainly got his attention, the patient, uh, but this got our attention as maybe this isn't such a crazy idea. Um—

And so, uh, we continued with that therapy, and uh, he, now one thing about these, you and I see this all the time, most of the time, the cancer doesn't just disappear or go away, especially when it's really advanced like that. But sometimes, it will, it will regress to the point where it kinda goes into a dormancy.

Dr. Stengler: Right.

Dr. Anderson: And this actually happened with him, and he was able, uh, after it was about a year of therapy the tumor had shrunk enough where his organs could work again. And he was able, by continuing with the dietary intervention and a few other things, um, to stay, in, in a dormancy period. And um, in the case of that particular patient, um, that—he was patient number one seven years ago, and he's still alive.

Dr. Stengler: Yeah.

Dr. Anderson: His oncologist told him, "Literally, with the size of your tumor," around their first meeting, you know, "You got maybe three to six months—

"Because you're just, you're running out of room for your organs." So, that, that one got our attention, and, and we had to keep with this model, though, of people, where nothing else had worked, and we tried natural things, didn't work. And standard.

Um, so then we got a series of, of patients, uh, sort of emboldened by the fact that this one worked, uh, and you know how it is, sometimes one thing works, and it doesn't ever work again. Uh, but we, we collected over the next six months, uh, a pretty good group of people where they had run the gamut of their standard therapies, and were told by the oncologist, "I can't—I've got nothing new. Can't give you anything else."

And there's nothing experimental—it's, you know, I—I mean they were out of options. Um, and then we had done vitamin C, or artesunate, or some of other combos, and—

Dr. Stengler: Yeah.

Dr. Anderson: It was just not going anywhere.

So, with different types of tumors, uh, basically, we had, um, uh, a number of them have similar responses to this first gentleman, and that is their labs that would show the variation if it was a lab, the labs would regress back towards normal. When the chemotherapy wasn't even doing that.

Um, if it was a matter of, uh, you know, other testing, we would follow whatever the testing was appropriate to follow with the patient. And then there were a couple of patients that were basically said—I would just like to not hurt as much and feel better, and maybe if my cancer wasn't growing so quickly, I could do that.

And so, we—you know, there, they were there for, uh, quality of life. So, we did those over an initial series of, of folks, and we report on in the initial series in the book, with that many since then—

Um, and we had a—the majority of them where they actually had regression of their disease—

Dr. Stengler: Wow.

Dr. Anderson:	And, and that really got our attention in the, uh, in the arena of—so, Dr. Warburg probably was onto something. We know that any one piece alone is not enough, because I had personally tried, say, the DCA alone in the past, and it just, it, it would slow it down, and then the cancer would just come back, or I would try the poly alone, and it would slow down again. I'd try the diet alone.
	Together, they started to work better.
	In 2014, I happened to be at a hyperbaric conference that I often am a speaker at, and I was listening to, um, what turned out to be one of the, uh, metabolic, uh, cancer therapy people that are publishing now. Dominic D'Agostino. And um—
	He was talking about work he was doing, exactly the same ideas, of stacking therapies to take advantage of the, the, the negative side of the Warburg effect. And I liked through, and I thought, "Well, okay, what's he doing different?"
	Well, he was doing the diet stuff, but he was also starting to add, uh, exogenous ketones, which is a supplement of ketones, so there's that. And uh, he was doing hyperbaric oxygen, which at the time, we were only doing for—in cancer patients for neuropathy, and side effects—
Dr. Stengler:	Okay.
Dr. Anderson:	Okay, because prior to about 2010, it was considered very bad to do hyperbaric oxygen in cancer patients, and so by 2014, we were moving towards it, but there, there wasn't still a lot of research, and we were being cautious. So that was another thing, and what, what he explained at that time, and, and since then, he and I worked together, and have spoken together—
	Uh, in conferences, was that the hyperbaric oxygen actually does more to take advantage of this, so it forces oxygen in places that it wouldn't normally go in a tumor, etcetera. So, I thought, "Okay, so he's, he's got the diet, we're doing that similar, the ketone thing as a, a supplement I had not thought of." And I thought, "Well, we can add that." And hyperbaric, we already had—we could certainly add that.

And what really was interesting was at the very, very end of his talk, he, and he showed—his, his work has all been with animals—

Dr. Stengler: Okay.

Dr. Anderson: Basically, what he showed is each therapy, when, you know, from diet to then adding ketones to hyperbaric to this, there, the animals who got the multiple therapies, the more therapies they—

They got, the less metastatic their disease was. So, that again, fit what we had observed, and at the very end, he said, "Oh," he goes, "By the way, there's a drug no one here has probably ever heard of, but if you add that in, it even makes it work better. We just didn't put that into our research, and that drug is called DCA."

And I thought, "Well, we're already doing that." You know. So, at that point, we expanded and took a step back, and said, "Well, we're doing a lot of what Dominic was doing, that he's finding success in his animals. We're finding success in people. And so, let's take a step back and combine them and see what we can do.

And so, if you look at the power of each thing on its own, it's got a little bit of power. But when you look at synergy, if everything is taking advantage of the weaker cancer cell, and its biology, and, the, the weak points of the biology—

Then if you put multiple inputs there, it can't kinda back out as easily. If you just do diet, diet can last a long time, but the cancers often find a way out. If, from my experience, if you just do DCA, the cancer cell can back out.

Dr. Stengler: Yeah.

Dr. Anderson: If you just do ketones, you back out. You've gotta kinda surround the cancer with as many metabolic things as you can. So, what we came up with, and what we've sort of evolved that to is a particular protocol that uses the, the DCA and the poly for their synergy, but in protection, um, some hyperbaric oxygen, uh, definitely the diet change, the ketone supplements, um, you know, all those things that we talked about.

But they're, they're done together. What we've noticed is that the doses that, that are required now that we i—that we use for the DCA—

And the poly MVA are lower than they used to be, because—

Dr. Stengler: Okay.

Dr. Anderson: We have synergy—

Dr. Stengler: Yeah.

Dr. Anderson: So, we're actually getting improved results from our original 2009 to 2014 research subjects

Obviously, nothing works for everything, but this is one where we reliably see at least some pausing of cancer or regression in many of the patients.

And so, it's, it's become a very, especially in aggressive cancers, it's become one of our, uh, big go-tos that, that we, uh, that we use. And um, it's, it's an area that is big—you know, very large universities are doing a lot of research in this area, because they're seeing that, yes, there is genetic things we need to get into and take care of, but if we don't do something about the metabolism—

Of the cancer, we don't—you know, we don't have a chance of getting ahead of it, uh.

Dr. Stengler: So it all comes down to this synergistic effect, by doing the combined therapy, the combined metabolic cancer therapy, so—and that's what we typically find in practice. Uh, most doctors involved in integrative oncology, it's not one—you know, sure shot treatment. It's, it's a combination where you get the best results, so excellent information.

Dr. Anderson: Yes.

Dr. Stengler: Yeah, thank you.

Dr. Anderson: Yeah, it's um, it's—and it, it dovetails very nicely, because people always wonder, "Well, what do I do next," etcetera. A lot of the other things that we talk about, especially some of the oral supplements and that sort of thing, uh, we use those as follow-up, and that becomes very important.

And the one thing I will say that I think the, the lynchpin in the whole system is the one thing you can't take out of it is the diet change.

Dr. Stengler: You've got to have that, yeah.

Dr. Anderson: And of course, the, uh, you know, people, that's the last thing they want to change, but—

What we found was when we look back at the folks who did it, those that did the best, did the diet the best. Uh, those that refused to do the diet might have felt a little better, but it didn't last terribly long. So I think that's pretty crucial.

Dr. Stengler: So, that's critical. Friends, if you're listening out there, which I'm sure you are, the diet changes are just critical. It's a limiting factor, as Dr. Anderson has said, and so, uh, in this series, you're getting a lot of good information on nutrition that fights cancer, and make sure you utilize that to your advantage.

So, uh, thank you again—

Dr. Anderson: Thanks.

THE CANCER VACCINE

— DR. BITA BADAKHSHAN —

Dr. Stengler: Well, I've got a great interview for you, right now. We've got Dr. Bita Badakhshan, and she's a medical doctor, has a lot of experience in conventional medicine, as well as integrative and holistic medicine. So, Dr. Bita, so, great to be with you, today.

Dr. Bita: Thank you for having me here, Dr. Stengler.

Dr. Stengler: And, of course, you practice at the Cancer Center for Healing.

Dr. Bita: Correct.

Dr. Stengler: And obviously, you guys see a lot, a lot of, uh, people with cancer. And so, I'd like to start off by having you tell the viewers just what your, a bit more about your background in medicine.

Dr. Bita: Sure.

Dr. Stengler: We're always interested when doctors, you know, start with the conventional background, and then get into more of the holistic and nutritional realm. So, tell us about that.

Dr. Bita: Yeah, that wasn't my plan, either, to go into holistic, but it's a very, it's actually interesting story. Well, after finishing residency in family practice in New York, when I moved down here, I started working at different urgent cares, privates, and also private, uh, internal medicine office, and also Kaisers.

I had four different practices I worked part-time in each. And, uh, during that time, I would see cancer patient who were doing, uh, alternative integrative treatments. And that was interesting for me, because I never heard of it, because at that time, I was trained and learned once you have cancer, you have to go surgery, chemoradiation—that's the only way. So, my first patient that I was impressed with the pancreatic cancer, that I saw she just came for a urgent care visit, but she'd been living with her pancreatic cancer for over three years. So I was, like, "Yeah, what's your secret?" she's, like, "You're not gonna believe." I said, "No, I'm pretty open minded. I like to learn. Uh, please tell me." So, she had, was diagnosed with pancreatic cancer, did the biopsy, but never did the surgery, never did the chemo, nothing else, just started taking enzymes, and IV therapies, and changing her lifestyle.

And then, at Kaiser, I saw another lady with Stage 4 ovarian, and I was, like, "Oh, wow, what's your secret?" *[Laughs]*

Dr. Stengler: Mm-hmm.

Dr. Bita: And she told me similar story, um, she was doing holistic, changed her diet, and didn't go with conventional. So, I thought, uh, these are a sign for me to look into this. That's when I started looking at natural holistic, to see what's out there, and started study it all on my own. And, um, next thing you know, I meet Dr. Connealy here, and then, um, I started learning. She be, has been my mentor, for a few years now, and I started treating cancer patient.

Dr. Stengler: So you must be pretty excited: you guys are seeing good results and helping, you know, people's quality of life, length of life, and, uh—

Dr. Bita: Absolutely—I love what I do, now. Initially, it was hard, because it's tough, what cancer patient is going through.

But after seeing good result and improving some of patient with Stage 4, I'm saying we're not here to cure you; is here to, you know, improve your quality of life, and decrease the pain. And, but in some cases, I've seen amazing result with Stage 4 breast cancer, who are in remission still; Stage

4 melanoma, the tumor in the lung of my patient is gone—uh, I mean, I'm sorry, tumor in the liver is gone. And we have prostate cancer match to the bone, which fully remission. So, we, uh, I've been seeing a lot of cases like that, and made me, you know, love what I do. *[Laughs]*

Dr. Stengler: Yeah, that's great. Now, I know today we wanna talk about, uh, some of your expertise in certain, a certain type of testing, uh, you use with cancer, cancer patients, people with cancer. And then, also, a very specific type of treatment you're seeing good results with. So, why don't you tell us, take your time and tell us about those things.

Dr. Bita: Sure. Sure. So, one of the labs we use it's called RGCC.

And it's, um, one of the highly-rated labs in the world, and, uh, their service 14 different countries, and I actually went to their lab in Greece. Their headquarter is in Switzerland, and they're doing amazing stuff, there. And, uh, one of the things we look at on our cancer patient is circulating tumor cell and stem cell.

Dr. Stengler: Mm-hmm.

Dr. Bita: So, I have patient who come here who had treatment of, uh, breast cancer or lymphomas, and they say, uh, "You know, I'm cured. I'm, I have, uh, you know, no cancer anymore." So, first thing I do is, "Okay, let me do your circulating stem cell and tumor cell, to see how much is floating." As we know, according to the oncologist journal, treating, uh, cancer with chemo radiation surgery doesn't really affect the stem cell; it doesn't bring the stem cell down. If anything, it makes it more virulent and more aggressive recurrence of cancer, so.

Dr. Stengler: Maybe, maybe, yeah, maybe just tell the viewers just maybe a, a basic definition of what a, you know, a stem cell is, just, yeah.

Dr. Bita: So, sure. So, circulating, uh, stem cell, it's initiated before even the tumor is formed. Once that tumor is formed, it's circulating tumor cell, which it sheds the circulating tumor cell into blood and lymphatic. That's what metastasis happens, like, patient come, "Dr. Bita, I had bilateral mastectomy. Why do I have recurrence?" It's because of the circulating tumor cell that are floating in the body, and because of the stem cell being positive. The patient is not fully in remission or fully cured from cancer until the stem cells is negative and circulating tumor cells are zero. So, that's what we look on—if I see a patient who says, "I got my treatment two years ago. I'm in remission. Everything is, uh, normal, scans are negative," I've usually look for that—we do that RGCC test, look for circulating tumor cell and stem cells.

And then, according to the number, it tells us their prognosis—the higher the number is, the worse prognosis, more increased risk of metastasis to other organs. Then what I do is, I do check other markers, too. Then I check their nagalase level, for example. Nagalase is an enzyme that is secreted by viruses and by cancer cell. What they do is they affect our white blood cell; they go attach to our microphages and lymph, lymphocytes and suppress them, deactivate them, so now they don't recognize cancer cell anymore to engulf them and, uh, destroy them. So, basically, our body loses that ability, and those circulating tumor cell and stem cells to keep increasing, and then they metastasize. So, your lower nagalase level you have, you're better, you're off, your immune system is better.

So, your higher-stage, uh, cancer patient is, your higher level of nagalase they have. So, I, that's another marker I follow through our therapies and treatments. And then, another thing we look at is the PHI ma, marker. PHI stands for phosphohexose isomerase, which is a marker of anaerobic, low oxygen; it's an enzyme of anaerobic. So, your higher the PHI is, the most risk of metastasis that patient have. For example, I had a patient who came with melanoma, had a skin cancer removed, said, uh, "I'm fine. I'm in remission. They said everything is clear, I don't need to be worried." So, the melanoma, so I followed him, but not that closely. This was beginning, it's few years ago—I didn't know the importance of PHI. And in the beginning, when we monitored his PHI, was pretty low.

Dr. Stengler: Okay.

Dr. Bita:	And, but his circulating tumor cell wasn't that low. Uh, this is, like, 2013, when we just started with all that, so, it took me a few years to *[laughs]* learn more.
Dr. Stengler:	Yeah.
Dr. Bita:	So, patient, um, his PHI suddenly—but my mistake was I didn't repeat it every two months, like what I do now, every six weeks. I waited three, four months; after four months, I repeated his PHI, suddenly it was jump, went high up there. So I'm, like, "Oh, something's going on. He's probably having a metastasis or something." He had a higher circulating tumor cell from beginning, so he was at higher risk.
Dr. Stengler:	Mm-hmm.
Dr. Bita:	So, anyways, what we did is we scanned his—he did have match to the liver.
Dr. Stengler:	Oh, okay, so it matched up.
Dr. Bita:	So, it did match up, but now we brought his PHI down, so he's fully in remission right now; he's doing amazing.
Dr. Stengler:	With the treatments you did, you've done here at the center, yeah.
Dr. Bita:	So, with the treatment we've been doing at the center and giving him SOTs now, he been doing great.
Dr. Stengler:	Oh, we need to talk now—yeah.
Dr. Bita:	So the SOT, so, what is SOT, now? So, the SOT is one of the therapies we add to our protocol here, which RGCC labs make us. SOT stands for supportive oligonucleotide technique. So what the RGCC lab do is, they look at patients, um—so, we send the, uh, patient's blood, the liquid biopsy, basically. So, they look at the circulating tumor cell and stem cell. And then what they do is, they make it a messenger RNA. They generate the SOT according to that patient's circulating tumor cell and, uh, stem cell. Then they give us that as a powder form, and we make it as a vaccine.
Dr. Stengler:	Mm-hmm.

Dr. Bita:	We'll inject it to the patient; it works in their body for four months, four, about three-and-half, four months. And then this vaccine is given every four months.
	As we know, circulating tumor cell, they lose ability to die; they can't perform apoptosis. The SOT binds to it; they cause the cancer cell death.
Dr. Stengler:	Mm.
Dr. Bita:	So, the best result is on earlier cancers, but we've been seeing prostate cancer, for example, Stage 4 matched to bone, just by changing diet and getting the SOT, shutting it off—no light up on the, on scan, so.
Dr. Stengler:	And I presume you don't see many side effects with that treatment.
Dr. Bita:	And it has no side effect.
Dr. Stengler:	Mm-hmm.
Dr. Bita:	The only thing is, if a patient goes through chemo radiation, the efficacy of SOT goes down.
Dr. Stengler:	Okay.
Dr. Bita:	Usually, SOT, what I recommend to my patient, not much to late stages; I recommend for early, like, if you remove your lump, you remove the tumor, you know how much circulating tumor cell you have, you go and attack it with SOT. One issue is, in the beginning, another thing we didn't know, when you give the SOT, because it attacks the tumor as well as circulating tumor cell, it causes inflammation.
	It can cause increased growth of a tumor.
Dr. Stengler:	Initially, before, yeah.
Dr. Bita:	Initially, yeah. So best result is on it, I feel like it's on patients who had the tumors removed, but we've been giving it otherwise, as well. And then, um—what else—*[Laughs]*
Dr. Stengler:	It's all right.
Dr. Bita:	Let's see—let me think—
Dr. Stengler:	Is there any other treatment you wanna talk about?

Dr. Bita:	Um, SOT—oh, let me talk about a case with, uh, head and neck [crosstalk] amazing result.
Dr. Stengler:	Good, yeah, go ahead. I'll just ask you a question, then.
Dr. Bita:	Any other patients, we could say.
Dr. Stengler:	Yeah. So, yeah, any other patient cases you'd like to share with the viewers?
Dr. Bita:	So, I have, one of my, um, early cases, which were we just started with SOT, um, he came in as a, uh, as a head and neck cancer patient, squamous cell carcinoma, with HPV.
	As we know, 70 percent of head and neck cancers, they are due to HPV virus.
Dr. Stengler:	Mm-hmm.
Dr. Bita:	And the reason I think the link between a viruses and cancer is because viruses produce that enzyme we talked, called nagalase. And nagalase is attached to our immune cell and suppresses our immune system, so that's what leads to the cancer from first place, too. But there also viruses, uh, attack our DNA, our genome, and they lead to cancer. So, as we know, lot of cancer causes are due to virus, lot of breast cancer patient are due to parasite, we see even parasite in prostate. So, parasite is coming a, one of the high reasons, as well. So, anyways, this guy came in, uh, he had his tumor removed, and he had cervical lymph node, he had one, uh, affected one of them, and it was removed. And he said, "I'm refusing chemo and I'm refusing radiation. What can you do for us?"
	So, we did his circulating tumor cell, and it was pretty high—it was 12-point-something, and usually you want it to have less than 5. Your lower, you're better.
Dr. Stengler:	Mm-hmm.
Dr. Bita:	Our goal is 2.
Dr. Stengler:	Okay.
Dr. Bita:	When the circulating tumor is greater than 5, there is higher risk of metastasis. But you could have a patient with 4.5

and have metastasis, too. So, his numbers was high, and his nagalase level was high, as well. And then, what we did, um, we gave him the SOT every four months, we gave him IVs in the beginning, we put him on antiviral therapy.

Dr. Stengler: Mm-hmm.

Dr. Bita: One of the ones that I love to use is EC AC-T, which is great. And, uh, we brought his nagalase, now he is normalized; is less than a regular person, is, like, 0.68. I just saw him, that's why I know his numbers. *[Laughs]*

Dr. Stengler: Yeah.

Dr. Bita: And then, he just did his MRI, and it was five-year MRI is still in remission.

Dr. Stengler: Wow.

Dr. Bita: Nothing, no tumors, nothing. So, he been getting his SOT every four years, and his latest circulating tumor cell was 6-point-something. So, we brought the CTCs down, but is not, still not perfect.

Dr. Stengler: Mm-hmm.

Dr. Bita: Since 2013, so he been getting, I don't know, his eight SOTs, like, every four months, been having a SOT. So, um, but, thank god, no metastasis, yet.

Dr. Stengler: Wow. And, uh—

Dr. Bita: *[Crosstalk]* don't think the goal is to really bring the circulating tumor cell down to 2, less than 2, then I'm relieved he's doing *[crosstalk]*. *[Laughs]*

Dr. Stengler: Wow, that's great. Did he have, did that patient have an oncologist, too, or is he just doing everything here?

Dr. Bita: He saw the oncologist initially, he got the biopsy diagnosis, he got the surgery, but then he refuse chemo and radiation.

Dr. Stengler: Right, right, wow, it's a great story.

Dr. Bita: So, one problem we have with chemo and radiation is they both affect the cancer stem cells.

Dr. Stengler: Right.

Dr. Bita:	And, uh—
Dr. Stengler:	Calavera's about that, the negative effects of that.
Dr. Bita:	Yeah, and it makes it more virulent and makes the cancer come back harder, and not responding to those chemo they did before or radiation before.
Dr. Stengler:	Now, how come, uh, in your opinion, why don't—I don't see my patients, their oncologists, uh, giving it, giving them that information. No one seems to know about that.
Dr. Bita:	There are, I mean, there are a lot of research out there, especially now, in the oncologist journal, that chemo can make the circulating stem cell and tumor cell worse, and they doing studies in breast cancer patient *[unintelligible]*. I think it's gonna get there; it just takes time.
Dr. Stengler:	Well, I agree that it's, it's a phenomenon that happens; it just seems the patients out there aren't being told that this is, you know, a risk.
Dr. Bita:	We have some labs in US that check for circulating tumor cells, but they're not as accurate, yet; they're not there, yet.
Dr. Stengler:	Yeah.
Dr. Bita:	They could find the DNA fragments, they could find the cancer DNAs, this, that, but they're not there, yet.
Dr. Stengler:	So, overall, having come from the conventional world, now, to integrative medicine, obviously, you must have a, a, a pretty good degree of confidence in what you're seeing with the integrative oncology.
Dr. Bita:	Yes, I do, but the hardest part is cancer cells are becoming so virulent, and cancer is becoming harder to treat now than before. And, um, you can't, you know, what I treat a patient with triple-negative, uh, before, it's very harder to treat them now. It's like the response even to natural sometimes is hard, you know. But, um, I love what I do, and the result we get, the best part is we don't harm the patient; none of the therapies are toxic to the patient. And sometimes I do recommend chemo, sometimes I do recommend surgery, but not radiation that much. *[Laughs]*

Dr. Stengler:	Mm-hmm.
Dr. Bita:	Radiation is one of the things I don't recommend that much, and, um, one of the reason is because of the genetic mutation it causes, and the, other cause of cancers. Like, I had a patient who came with history of breast cancer, had chemo radiation, and, uh, now, she had leukemia because of the radiation she had. And then she had to go through chemo; unfortunately, I saw her twice then she passed. She did not have any white blood cell left; the white blood cell was wiped out.
Dr. Stengler:	Mm-hmm.
Dr. Bita:	So, um, radiation I don't touch, but, uh, *[laughs]* chemo, sometimes we have to, sometimes we do need to do surgery. But the key is to not go jump into surgery, that's what I tell patient. The whole process, what we do here, you prepare the body for surgery. Like, if someone even gonna have a knee surgery, for example—it's not related to their cancer—if they don't prepare the body for it, it's gonna make all her immune system—
	—immune cells go and heal to that, heal that area, and circulating tumor cell in the blood keep increasing, and increases risk of metastasis other places. So, before any kind of surgery, even if it's not related to their tumor or cancer, we prepare them. We do couple weeks of, like, right nutrition, IV therapies, detoxing, and giving them Tagamet or modified citrus pectin, stuff to decrease the metastasis.
Dr. Stengler:	Right, right. Well, that's been great information—I know the viewers are gonna really appreciate this. And thank you for all the, you know, patients you're helping.
Dr. Bita:	Thank you for having me, here—it's great pleasure.
Dr. Stengler:	Yeah, thanks a lot.
Dr. Bita:	Thank you.

PATIENT STORY

— LARRY F. —

Dr. Stengler: Well, hi everyone. I'm here with, uh, my patient Larry.

Larry: Yeah.

Dr. Stengler: Great guy. I've known him for years. How many years have we known each other now?

Larry: Uh, quite a few.

Dr. Stengler: I mean, I think we're going back our kids were—

Larry: Yeah. Yeah—at least 10, 12 years.

Dr. Stengler: Yeah.

Larry: At least.

Dr. Stengler: Yeah.

Larry: Somewhere around there.

Dr. Stengler: Yeah.

Larry: Yeah.

Dr. Stengler: So we kind of have a story with you.

Larry: Yes.

Dr. Stengler: Couple years ago, um, I was seeing you and though maybe you had some allergies going on and you had some hoarseness in his voice and, you know, took a look in there and couldn't see much, you know, problematic.

Larry: Yeah.

Dr. Stengler: And treated you and you didn't get better. So then I sent you to an, uh, ENT doctor. And you went to the first one and he didn't really find anything wrong. Right?

Larry: Said—*[laughs]* He said I had indigestion. *[laughs]*

Dr. Stengler: *[unintelligible]* said forget—indigestion. Okay, acid reflux and then—

Larry: Yeah, acid reflux. *[laughs]*

Dr. Stengler: Acid reflux didn't help treating that.

Larry: That didn't work.

Dr. Stengler: And I said, "No, there's something strange going on." You kept having the hoarseness and—

Larry: Yeah.

Dr. Stengler: So we sent you to another specialist and what did he find?

Larry: Well, the second specialist—

Dr. Stengler: Yeah.

Larry: actually said the same thing.

Dr. Stengler: Oh!

Larry: Uh, that, uh, "You have, uh, acid reflux or something." I said, "Uh, can't be."

So—and so I came back to see you again you said, "Well, I'll introduce you to someone." You introduced me to Dr., uh, *[unintelligible]* say his name?

Dr. Stengler: That's another specialist? Yeah.

Larry: Yeah, specialist.

Dr. Stengler: Mm-hmm.

Larry: And she looked and she said, "Um..." She did a, you know, ran a tube up my nose and down my throat and she says, "You'd better go have that, uh, uh, scanned. A CT scan.

Dr. Stengler:	Mm-hmm.
Larry:	Which I did and she suspected cancer, a tumor, and as it turned out yes I did. Uh, I was diagnosed with a squamous cell carcinoma on the base of my tongue and, of course, um, the only, uh, alternative we had then was, uh, radiation and, uh, chemotherapy. Which I did for—well, I started in January of 2016.
Dr. Stengler:	Mm-hmm.
Larry:	concluded in May of 2016.
Dr. Stengler:	Mm-hmm.
Larry:	And then we started a program, uh, with you then.
Dr. Stengler:	Yeah.
	So now, of course, I mean, part of the story with you was you, of course, were doing the radiation therapy, you know, to your throat and they told you, yeah, you'd have some hoarse and some stuff like that. But you came in to see me maybe, uh, a week or two after—
Larry:	That's right.
Dr. Stengler:	Um, well, a few weeks after you'd been into the process and you could barely swallow and it was a little more severe than, uh, you had known. Right?
Larry:	Yes. Yeah.
Dr. Stengler:	Yeah.
Larry:	Yeah, I was having difficulty swallowing and, uh, I had no appetite whatsoever. Uh...
Dr. Stengler:	Lost how much weight?
Larry:	I lost a lot of weight. Lost at least 30 pounds.
Dr. Stengler:	Yeah.
Larry:	Because, uh, I wasn't eating. Because I didn't—I had no urge to eat.

Dr. Stengler:	Mm-hmm.
Larry:	Although I knew I needed to eat. So that's why we got together and—
Dr. Stengler:	Yeah. I remember you were in with your—one of your daughters and your wife and everyone was extremely concerned, understandably.
Larry:	Yeah.
Dr. Stengler:	And, um, you were weak, because you couldn't get any nutrients in you, couldn't swallow, so we, uh, put you on some shakes. We did some IV's—
Larry:	We did.
Dr. Stengler:	I think several days a week, just to keep you going.
Larry:	Just—
Dr. Stengler:	Some nutrients and fats!
Larry:	Yes.
Dr. Stengler:	Actually fats, you know, IVs of fats as well to get some nutrients and some calories in you. And it, basically, were under the gun, because if we couldn't sustain you they would had to put a tube in your stomach and—
Larry:	That was—I can remember.
Dr. Stengler:	I can remember the—yeah, that was the alternative. So you were coming almost every day and we're doing the IVs for a couple weeks just keeping you going until your throat could heal up.
Larry:	Yeah. I didn't want tube—I did not want that tube in my stomach. *[laughs]*
Dr. Stengler:	Right. So we were able to keep you going and finally things healed up and you—
Larry:	You did and, and—
Dr. Stengler:	Got better, so... yeah.
Larry:	We did. Course there was another fellow that helped a lot.

Dr. Stengler:	Mm-hmm.
Larry:	Probably—
Dr. Stengler:	Yeah, *[unintelligible]*, yeah, yeah.
Larry:	He was the man, yeah. Yeah.
Dr. Stengler:	Absolutely.
Larry:	Faith in God.
Dr. Stengler:	Yeah.
Larry:	It's—yeah.
Dr. Stengler:	Yep, good point.
Larry:	Yeah.
Dr. Stengler:	Very important point.
Larry:	Yeah. Amen. Yeah.
Dr. Stengler:	So, um, yeah, so now you do, like some intravenous Vitamin C and some ozone therapy just, you know, as a help your immune system inflammation.
Larry:	That's—exactly.
Dr. Stengler:	About once a month, every couple months. It's been a couple years now since you had the cancer, right?
Larry:	It has, yeah. I was, uh, May of 2016, so it's coming up on two years.
Dr. Stengler:	Mm-hmm.
Larry:	And, you know, after that initial program we were on with you for, I guess, about six months.
Dr. Stengler:	Right.
Larry:	Uh, until I finally was able to, you know, come back. I mean, although I was, you know, ambulatory, I was out walking around and things, I wasn't, I wasn't doing an exercise and I had no strength.
Dr. Stengler:	Mm-hmm.
Larry:	So for about six months—and finally slowly we came back!

Dr. Stengler:	Yep.
Larry:	And this is a C drips and the ozone, uh, really have, have worked, I'd say, miracles, really.
Dr. Stengler:	Yeah. Well that's good.
Larry:	Yeah.
Dr. Stengler:	I know you, you've had a couple follow ups and they say everything continues to be clear, right?
Larry:	I've had a couple follow ups. As a matter of fact, uh, just last week I did, uh, another—they, they put me on, uh, new CT scans every six months.
Dr. Stengler:	Mm-hmm.
Larry:	Uh, just to monitor.
Dr. Stengler:	Mm-hmm.
Larry:	And see and, uh, last week and the doctor called me on, uh, last Friday and said, "Everything's cool. Everything's good." *[laughs]*
Dr. Stengler:	Yeah, that's great.
Larry:	There's no, no resurgence of a tumor, there's nothing. It's all good. So...
Dr. Stengler:	So it seems like it's a perfect example of that concept of integrative oncology. You know. In other words you got the conventional cancer treatment.
	We supported you and got you through that.
Larry:	Yes.
Dr. Stengler:	And then we're doing the preventative part on our, our side with the nutrition and the IVs and all that. Because in conventional medicine the other—once you're done your radiation, chemo you're kind of on your own type of thing. Right?
Larry:	Yes. Yeah.
Dr. Stengler:	Yeah. But—

Larry:	So—with, with your intervention, uh, and your expertise, uh, has made the difference completely. I'm... I wouldn't be here, probably, if not for the—
Dr. Stengler:	Well, you're a great patient. I mean, you always do all the treatments, you don't complain, you're very much, you know, uh, proactive in your health and you—you've been like that since I've known you for 15, 20 years.
Larry:	Yes, I believe we have to be that way. Right?
Dr. Stengler:	Mm-hmm.
Larry:	Uh, I mean, we can have a, have a plan, but if we don't follow the plan, uh, it's just a dream.
Dr. Stengler:	Mm-hmm.
Larry:	Right? So went on the plan. I had a positive feeling for it, because I had faith, faith in you, faith in God.
Dr. Stengler:	Mm-hmm.
Larry:	And so I can only say here I am.
Dr. Stengler:	And you're—and you're in good shape for your upcoming, uh, daughter's wedding.
Larry:	That's right. *[laughs]*
Dr. Stengler:	So there you go. Everything's good! *[laughs]*
Larry:	Everything's good. *[laughs]* Everything is good.
Dr. Stengler:	Alright.
Larry:	Yeah.
Dr. Stengler:	Well thank you. Thanks for sharing that with our, uh, viewers.
Larry:	My pleasure.
Dr. Stengler:	Okay, thank you.
Larry:	My pleasure.

EPISODE 4: THE FOOD/DIET CURE

17 of the Most Powerful Anti-Cancer Foods (and Supplements)—and How to Easily Work them into Your Daily Routine

THE CHRISTMAS MIRACLE CURE

— DR. NASHA WINTERS —

Dr. Stengler: Welcome to Outside The Box Cancer Therapies. Today, I'll be speaking with Dr. Nasha Winters. She is a visionary and CEO of her own company as well as a best selling author, lecturer, and she has more than 25 years of experience in the healthcare industry. She is a thought leader in personalized precision medicine and Dr. Nasha works to educate clients, doctors, and researchers worldwide in how to apply integrative oncology philosophically and therapeutically.

Dr. Winters is board certified and licensed in acupuncture and oriental medicine from the International Institute of Chinese medicine in Albuquerque, New Mexico. She has a doctorate in naturopathic medicine from Southwest College of Naturopathic medicine in Tempe, Arizona and as well, she has received her fellow of the American Board of Naturopathic Oncology. A diagnosis of cancer in 1991 redirected her focus from pursuing conventional medicine to exploring, at the time, the emerging field of psychoneuroimmunology.

Her interest in all things related to health landed her in a rich learning environment from naturopathic and Chinese medicine to ayurvedic medicine and beyond, further rooting her in a scientific but holistic trained centric approach that leaves no stone unturned. She believes that there is no single cause, target, or treatment for chronic illness and cancer and it takes a well rounded understanding of the whole person to have the greatest impact on this multifactorial process.

She is the co-author of the metabolic approach to cancer, integrating deep nutrition, the ketogenic diet and non-toxic bio-individual therapies. She is in private practice in Durango, Colorado. Well welcome, Dr. Winters. Again, it's great to be with you.

Dr. Winters: Thank you so much. This is a joy to be here.

Dr. Stengler: Excellent. Well, I'm sure all the viewers are very interested to know about your personal story.

Obviously, a lot of people watching this series have cancer, have a loved one who has cancer. Maybe they've had cancer in the past and they're gonna be very inspired to hear about your personal so tell us about the beginnings of what happened with you. You had cancer a number of years back and what happened? What kinda cancer and how you came through all that?

Dr. Winters: Wonderful. Well, first of all, I can remember a time not so long ago as I'm sure you can, where we didn't—we're—a lot of people hadn't been touched directly or indirectly by cancer. I've watched that unfortunately change drastically in the last 25 years and, um, today, even while we're speaking today, 1,600 people in the United States will die of cancer.

Dr. Stengler: Mm-hmm.

Dr. Winters: And 1 in 2 men and 1 in 2.4 women will be diagnosed with it in their lifetime. So I hear that and it kinda sends shivers down my spine but back in 1991 when I was diagnosed with cancer, I was kind of, uh, an island, especially being young with cancer.

I was 19 when I was very, very sick and spent about a year in and out of emergency rooms and doctors offices and because I was so young, it was sort of that, uh, zebra concept. You know? Everyone kept looking at me, thinking, "There's no way she can have anything but maybe IVS or an ectopic pregnancy or it's just mentally ill." I mean, honestly, those were the types of labels being put on me at that time. And so over time, the doctors just finally kind of ignored me even more. The more they saw me, the more they disregarded me and so I, uh, stumbled upon, um, an ER doc who was someone I hadn't seen before who took it upon himself to do a little deeper investigation.

He actually finally did, um, order—ordered a CT scan—or excuse me. An MRI. An that time, that's what we had was an MRI in '91 and then did some more thorough blood work and it was a shock, as you can imagine when he had to come in and tell the women, or the young women at that time who was the same age as his daughter, that I had a terminal stage four, um, ovarian cancer process happening, um, that had been brewing for quite some time.

Because cancer, we don't go to bed and wake up with it. It—it took some time to get there and previous to that, I had two bouts of cervical cancer at age 14 and 16 where everyone was just like, "No big deal. Just burn it. You know, cut it out there. No big deal." We didn't know the things back in the late '80s and early '90s that we do today. We were thinking HPV infection. We weren't—so we weren't think Rocka genetic mutations. These are the types of things today we see in clinical practice if we see some-one presenting with odd stuff like myself at that time. We think a little bit differently.

But no one knew then and so at that time of diagnosis, I was so ill, I was in end organ, um, stage failure. My kid-neys and liver were failing. I was filled with ascites fluid. Looked about 9 months pregnant, actually more like ten months pregnant at that point. They couldn't take the flu-id because I was so hyper bulimic already that they were afraid they'd mess with my, uh, fluid balance and ultimate-ly kill me in the office.

So they were able to such little bits out over a period of a few weeks and basically, send me to a palliative care team. Um, and that time, we didn't have hospice in my commu-nity, um, and so that was as good as it gets and they really offered an option of palliative chemotherapy online that even told me it was just a matter of weeks or months that I had. So thankfully, being uh, a pretty, uh, determined and stubborn person, I wasn't gonna take that for an answer so I thought, "If I'm gonna go out, I'm gonna go out with knowledge. Okay?"

[Laughter]

Um, somehow, I could intellectualize my self at a lot of things and traumas at that time in my life, which was part of my why I got cancer to begin with.

Dr. Stengler: Right.

Dr. Winters: Um, but it helped me. It was a survival mechanism for sure. And I ended up picking up the first book that jumped at me off the shelf at the library, *Quantum Healing* by Deepak Chopra, which was very new and innovative at that time. Um, and it changed my life.

It changed my major. It changed my—my whole trajectory, uh, which puts us here having this conversation today.

Dr. Stengler: Wow. So basically—how old were you then when you had your diagnosis?

Dr. Winters: I was officially—I turned 20 on September 30th, 1991 but I had been sick for a good year before that, really, really sick. In and out of the hospital getting progressively worse. My actual diagnosis came on October 21st—

[Crosstalk]

Dr. Stengler: Oh, okay. Because you look—you look so young. I—I thought, "Wow. The numbers don't add up." Uh—

[Laughter]

Dr. Winters: Yeah. I just turned 46 and I just celebrated 20—basically 26 years out with this diagnosis.

Dr. Stengler: Wow. So that's quite the story. So basically, you got the diagnosis of a serious advanced cancer. Essentially told there wasn't much that could be done for you, try and make you more comfortable. Um, you did research. You got motivated. You got inspired. So take us through the transition then once you became educated. The types of therapies you started to use just in general because we're gonna get in more detail and all of these therapies you have an expertise in.

Dr. Winters: Perfect. So at that time, you have to remember, this was the time of the Dewey Decimal system. There was no internet. There was no Facebook. There was no Dr. Google out there. Um, I was a pre-med student. I was very interested in the sciences. I was a pre-med student working in my library at my college. So I started to spend all my extra time reading through old textbooks and so I was interested in understanding the biochemistry and the physiology of what was happening in my body at the time. And at the same time, I was starting to get into the groovy Deepak Chopra stuff as well, the psychoneuroimmunology side of things but the chemistry was still where I was digging.

The biology is where I was hanging out and that's when I first ran across the work of AutoWarburg, um, from the 1920s fame who, um, is where we're gonna be going in our conversation here in a little bit. But I was struck by that that this resonated with me so much of what I was reading—

About what happened in my body, what was happening was basically a metabolic process gone awry. And that if it went out of balance, then therefore, there was a way to bring it back into balance. Now, again, I'm young. I'm a young budding scientist at the same time. I start experimenting. What else can you do? A living laboratory. Right?

Dr. Stengler: Right.

Dr. Winters: So I went 100 percent vegan. 100 percent but you have to remember this—in the '90s, my I—idea of a vegan was iceberg, um, iceberg lettuce and, uh, loads and loads and loads of grain. You know, pretty much rice and iceberg lettuce. That's what I was trying to sustain myself on. That, I think on some level, was a step up from the diet I had been eating so highly processed.

I actually started to add in some green things. My husband, at that time was my boyfriend, chopped up, uh, like

	broccoli and red bell peppers to put into my boxed macaroni and cheese. Right?
Dr. Stengler:	*[Laughs].*
Dr. Winters:	They even had a—a vegan version at that time. It was crazy of how I was basically doing a processed vegan diet but it was still a step up from where I was. And then overtime, I learned, "Wow. Maybe a more holistic real food based vegan diet and then a lot more vegetables." And then it kind of morphed over time into vegetarianism and now, more into the time where I am today with kind of a—a plant based, ketogenic, cycling type of diet based on real food is where I've evolved to in 26 years.
	But each step I took seemed to help shift something in my metabolism, in my chemistry, and it seemed to buy me enough time to figure out or get to the next stepping stone of my own healing process.
Dr. Stengler:	Wow. So started—the base started with nutrition and you worked from there.
Dr. Winters:	Absolutely. And simultaneously on the nutrition path, I did start to adjust—address the psychosocial path and so I was very much working on the psychology because we didn't have knowledge of this at the time
Dr. Winters:	Um, on top of these little changes and learning. I met an acupuncturist who helped me with my pain management and the digestive issues because I was having blockages and other problems, as you can imagine, with that much tumor burden.
	Um, so as you can see, it was no one thing. I was learning as I went along and I just happened to frankly, in those first few years, get lucky enough to stumble upon the next aha moment to help me bring my terrain back into balance. I wish I had me now 26 years ago *[laughs]*. You know, we could do this process and it won't take—it wouldn't take me 15 years, you know, to do this with somebody else like it in some ways did for me.
Dr. Stengler:	Yeah.

Dr. Winters:	Um, but even for me just to give context, I had another huge breakthrough in 2010. So a full, you know, not, you know, 19 years or whatever. Or excuse me, uh, yeah 19 or so years into this process learning that I was, um, still having way too much carbohydrate in my diet. I had a completely messed up thyroid. I was about 40, 50 pounds heavier than I am now. Terrible sleep patterns. My hormones were all over the map.
	No matter how good I was doing everything on my more vegetarian diet and all the tools and tricks of the trade of naturopathic medicine, it wasn't enough. I wasn't going deep enough on the metabolic processes and that's when I really started diving in and about that same time is when folks like Dr. Thomas Siegfried started bringing his work to—to the mainstream. Again, I've been a research all along so starting to hear murmurs of other people looking at other ways to do pushback on a tumor burden was very powerful for me and I'm still—still on the journey.
Dr. Stengler:	Oh, absolutely. Well, that's powerful because here, you have the—you know, you've been the patient. You've been the researcher. Now, you're the doctor helping thousands of people so this is phenomenal and I—I know our viewers are gonna be very excited to hear the rest of this interview. Well, Nasha, as you know, uh, I was doing some research before writing the book with Dr. Paul Anderson, our book *Outside The Box Cancer Therapies*, and I found there were very few books out there which were comprehensive in integrative oncology. And I'm sure you've found the same thing.
	And lo and behold, one of the very few books I came across was your book, *The Metabolic Approach to Cancer* and it is phenomenal. Very well done.
Dr. Winters:	Well, when I think about the metabolic approach to cancer, um, and what is the—the base camp of why this book came to fruition is understanding that, um, there are—I—I guess I'll just kinda dive in. To me, the way I think about it is we're a bucket. Okay? And into that bucket are droplets of critical factors, you know, things that are coming in

from our environment, things that are coming in from our predecessors, from our ancestors, or our epigenetics, our genes, things coming in from our food, our soil, our water, our sunshine, things coming in from the relationship we are involved in. I mean, basically, that bucket is being filled all of the time with information coming into it.

Over time, that bucket may get sloppy. It may get mucky. It may get too much of the wrong elements in there. Um, and so when that happens, what it does is it basically makes, uh, the processes within that bucket less efficient and effective. And when we get, uh, less efficient and effective, you know, we just stop. We—we just kinda get stuck. We stagnate. So from ancient Chinese medicine, blood stagnation, blood and stagnation, Chi stagnation has a pathology, you know, part to it. Um, even in when we get a blood clot in—in a disease process, that's an ultimate stagnation.

Dr. Stengler: Hmm.

Dr. Winters: You know, tumors are considered kind of big stagnant pools of—of, um, you know, muck as well but basically, that's what I—*[unintelligible]* seen this with my clients. It's like what gummed up the works and how can we get it flowing again? That's more of the kind of, uh, macrocosm concept of it.

But when you get down to the absolutely fundamental building block of these processes, that comes down to those little powerhouses, the mitochondria that are within each and every one of our cells. And again, reflecting back to my first few moments in the library after my own diagnosis, stumbling upon the work of people from the early 1900's and into the mid 1900s that were starting to see cancer as a metabolic mitochondrial disease versus a somatic genetic disease, that resonated with me so much more, um, than anything of just a one cause, one effect, one treatment type of approach. So that's where I started spending my time for my own healing process and then had the lovely opportunity to quote on quote, practice on many, many, many patients over many, many years to understand that if I could correct that, uh, the composition of that bucket, then we can see some pretty miraculous outcomes.

And so that whole writing of this book, *The Metabolic Approach to Cancer*, is really 25 years of my understanding of my own process and that of thousands of other patients I have had the privilege to witness their process, um, and how we've taken them from point A to point B, um, by addressing that—that mitochondrial material.

Dr. Stengler: Right. So in essence, for the viewers, there's different theories as to why people get cancer. And people like yourself, myself, we believe often it's multifactorial but you can simplify it in some ways. It comes down to cellular health. We now know, you know, for the viewers out there, if you take a typical human cell, I mean, it's like a small American city. All the activity going on in it. I mean it's—it's unbelievable really.

You know, there's a lot of focus in oncology today on genetics and certainly genetics can play a role in someone's pre—predisposition to cancer and other chronic diseases.

However, I think from reading your book, you're similar to me. Genetics can be a cause but really, if you look at the science, in terms of being a, uh, a significant factor in the initiation of cancer, it really is still a small percent. I mean, if you look at the American Cancer Society and take breast cancer for example, which is very common, I mean, it's still a very small percent of breast cancers, which are strongly genetically related.

We have this role of epigenetics. We have how nutrition and foods, uh, can influence the information our DNA expresses. Can you tell the viewers more about what we've learned with advances in nutritional science in the last decade?

Dr. Winters: Oh, my gosh. It's *[laughs]*—again, being someone's who's been on this journey for myself and thousands of others and I—I know my colleagues like you and Paul who've been at this for a while, we have just seen such a renaissance in medicine. It's so much fun to be part of medicine right now. Um, because there's a lot of things we've seen as vitalistic practitioners that the science is catching up with and showing us.

But ultimately, we still kinda took a wrong turn in Albuquerque back in the '40s and '50s when we started to put all of our eggs in the basket of genes being the cause and effect and we spent an enormous amount of time, money, energy on researching the—the genome project and came up—well, frankly, a bit short because we were really hoping and expecting to see, "You have this one gene mutation, you give it this one treatment and all is good in the universe." It does not happen that way.

And if you take it back even further, when we talk about the gene or the somatic theory of cancer or even any chronic illness, there are all kind of on the spectrum for me. Um, where these scientists are looking, they're looking at the nuclei within the—the—the cell, within the mitochondria of that cell and so if they take that, um, damaged, sick nuclei out of that sick cell and they put it into—a cell that's healthy, okay, into the cytoplasm of the healthy cell, that healthy cell does not get cancer. If that—if it was truly a genetic case, you could easily transmit those—that genetic material from the nucleus from one cancer cell into a healthy cell and therefore turn on cancer. That's an incredibly simplistic explanation of this but that's what it would—would happen if that was in fact the case. But what really happens and we have some amazing folks like Dr. Siegfried and, um, Dr. Mina Bissell and, um, Darlington's work, I believe is his name.

These guys started doing things called these mitochondrial transfers and they were able to then take the nuclei of a cancerous, you know, cell, put it into the—into a cell of a health non-cancerous cell and cancer doesn't take place. In fact, they were able to see that the cell repaired, that it healed. Okay? That it became functional again.

You can also then take the healthy nuclei and put it into the cytoplasm of a cancer cell and over time, you will actually create cancer. Okay?

So that kinda gets everyone's brains going, "Wait a minute. So I can take cancer cells and put them into healthy cells and not cause cancer but I can take healthy cells and put them into sick cells and make those cells sicker." That idea is that okay, it's not in the DNA nuclei. It's in the soup that that nucleus swims in, the cytoplasm. Okay?

And so we know how to clean up that cytoplasm and we know how to keep the mitochondria happy and we know how to turn that frown upside down of a cancer cell and put it into a healthy cell environment.

Dr. Stengler: Right. Well, that's very empowering to the viewers because again, there's much people can do to change their genetic destiny, so to speak, so that's great news. Now, one of your expertises is that ketogenic diet. And I bet if I went out and pulled a thousand medical doctors, a thousand oncologists, uh, what is the ketogenic diet? I'd be willing to bet a very high percent of them could not define what it is or be aware of some of the groundbreaking research that's been occurring in recent years. So please tell the viewers what it is and what makes it such a powerful nutritional approach to cancer?

Dr. Winters: There's actually much more mythology around it than there is reality and up until about two months ago—there was not really a good primer out there that's just cancer specific around the ketogenic diet. There's been a lot of research around its use and epigenetic—or excuse me. In, um, epilepsy, neurological disorders, um, weight loss, you know, per—human performance. There was a lot of great discussion on that building in the last few years. Um, but cancer was still a different animal and it—and it is. It needs to be—it needs to be approached different in the patient dealing with cancer than in someone just wanting to do this for a little bit of weight loss or longevity or brain enhancement because the metabolism in the healthy body is different than the metabolism in a cancering body.

So what a ketogenic diet is is basically our bodies were built to function on two main fuel sources at any given time. One is the burning of sugar, sugar metabolism, and the other is the burning of fatty acids of these ketones.

Um, and so we—when we are in, uh, a starvation period, when we are in the—the deepest part of winter, when we don't have berries and, um, seeds and things to pick from nature and we're just kind of hunkering down and going for long fasted states of time, we need an alternative fuel source that number one, helps us stay alive, number two, helps us find our next carbohydrate rich meal, number three, keeps us, um, you know, burning efficiently and effectively and not loosing our mind in the process of it because our mental capacity can go down the tubes when we're hungry. Okay?

In just 100 years, we went from about 30 grams of our diet being carbohydrate to about 80 to 90 percent of our diet today as carbohydrate, um, in some cases. And so that switch over has made us much more metabolically inflexible to tap into that alternative fuel source at need. And with that has come a lot of chronic disease and the main diseases that are plaguing us today are neurological diseases, cardiovascular disease and cancer and cancer's expected to outbid the, uh, first place, uh, mortality rate of cardiovascular disease but we're expecting that the neurological diseases are what are actually going to bankrupt our healthcare system.

And so when you look across the board at the common thread of all of these conditions, it is an inappropriate metabolic, mitochondrial fuel process and it's become inflexible.

Dr. Stengler: Right. So essentially, tell the viewers how cancer cells prefer, you know, the sugar for fuel. Um, the ketones produce by the higher good fat diet, the low carb diet. I think you'd say on the lower end a protein but maybe lower to moderate. Um, how that's destructive to cancer cells, how their mitochondria can't get fuel from those ketone bodies and again, why the ketogenic diet then, uh, can be so effective.

Dr. Winters: First of all, cancer cells are little sugar hubs. They have a preferential fuel source. They want that sugar and as they start to ferment and move away from respiration, the glycolysis that starts to speed up their need to be even more sugar centric. Okay?

We also see that a lot of tumors and tumor cells have, uh, many more insulin receptors on their cell wall than our healthy cells. So they also become, um, a place that each time you dump glucose into the system, you also have to respond with insulin and so we end up having kind of this increased, um, metabolic rate of the body being able to gobble up—those insulin receptors are gobbling up the sugar even more forcefully on those tumor cells and tumor, um, you know—tumors themselves to try and get as much glucose into the system as possible.

So it becomes kind of a—a fight for nourishment, for nutrition. Now, interestingly enough, they do not have the same ability and majority of cells because there's—there's some studies out there that suggest that there may be a couple of cell line studies out there that could actually use ketones as a fuel source

Um, but basically, the ketones are not a preferred or even a—a usable resource for the cancer cells. So the great thing is our—is our other cells in our body, our healthy cells can flip in and use the ketones very effectively, especially, um, our heart, our muscle, our brain are very much able to run entirely on ketones. Okay? Cancer cells are not. So one of the things, of course we can starve them with that mechanism that's but one of the processes but—

What we're also seeing is that we embolden or strengthen the quantity and quality of the healthy mitochondria in the face of ketones and in the lower carbohydrate environment or even fasted environment by a mechanism called autophagy. Okay? So we're basically sweeping out the garbage, making room. You know, taking out the garbage so we can make room for something new, something good. Something to grow positively in the healthy cells.

Um, and so when that happens, we are sort of outnumbering, if you will, you know, that the power, the vitality, the function of our healthy mitochondria to the unhealthy mitochondria and helping induce what they call mitophagy, so kind of break down of those damaged mitochondria in those, um, cancer cells. So we're kind of strengthening one side of the equation while weakening another. And a lot of research is now pointing to the fact that a ketogenic diet will enhance all of our therapies across the board because it acts like basically a Trojan horse.

So it's going to make those cancer cells much more vulnerable so that whatever you put in behind them, whether it's chemotherapeutic agent, whether it's a PD1 inhibitor, whether it's intravenous vitamin C, those cancer cells are gonna already be a bit weakened and, um, and vulnerable to whatever therapies you put in.

Dr. Stengler: Right. And that's excellent, excellent information. You've probably heard it 100 times as—as I have, probably thousands where patients are seeing their oncologist and there's obviously value to that. They need to be monitored and get certain lab tests and certain types of treatments, uh, depending on what's going on with the person but, um, you know, I've had so many patients tell me that their oncologist has told them just to relax. "Diet has no effect on your cancer. Eat what you want. Enjoy your life." Um, it just seems to fly in the face of good science. I mean, our cells don't work by magic. You've talked about, you know, the effect of cancer cells, how they love sugar and so forth, how insulin, when insulin spikes—

It's even considered in conventional medicine to be carcinogenic. No one argues about that. Um, so it's—it's—it's concerning. Oncologists still are about 30, 50 years behind when it comes to nutrition and as a result, people are not getting the best results they could beyond cancer. Whether you had heart disease or any kind of chronic disease for sure. Okay, Dr. Winters, in your book, you had a really good section on foods that people should remove from their fridge and freezer. Would you mind reviewing that for—for the viewers here?

Dr. Winters: Absolutely. Well, first of all, I wanna just come back around to what you brought up about how a lot of oncologists are still misinforming their patients.

Dr. Stengler: Oh, please, yes.

Dr. Winters: Because I think that that sort of leads to well, why is it so important to do a little bit of a pantry or a refrigerator overhaul is that, um, we are being told or a lot of the patients— in fact, I had someone yesterday who's UCLA doctor, very smart doctor, told them that sugar has nothing to do with cancer despite the fact that they were reviewing the patient's pet scans results at the time, which is a test that—

That takes glucose into the cells and looks at it *[laughs]*, you know, to see where the cells are most active, where it lights up. It's based on sugar metabolism.

Dr. Stengler: That's amazing. That is true. I mean, if you got activity of cancer cells, they're sucking up the sugar and that's how find it—you find it on the test.

Dr. Winters: Exactly. And they're even got a new test coming out which we should have access to in the next year or so of using MRIs instead of the old gadolinium and some of the other heavy metals. They're actually starting to use sugar, um, isotopes in the MRIs that are coming around. So those will be maybe a little less toxic for our patients but again, they can say out of one side of their mouth, "Wow. These are great tests. This is how I know what's going on in your body," and at the same time, saying, "Sugar has nothing to do with it. Please just kinda let that wash over you with some common sense *[laughs]*." So that's huge.

Number two, I just got back last weekend from an amazing conference in, um, uh, at Hopkins, uh, co-presented by Hopkins all about the metabolic approach, you know, to cancer.

And the whole thing was not about naturopathic interventions per se but it was all about how we use ketogenic diet as the base camp of any of our therapies, whether it's breeded therapy or other, uh, radiotherapies, um, surgical interventions, chemotherapeutic agents, targeted therapies, hormone blockade and all of these researchers and clinicians are out there saying, "You are going to have such better outcomes, such better cytotoxic response while having less side effects if you implement a ketogenic diet along with these conventional therapies." That, you could have pushed me over with a feather, um, seeing that happening in a such a, uh, an environment.

So that does lead to us to say, "There is a bridge happening of us starting to understand that food does matter and think of it—you—even if you're not quite attached to it being the end all be all cure all, at least know that it's going to help any of your therapies work better. So thinking of it as kind of a foundation for anything that you do.

Dr. Stengler:	Right.
Dr. Winters:	So when you start to go to the foundation, you have to start simply by going to your refrigerator, your freezer, your pantry and start there. Um, sadly enough *[unintelligible]* a lot of people don't even shop, grocery shop and cook their own food which is I'd like to see that turn around as well because you have much more control over what goes into that—into your body if you yourself are purchasing it and putting it into your fridge, freezer, and pantry. But if you had to start, you'd wanna go through and start getting rid of any liquid sugar. You know? Liquid calories.
	So I tell people like, "Get rid of anything—" you know, even had somebody the other day say, "Well, what about—this green tea has a little bit of sugar." I'm like, "Well, you just got rid of some of your—you could have had a piece of squash *[laughs]*, you know, instead of sipped two sips of that tea. You could have had more nutrient density had you not just drank your carbohydrates for the day." So start to get those off the table first. In fact, even the pediatric association is telling people to stop giving their kids juice.
Dr. Stengler:	Right.
Dr. Winters:	Good. You know, we're seeing this happening in fields outside of oncology, which is beautiful.
	So the soda and sugary drinks, get them out of them. Um, you can make your own Stevia flavored if you need to still—if you need that bubble or if you need that sweetness in life but I'm still encouraging people that if you're still craving sweets that much, that maybe you need to look for finding sweetness in your life in other places outside of your palette. So that's quite potent at that kinda gets people a little started as well.
	Um, getting rid of the not—what I tell people, get rid of the four legged super fund sites that are, um, walking through your—your pantry and your refrigerator and freezer." So that means your eggs, your dairy, your animal protein, your poultry, your, um, your fish, because if you've not got a quality—do you not know where those food items come

from, you are causing more harm than good. So that's one of the big misnomers of the ketogenic diet out there in the world is everyone's still thinking Adkins, which is very high protein ketogenic diet. Keto—keto for cancer is actually, like you said earlier, a low to moderate protein.

In fact, most people do better on a lower protein but to me, the quality is key. Because if you have an animal that has been grass-fed and then corn finished or corn fed and finished, their levels of insulin growth factor are going to be so much higher in that meat that you're going to eat that and therefore, stimulate your own growth factors. Not the mention the numerous chemicals we're throwing into them in antibiotics and herbicides and pesticides and the [unintelligible] that's now labeled a known carcinogen in their feed. You name it, that's going in there.

Processed foods. I mean, I think my story of how I got cancer is really, you know, multifactorial but I certainly was feeding the heck out of it with my boxes of Captain Crunch cereal, uh, my—my—my favorite breakfast was cinnamon toast on super crust white bread, you know, that I toasted and made my own white sugar cinnamon concoction. Probably wasn't even real cinnamon at that time [laughs]. You know, boxes and boxes of mac and cheese.

I mean, there was—basically, if it comes—if it comes from a factory, don't eat it. Okay [laughs]? That's sort of that place of getting people back to food as its original source. Did it come out of the sky, the—the ground, the tree. The, you know, the—the—the—the—the pasture. Where did it come from? Know and get it as close to that source as possible. And then, um, the non-organics [unintelligible]. We've really come a long way in understanding. We used to kind of poo poo that and say, "Oh, there's no difference between organic and non-organic." We said that because there just weren't the studies but the studies are coming now.

And we're actually shown a few in the last couple of years that shows the nutrient density is in fact higher in a organic pro—produce and that we definitely are getting a heck of a lot more than we bargained for chemical wise in our non-organic produce. And things like the environmental working group gives us an annual update every year of the clean 15—or excuse me, the clean—yeah, the clean 15 and the dirty—they used to call it the dirty dozen but now, it's the dirty 30. So, you know, it's like, oh, goody. We keep adding to this.

So that's the big one where to start from your fridge and freezer and the same goes for your pantry. You know? Flour products have really taken over and they're much wasted carbohydrates. I want people to get their carbs from their vegetables. You are gonna get plenty of your carbohydrates from your, um, starchy vegetables and even your non-starchy vegetables meet all of your carbohydrate needs and then some. And so we don't have to have a piece of bread or a big, huge baked potato or a bowl of pasta with every meal. That's not normal.

And so coming back to adding an extra dose or two of vegetables to your platter versus a—a processed flour based product is going to do your, um, mitochondrial metabolic function a world of good. And I think those were the big ones. Little bit on the oils. I think you—uh, the inflammation is always a key here and so we've gotten really, uh, away from quality fat since the 1970s. We've kind of, again, took another wrong turn in Albuquerque but, um, at this point, you really want to avoid canola mostly now because it's GMO. Um, you also wanna avoid, um, high heat to things like your olive oil. So you've got this beautiful oil but once you heat it too much, you've now kind of ruined its medicinal quality. So looking at the quality of fats, the form of fats, um, and then the other one I see still show up a lot in my colleagues' practices is a lot of people are still using flax oil and you really wanna get away from that. It goes so easily rancid and oxidizes so easily and you just add that to an already oxidized body and you just kind of—

It's like rusting the system exponentially. So those were kinda the big take homes, I think, of the pantry, fridge, and freezer overhaul.

Dr. Stengler: Oh, that's great. Great. A great review. You know, I tell my patients with cancer and other chronic diseases, you know, it can be stressful for people to make these dietary changes sometimes, But if you have something like cancer or some other serious disease, I mean, you've gotta focus on your diet. Um, it's just critical. You don't have time to be taking, you know, a year to adapt to a new diet. You've gotta be motivated. You gotta take the information like you provided and apply it because this is what's gonna keep you off experimental drugs, more surgeries, and these types of things.

Dr. Stengler: Excellent. Um, you're one of the experts on mistletoe extract. And, um, that's been around for a number of years. I'm gonna read some interesting information. I've written about this in the past and I've used it in my practice as well. It's a phenomenal botanical.

The mistletoe extract has become one of the most well studied compounds in complementary cancer therapy. It actually has more than 120 published studies. I always talk to doctors and, "Oh, these things you guys recommend don't have studies." Well, here's another example where that just isn't true. Uh, it's widely used in Europe. We know it's used a lot in Germany, Austria, Switzerland. And in fact, in Germany, a high percent of cancer—can we do that again? In fact, in Germany, a high percent of cancer patients are treated with mistletoe extract in some form.

And even according to the national cancer institute here in America, they set—they, uh, quote say, "n certain European countries, preparations made from European mistletoe are amongst the most prescribed drugs for patients with cancer. And so the point I wanna make is these are oncologists as well as holistic doctors in these countries recommending mistletoe for a variety of different types of cancer.

So tell us what you know about mistletoe and some of your experiences with it.

Dr. Winters: Perfect. So first of all, it is mistletoe therapy as an injectable in the adjuvant support for cancer patients has been used for 100 years as of this year.

If you look at it, it looks like a ball kind of growing up in the limb structure of trees. There's over 3,000 species but for the cancer purposes, the pine, the fur, and the apple are the most common that have the lectin content that have an anti-cancer property.

Dr. Stengler: Right. And we should—and I should point out just for our viewers, um, there are, of course, types of mistletoe, which are toxic.

Dr. Winters: Such a good point. Because that is, it's funny. Because I've even had folks say, "Well, I'll just go out and harvest it and make my own tincture." It doesn't work that way because even the way it's harvested, they take some of the leaves from the summer and the berries from the winter and they centrifuge them in a way with, like, a pulsing kind of comeopathic approach from the anthroposophical philosophy and it's done in a standardized, FDA like approved, you know, pharmaceutical, uh, manufacturing facility. It is incredibly rigorous in its testing and its, um, application.

As of February of 2017, there is a trial going on at John's Hopkins. I helped advise and still give some advance on—on their trial for solid tumors that have failed two lines of therapy. Um, there's still, uh, signing patients and they'll basically, um, right now, it's a safety study despite the fact that there are thousands actually of studies showing its safety worldwide but we've not really done the full studies in this country so it's a big step, I think, in our world.

When I think about this medicine, you know, a lot of people will come to you and think, "Oh, I'm just gonna take mistletoe and that'll do it. You know?" Please don't get, uh, seduced by the idea of one treatment. Just like ketogenic diet in and of itself, yes. Can it help—does it impact all of the terrain ten that I talk about in my book?

Absolutely. Does it have efficacy in—in directly impacting every one of the ten hallmarks of cancer? Absolutely. We've seen that in study after study but it is never really meant to be used as a standalone therapy. It's meant to make other therapies work better. Similar conversation with mistletoe, it's always been used as an adjuvant to other therapies. Um, and you noted so beautifully that about 85 percent of all cancer patients in Germany will use mistletoe at some point in their treatment, whether it's around their surgery, their chemotherapy, their radiation or the—or the follow up. Okay? So it really is and also doesn't impact the *[unintelligible]* pathway so there's no contraindications for its use with even pharmaceuticals or other natural therapeutics.

Because it's so lectin rich and those lectins are very vulnerable to, um, degradation, mixing it with other therapies and other chemo—you know, other bags and what not, nutritional IV bags, will degrade the anti-cancer lectins.

There's only one, um, uh, way to do that with some IV mistletoe or excuse me, with IV vitamin C but that's a whole nother training for people who already understand how to use this appropriate. Because even if you have some of the other minerals in with that IVC bag, you will destroy the ability for the mistletoe to do its job. So it has to bypass the digestion for it to have the efficacy to make the major changes that it does to immune regulation, anti-angio genesis, lowering inflammation, harmonizing. Again, the other therapies, similar to what we talked about in ketogenic, it will enhance the other therapies. It also is one of my most favorite ways to bolster the bone marrow.

Dr. Stengler: You know, as holistic doctors, we put a, uh, a very strong emphasis on the quality of life for patients with chronic diseases. You know, for all patients, uh, especially people with cancer. Sometimes, people are just look at length of life and all that but obviously, quality of life is—is critical. Now, in mistletoe, as you know, uh, they have studies proving what you just said. So for example, you did a study, a quality of life study of 270 breast cancer patients who'd underwent chemotherapy and it was a German study.

It was published. Physicians rated improvements and general well-being in 87 percent of patients. Mental health improved in 71 percent. Disease coping, 50 percent. Uh, the patients getting the mistletoe also reported improved appetite, sleep, less pain. Um, so that—you know, those are phenomenal results, which, you know, you and I see with patients using this phenomenal plant.

Um, so I also wanna mention, uh, you know, there's so many studies we could talk about. One study I found very, uh, impressive. Patients with cancer of the colon, rectum, stomach, breast or lung who took mistletoe extract, form known as iscador in addition to conventional therapy—so here, we got the integrative therapies again, um, so they reviewed, you know, the patients who participated in the study and those who got the mistletoe extract in addition to the conventional treatment, uh, lived 40 percent longer than those who just got, you know, the conventional therapy alone.

So that's, you know, that's powerful.

Dr. Winters: It is. It is. And, you know, we—we spend millions on dollars on therapies that can extend our life by, you know, a few weeks to a few months and yet, we have a therapy that's been around for 100 years that's relatively affordable, completely safe and effective to couple with all of our other therapies, conventional or otherwise, that has the potential to give you quality and quantity of life. It's just sad to me that it's not more widely available.

Dr. Stengler: And again, for our viewers, it's up on the screen but the medic—the *Metabolic Approach to Cancer* integrating deep nutrition, the ketogenic diet and—non-toxic bioindividualized therapies by Dr. Nasha Winters and her co-author, Jess Higgins Kelly. So excellent. Well, you have provided phenomenal information to our viewers. I mean, I'm not just saying that. It really is true. You're doing great work. You got a great book. I know your patients love you and so again, thank you for all your great information. And for the viewers out there, if you want to get more information on Dr. Winters, maybe you ought to consult with her. Um, go to her website, optimalterrainconsulting.com. We'll put it up on the screen and again, her book, *The Metabolic Approach to Cancer.* Just excellent. So again, Dr. Winters, thank you for all your time in this series and we greatly appreciate it.

Dr. Winters: Thank you so much. And—and be well.

Dr. Stengler: Thank you.

FOOD TO INCLUDE AND FOOD TO AVOID

— DR. FRED PESCATORE —

Dr. Stengler: Well, hi everyone. Today we have a great video for you. We're with Dr. Fred Pescatore. He's one of the most sought-out natural physicians in the country, and you've seen him probably in the media. He's been on several of the well-known cable TV shows. Um, he's also—a lot of people know him as an author of *The New York Times* best-selling book, *The Hamptons Diet*. As well, he had another best-selling book on children's health: *Feed Your Kids Well*. Very important as well. And he's written several other books. He's got a great newsletter.

He's got a private practice in New York. He also, in terms of what we're talking about today, wrote a book called *Cancer-Free for Life*. And so, Dr. Pescatore has got over 30 years of knowledge in this area. He's traveled around the world, many different countries, seeing how they do medicine using natural techniques. So, uh, Dr. Pescatore, thank you so much for being with us today.

Dr. Pescatore: Ah, thanks for having me. It's, it's gonna be great to be here and to be able to discuss things like this. It's gonna be fun.

Dr. Stengler: Absolutely. Well, maybe tell us a bit more about your background.

Dr. Pescatore: Well, it's sort of interesting. I mean, it—I stumbled onto this field, like I think most people do.

Dr. Stengler: Mm-hmm.

Dr. Pescatore: Uh, simply right out of, uh, right out of residency training, and I happened to get hired by Dr. Atkins. You know, Dr. Rob? You know, the famous doctor Atkins?

Dr. Stengler: Right.

Dr. Pescatore: And, uh, and then it changed my whole way of thinking about medicine, and so it made me like medicine again. It made me want to do medicine again, uh, because I was really on the verge of quitting—

Dr. Stengler: Hmm.

Dr. Pescatore: —and getting out of this field altogether. But, um, I'm glad he was there, and I'm glad I stumbled upon him. And how I got into integrative oncology was really when I was working with him.

Dr. Stengler: Oh okay.

Dr. Pescatore: And, uh, we used to do a lot of oncology. We had an entire floor. We had a six-story building in Manhattan, and we had one floor de-devoted strictly to oncology.

So, we used to do things like hypothermia and intravenous therapies, and, uh, all sorts of things from all over the world when you still could do those things pretty readily, and—

Dr. Stengler: Wow, I didn't know that. Of course, people always thought of him and, you know, you to some extent in terms of, you know, diet and weight and all that. But you guys have been doing this for a long time. You're way ahead of the curve there.

Dr. Pescatore: Oh, we've been doing it forever.

Dr. Stengler: Yeah.

Dr. Pescatore: But see, the bottom line is diet affects everything.

Dr. Stengler: Right.

Dr. Pescatore: Right? So—

Dr. Stengler:	Right.
Dr. Pescatore:	—if you can't get the diet right, not—no amount of supplements, no amount of intravenous therapies, no amount of anything really is gonna help your body to help heal itself if you don't have, if you don't have your diet in order. So, so, I don't mind being referred to as a diet doctor a little bit because diet really is the fundamental of health. I mean, if you don't have your diet right, it's all off.
Dr. Stengler:	Yeah.
Dr. Pescatore:	I mean, look, we know that, uh, we know that at least 11 to 13 cancers now are directly attributable to sugar. So, and I've been talking about the negative effects of sugar for 30 years now.
	So, you know, it's something as simple as that, which I think is the message that people don't get. Like, they know that tobacco causes cancer, and they know the sun can cause cancer. What they don't realize is that, you know, that candy bar you're eating every day is also causing cancer.
Dr. Stengler:	Right, good point. Well, maybe tell the viewers, I mean, people understand to some degree how diet can relate to cancer. Like you said, I don't think the general public, a lot of practicing physicians realize the critical importance of good diet in preventing and treating cancer. Maybe just talk a bit about, you know, what's going on with the immune system, you know, the cellular environment, uh, things like that when the nutrition is good versus, you know, not being good.
Dr. Pescatore:	Well, I mean, when you're eating something, you're creating an environment inside the body. And so, that environment will either be a healing environment, or it will be an illness env- uh, uh, enhancing environment. And so, that's why it's so important that we look at everything that we eat. So, for example, I talked about sugar.
	We know that sugar decreases, suppresses the immune system. Uh, it suppresses the ability of the white blood cells, which are the cells that go and, like, scavenge for any, uh, any intruders. Uh, so it damages them. One teaspoon damages

them by, like, 56 percent, and 2 teaspoons damages them by about 83 percent; and the average American consumes anywhere from 33 to 40 teaspoons of sugar every day. So, I think that's something really people should pay attention to.

I think when you're looking at are you having, are you having meat that's been, uh, you know, grass-finished, or are you having, you know, meat from—that's just regular old meat from the grocery store? And by meat, I mean chicken. I mean the whole gamut of protein.

Dr. Stengler: Right.

Dr. Pescatore: Uh, so, it's really important that you know whether there is antibiotics in your food, whether there's drug hormones in your food, all of which can lead to very detrimental effects in your health. And that's not to say that vegetables you don't have to worry about either because with the huge glyphosate issue in this country, which is a very dangerous chemical and very dangerous neurotoxin.

So, just to bring this home is that we produce cancer cells every single day. As we speak, we're producing cancer cells in our body, and a healthy, intact immune system—if we have a health, intact environment—goes around, gobbles them up, and gets rid of them. It's when we lose that ability because we have all of these toxins, whether it's from what we eat, what we drink, what we're taking, what we're not taking, what supplements we're not taking.

Just whatever it happens to be, stress, however, you deal and manage with that—all of that is creating a toxic environment in the body where these cancer cells can then take hold.

Dr. Stengler: Right. So, take us through. Say, a patient comes to your clinic, and you're talking to them. Obviously, you're gonna put a lot of emphasis on the things you just talked about, getting the diet on track, handling stress, detoxification. Tell us a bit more how you look into helping these people, um, to either prevent or, or battle cancer?

Dr. Pescatore: Well, really what we're doing to look at is, you know, patients will either come in with cancer—

Dr. Stengler:	Mm-hmm.
Dr. Pescatore:	And I either take a role that helps support them in whatever they're doing. Some patients will come in and say, "I will not do any chemotherapy, radiation, surgery. Just will not do any of that stuff." So, so I have multiple different roles to play here. So, yes, we start everybody on a good diet, but the other thing we do is, uh, look at all the inflammatory markers that might be going on. We look at the health of their immune system.
	The inflammatory markers are super critical because what you're eating actually affects whether there's more oxidative stress, less oxidative stress, all of those types of things, which can damage how your body is fighting the cancer. And then I put together an oral nutritional supplement program for everybody looking at, you know, going by what I've seen in the bloodwork.
Dr. Stengler:	Right, right.
Dr. Pescatore:	What are maybe some of your top supplement recommendations? I know everyone's different, but in terms of helping the immune system and so forth, are there some, like, key ones you see routinely used with your patients? I know you're very individualized, which is the best way.
	Are there some kind of ones you see commonly used with patients, just in a general sense?
Dr. Pescatore:	Sure, there are definitely, definitely the big ones, right? I mean, you have to get rid of inflammation. So, um, and help support the immune system. So, I think the best—one of the best ones to use would be—and it's one of my favorites, and it's called ME-3.
Dr. Stengler:	Hmm.
Dr. Pescatore:	Um, it goes under the brand name Reg'Activ, but, um, what ME-3 does, it's, it's actually a single source—it's a single, um, strain probiotic. And what it does is it actually enhances the body's ability to produce glutathione. So, they have isolated a bug in our body, a bacteria in our body that produces glutathione, and glutathione is one of

the most important antioxidants in the body.

It helps detoxify the liver, um, which is critical if you have cancer, but it's critical if you have anything, if you ever want to maintain your health. So, that's one of my favorite ones that everybody goes on. I also put somebody on—I also put people on something like AHCC, which is a mushroom extract. That's my favorite mushroom extract.

But there are many, many other mushroom extracts that, that help to regulate, uh, you know, that are biological response modulators and things like that. I also like putting people on anti-inflammatories like curcumin, turmeric, however you wanna—whatever you wanna call that spice. Um, it is a wonderful supplement for so many things and has so many different properties to it, including as an anti-cancer property as well as an anti-inflammatory property.

Um, then I also look at again, we look at people individually. So, are they experiencing things like chemo brain? A lot of people get chemo brain.

Dr. Stengler: Right.

Dr. Pescatore: So, so, a lot of times people will come to me to, to clean up after what conventional medicine has done to them. So, I like to use—you know, for chemo brain, I like to use things like alpha-GPC and this, this supplement called bluenesse, which is a lemon balm extract, acetylcholine, all of these great things that help sort of clean up the brain.

Dr. Stengler: Right.

Dr. Pescatore: Because chemotherapy—I can't tell you how many patients I have come in that just can't think after having chemotherapy, and it doesn't last for a week. It lasts for months and months and months, and that's why I tend to focus on sort of, uh, definitely focus on chemo brain. Definitely focus on the anti-inflammatories, and definitely focus on the immune-enhancing supplementation.

Dr. Stengler: Yeah, good.

Dr. Pescatore: So, that's where the ME-3 comes in. That's where the anti-inflammatories like curcumin comes in, and then all of the brain stuff like bluenesse and, uh, alpha-GPC and, and that sort of thing. So, there are many, many, many ways of, of, of exploring this, uh, alt-, uh, a different approach to integrated oncology that oncologists just don't look at, and it's a shame really.

Dr. Stengler: Yeah, that's great. You know, one of the things in this series that we haven't really addressed and maybe you talk about it a bit, of course, patients undergoing chemotherapy, radiation—maybe they've had surgery or just the stress of it all—fatigue, you know, is very, very common. What are some of the things you like to do to rejuvenate their, you know, energy levels, um, with, uh, nutritional natural medicine?

Dr. Pescatore: Well, I think a great way of, of, uh, dealing with, uh, energy levels is really getting to the bottom of it, which is really mitochondrial support.

Dr. Stengler: Mm-hmm.

Dr. Pescatore: So, you need mitochondrial support, and you need adrenal support. So, for mitochondrial support, I like robobeet, which is, uh, sort of a newer, it's a nutritional supplement that actually works well as sort of an oak tree extract. And then there's also something that I like, um, called ribose, which people talk about. These specifically work on the mitochondria. You can use medium-change triglycerides oils to work on the mitochondria as well to just give them—because the mitochondria are the actual fuel cells in your cells.

So, if they're—if they don't have any substance to work on, then they are not gonna be able to do their job, which is to provide, to provide energy for you. So, that's why it's so important that you provide energy to the mitochondria. Glutamine is an excellent product. It's an amino acid. Glutamine has been shown many, many times to just help the healing process. It helps the gut to heal, and you've gotta keep a healthy gut along with all of this.

And we could spend an entire hours and hours and an entire summit talking about gut health, but, um, you really have to keep your gut healthy. You really want to keep your mitochondria healthy. So, that's why things like robobeet and, um, ribose, uh are—and, and glutamine are my three, uh, specific ones that I use for energy levels for that.

Dr. Stengler: Well, that's great, and probably like me, you find for people who really need a for a period of time to bring 'em up really quickly, like you talked about before, the IV ozone, the IV B vitamins—

Dr. Pescatore: Yeah.

Dr. Stengler: —and all of that. Those are just kind of a given, right?

Dr. Pescatore: Absolutely. I mean, IVs are something that I think are so critical for anyone who has cancer, and you can get—you can really restore people very quickly. And you could really help them diminish the side effects of the chemotherapy, radiation therapy, and that sort of thing that they're getting, um, without causing any harm. And, of course, your conventional oncologist and your conventional radiation oncologist is gonna say, "Don't do any of that." But you know what? It's your body.

So, you have the right to do whatever you want and what's gonna make you feel better, and I know those things will make you feel better.

Dr. Stengler: You know, and things that have—as you've witnessed over the past 30 years, I mean, the scientific validation of the things we're talking about, I mean, it's beyond the point where there should even be debate about it. But, like you said, we still, you know, have these issues with the oncologists who aren't familiar with the science on the nutrition and the supplements and the IVs and all of that.

So, you've seen this change. Are you finding a gradual change in the oncologists' approach or acceptance of this, or do you find it still pretty slow-going overall?

Dr. Pescatore: I think it's extraordinarily slow-going with the oncologists, um, because, you know, you have to realize oncology is mostly cookbook medicine, right? So, "If you have X, we're gonna give you Y. We're not gonna deviate from Y because we don't know what the deviation means." And most of these places really only care about their statistics. They don't really care about you.

So, the, the one question you have to ask if you're, uh, if you're someone with, with cancer, is you have to ask, "Will this increase my survival time?"

Dr. Stengler: Right.

Dr. Pescatore: Not, "Will it decrease my cancer? Will it de- increase my survival time?" And you'll see funny expressions on the oncologist's face because they can't answer that because they really don't have good survival time studies, which is unfortunate. Because that's really—if you're gonna get any disease, you wanna know if you're gonna live longer, and that's really—you don't do anything unless you're gonna live longer. And, um, I guess I kind of lost the point of the question there, but, uh—

Dr. Stengler: Oh yeah, just how the oncologists, they're still slow to—

Dr. Pescatore: Oh -

Dr. Stengler: —getting on board here.

Dr. Pescatore: Uh, uh, you know, they're, uh, they've gotten around to giving people vitamin D.

Dr. Stengler: Right.

Dr. Pescatore: You know? So, so, slowly but surely. I mean, they're even recognizing that some people do have gluten issues even though they don't have celiac disease.

Dr. Stengler: Right.

Dr. Pescatore: So, we're getting there, and, and my goodness in this, these 30 years to—when I started putting people on gluten-free diets and yeast-free diets 30 years ago, it was unimaginable what they had to go through.

And now, at least we're getting some support, and the support always comes from the grass roots. That's why I like doing things to, direct-to-consumer because if it wasn't for the consumers, we'd still be in uber dark ages. We're in the dark ages as it is, but we would like not even see any light.

But it's, it's a really good thing we have avid consumers and avid—and people who are out there who want this information.

Dr. Stengler: Well, that's a good point; the grass roots. You know, we've got some studies now showing about 75 percent—it ranges from 50 to 75 percent—of people with cancer are using some kind of integrative therapy: nutrition, supplements, acupuncture, whatever. So, the majority of the population wants this.

Dr. Pescatore: Well, they also include prayer in that.

Dr. Stengler: Oh, good point, good point.

Dr. Pescatore: That's a topic for another day as well.

Dr. Stengler: Yeah, good point. Maybe lastly, I'm always kind of amazed—you'll see new cancer drugs being promoted as breakthroughs, and then you look at the literature, and they extend, you know, a lifespan by two or three months with all of the, the quality of life problems you get with them. I mean, it's, it's quite a marketing machine going on there.

Dr. Pescatore: And the cost.

Dr. Stengler: Hmm.

Dr. Pescatore: I mean, let's not forget about the cost of these things. I mean, the cost of these drugs. I just wrote a newsletter about how the cost completely defy any market means whatsoever. I mean, the costs are just—it's really crazy, and I really hope people would sign up for the newsletter just to get that one bit of information because it's ridiculous. I mean, you would think that the, the cost of these things would be coming down. Um, and, and you're right, and how they get that little bit of, of extra life span is powering the study larger, which means they basically include more people.

So, if you include more people, you're gonna get the outliers that do really, really well. Um, so, if you power a study high enough, you can get it to say whatever you want, and even that, that then makes the difference statistically significant so then they can go and, like, shout or spread that out on television and tell you that you should be on this drug, not that drug, and all of this other stuff. They have their, their evil ways, those—

Dr. Stengler: *[Laughs]*

Dr. Pescatore: —big pharmaceutical companies.

Dr. Stengler: Well, well said. Well, Dr. Pescatore, excellent information. What's the best website for people to, you know, get your newsletter, more information on your practice and products? What would you recommend?

Dr. Pescatore: If they go just to DrPescatore, P-E-S-C-A-T-O-R-E dot com, you can check out my practice. You can sign up for my free newsletters. You can do anything you want from, from there, that one, uh, landing page will take you wherever you wanna go.

Dr. Stengler: Perfect. Well, thank you again for your time today.

Dr. Pescatore: My pleasure. Thank you for having me.

Dr. Stengler: Thank you.

FIGHTING INFLAMMATION

— DR. ISAAC ELIAZ —

Dr. Stengler: Well, welcome everyone. We have a great video today with Dr. Isaac Eliaz, and he's an integrative medical doctor. He's also a researcher, a product formulator, and he lectures around the world on natural ways to help with detoxification, to help prevent and fight cancer. So, very highly-educated, and he's been a pioneer in holistic medicine since the early 1980s. He's published numerous peer-reviewed research papers on several different aspects related to integrative health.

But today, a lot of our focus will be on his expertise in the, in the area of inflammation in cancer and a very interesting treatment using modified citrus pectin. And he's done the research on this product, which a lot of us integrative doctors use in our practices. So, um, it's great to have you with us, Isaac. How are you doin'?

Dr. Eliaz: Thank you. I've been good. It's great to connect again and be on this program. I am really hap- happy for the opportunity.

Dr. Stengler: Excellent. Well, you know, in this video series, um, "Outside the Box Cancer Therapies" we're talking about many different aspects, you know, of cancer and what's going on. You know, from environmental toxins to nutrition to stress to hormone imbalances to immune problems. Um, there's always an underlying factor with cancer and other chronic diseases, and that's inflammation. Can you talk to the viewers a bit about inflammation? And then we could get into some of the ways we objectively can measure that with inflammatory markers.

Dr. Eliaz: Yeah, of course.

Inflammation is a normal, uh, reaction of the body to addressing multiple issues from infections to injury to abnormal processes. And, uh, so inflammation is necessary on a very short-term basis. The problem is how, is how long the inflammatory process continues, how significant it is, and which direction it is going. So, one of the issue that as inflammation keeps on going, it creates damage to the tissues.

Dr. Stengler: Mm-hmm.

Dr. Eliaz: And creates fibrosis and create degenerative effect. So, if we look at inflammation, it is the hallmark of every chronic disease, and it specifically will drive cancer to metastasize, to grow faster, to mutate, and to change the metabolic environment of the cell. So, if you want to live a longer life, if you want to live a healthier life—you have to be aware of the issue of chronic inflammation, and you have to address it really on a daily basis.

Dr. Stengler: So, it's like one of those things in life where a little bit is good; too much is bad. And it's like you—

Dr. Eliaz: Right.

Dr. Stengler: —said, the good thing is we have a lot of control, uh, in our choices and how we can help to modify and control inflammation.

Dr. Eliaz: Absolutely, absolutely, and part of it is that we live in an inflammatory lifestyle, you know, in—from the point of view that if we look at inflammation, inflammation is heat; and heat, in simple physics, relates to thermal energy, relates to space, to kinetic energy. We are moving very fast, right? Our, our time span and attention span, if it was hours or days 200 years ago, it's measured in seconds now, right? If you don't get—

Dr. Stengler: Oh, yeah.

Dr. Eliaz:	—a text back in three seconds, what happens? Somebody's not listening to me. So, our attention span, as our time contracts, the same activity is done under greater pressure.
	And this causes inflammation. So, we live in an inflammatory environment, which means, Mark, we have to be much more careful about protecting ourselves because in this baseline, then EMF and radiation and stress and toxins and pollution and the intention—they all accumulate together, and then the heavy metals come in.
	And that's why, for example, if we look at cancer, we talk about, a lot about genetics. While epigenetic is probably much—it's much more important, but really, cancer is a lifestyle disease.
Dr. Stengler:	Mm-hmm.
Dr. Eliaz:	It's the American Cancer Society—who would believe—you know, we have been in this a long time. Who would believe that the American Cancer Society will come with a statement that 90 percent of cancers are caused by lifestyle?
Dr. Stengler:	Right.
Dr. Eliaz:	If we said it in public 20 years ago, we would be executed, you know?
Dr. Stengler:	*[Laughs]*
Dr. Eliaz:	And now you've got the American Cancer Society realizing, "Wow, it's a lifestyle issue." So why? Because it's driven by inflammation.
	So, if we look at this pathway, we are—we want to—I—we want to ask ourself, "What starts it? What puts our body into an inflammatory kind of emergency state?" Well, there is a medical term for this, and it's called an "alarmin." A-L-A-R-M-I-N. There is certain compound that are alarmin.
	They put the body into this straight emergency mode. That's what also happen in sepsis. And then from there on, it's downhill. So, the, the conductors of the orske- orchestra, the alarmin, is called galectin-3.
Dr. Stengler:	Yes.

Dr. Eliaz:	And this is where my lit- my research has been for 22 years that we started with cancer, but nobody imagined that galectin-3 is such a central molecule when we started our journey. No, even now, very few people know about it, but to give a sense, there are about 5,000 published papers, scientific papers on galectin-3, more than 1 paper a day. And on our *[unintelligible]* there are more than 40 published case- uh, papers. You know, there is a paper coming in every week or two. Uh, so it's finally coming to the attention, and if we know what is the master compound that starts the process, if we can regulate it, you can imagine the health benefits from a therapeutic point of view and from a preventative point of view.
Dr. Stengler:	Uh, tell the viewers, you now, where galectin—where it's manu- what it is exactly, where it's produced in the body, how blood work can be done to measure to it, and then how it helps to assess a person's risk.
Dr. Eliaz:	So, galectin-3 is a protein. It's a, it's a, it's a carbohydrate-binding protein, which means it's a protein. So, it has an arm, and it has this kind of thing at the end, and here it binds to carbohydrates.
	But these carbohydrates, because of the structure of the galectin-3, are usually tied to protein, glycoprotein or oxidized glycolipids. So the, the, the ligen that it binds to are, are the molecule that can help in the repair process. So, galectin-3 inside the cell is important. It helps embryogenesis, development of cell. The problem is on the—the problem is on the cell surface and the circulation because what happens, once galectin-3 binds to one of these ligens, which is part of the process of inflammatory ligen, sticky molecule ligen that create metastases, uh, growth factors like VGF.
Dr. Stengler:	Yeah, yeah.
	There is a, is a significant study when they look at centenarians, people whose average age was 104, and they compared them to health control between 70 and 80 years old. So, out of the 70, 80, a few of them are gonna make it to 104, right?

Dr. Stengler:	Mm-hmm.
Dr. Eliaz:	The levels of the galectin-3 in the people who make it to 104—and galectin-3 goes up as we age, very significantly. The centenarians had, uh, much lower levels of galectin-3 than the average population at 70 to 80, dramatically lower. So, we know high galectin-3 means trouble.
Dr. Stengler:	Mm-hmm.
Dr. Eliaz:	And so, when we measure it in the blood, we don't measure it to decide if we need to address it. Everybody needs to address galectin-3. The only reason to measure it in the blood is if it's very high, you will need more modified citrus pectin because there are more galectin-3s that you need to blow.
Dr. Stengler:	Right. So, it's really a marker hopefully more doctors will start using to assess people preventatively or if you've got active disease to see if they need to be more aggressive with their therapies, and, and seeing if they're responding. Would you agree with that?
Dr. Eliaz:	Absolutely. So, I think if we look at, eh, if we look at the importance—so, this—so we talked about this, this, this protein, eh, eh, galectin-3—and how it's involved in literally every inflammatory process, every coronary—including infection, including sepsis, including autoimmune disease, including *[unintelligible]* rejection of transplants. It's what drives it. Well, all of us, our body as it ages, gets more inflamed, and that's why—when we really need to address it. So, if we live a healthier lifestyle and we lower inflammation, naturally, our galactin-3 will come down.
Dr. Stengler:	Mm-hmm.
Dr. Eliaz:	But as we age, as we're exposed to heavy metals, as we're exposed to stress, all of us are, it's an issue. But so really, if you asked me, "What is the most important supplement for somebody to take?"
Dr. Stengler:	Yes.
Dr. Eliaz:	If you look at my charts in my patients, six, seven, eight, years ago, ten years ago, I recommended modified citrus pectin, and it wasn't the first one I recommended. There

	were other things.
Dr. Stengler:	Mm-hmm.
Dr. Eliaz:	And maybe when we talk about modified citrus pectin, before I continue, let me say what is modified citrus pectin.
Dr. Stengler:	Yes, please.
Dr. Eliaz:	Makes sense. So, pectin is a long chain of carbohydrates of galec- of galacturonic acid, of sugars. It's a very high molecular weight, and it is sterified. It's not free. And it cannot get absorbed, and it has some benefit in the gut. It's a fiber. It can absorb some cholesterol, et cetera.
Dr. Stengler:	Like apple skins, for example would have pectin?
Dr. Eliaz:	Yeah. That's why ne, one apple a day keeps the doctor away.
Dr. Stengler:	Mm-hmm.
Dr. Eliaz:	But the effect is in the gut. When you break into a low molecular weight in a specific structure, it gets absorbed into the bloodstream, and there it, it has benefit. So, the person who discovered lectin, this idea of modified citrus pectin and started the discovery of lectin in the '80s, Dr. Avraham Raz, who is also Israeli—we are collaborating now on research.
Dr. Stengler:	Oh okay.
Dr. Eliaz:	And, uh, I developed the first available modified citrus pectin, and I made some of the key discoveries.

So, modified citrus pectin is effective for—I did a lot of research in cancer, of course, but I also discovered that it's effective for immunity, dramatic, more than pretty much anything, including medicinal mushrooms. It's a very good chelator of heavy metals, but most important, is the galectin-3 blocker. It blocks and stops excessive inflammation and fibrosis. We know that pectin is full of these, and I developed a specific modified citrus pectin called PectaSol-C. It's important to emphasize the name because of the concept of *[unintelligible]* science. As it has become popular, every pectin is modified when it's extracted from the peel of the citrus fruit or other fruits.

So, anybody can put something in a jar and call it modified citrus pectin, and when it comes to the health benefits, really, people need to stick with, uh, what was researched for over 20 years, which is really the PectaSol-C.

Dr. Stengler: Mm-hmm.

Dr. Eliaz: So, if we look at the modified citrus pectin and its, and, and, and its benefits, we can—I—we now have multiple studies from *in vitro* to *in vivo* to human clinical trials, showing very significant benefits for modified citrus pectin. For example, the study in, in ASCO, in, uh, in, uh, in, in February of, uh, just I presented in, in, in February of 2018 is in biochemical relapse of prostate cancer.

So, this is the third study that we have done, and it confirms the results of the first two studies. It was done in Israel by Dr. Daniel Katzman, who is a renowned neurological oncologist, and the patients were from multiple centers. This, this, this internal report is on 35 patients. Now, already there has been 50 patients, uh, close to 50 patients are enrolled.

And what we found was, was these people with biochemical relapse, the modified citrus pectin stopped or slowed down the progression in 80 percent of the patient, 80 percent. Sixty-two percent of the, of all the group, it completely either stopped it or got it better over 6 months period. Why is this amazing? Because it's not hormonal therapy. It's not something that changes every *[unintelligible]* and then the cancer will grow, uh, faster later. Every day that you slow the process with modified citrus pectin, you are prolonging somebody's life.

Now, the galectin-3 mechanism is not exclusive for prostate cancer. It's present pretty much on every cancer. It's just that with the PSA and biochemical relapse, when you remove the prostate before, either with radiation or with surgery, it's easy to follow up. So, what's so fascinating, if you look at the results *in vitro*, or you look *in vivo* in animal, or you look in humans, the best results are in humans which is—we know it's very unusual, right?

We have studies about procurement, and it looks great in animals, but, you know, maybe here and there it helps somebody. Why? Because of the multiple mechanisms.

Dr. Stengler: Right.

Dr. Eliaz: For example, in the immune system, if you make—if you take T cells, and you present them in an environment with galectin-3, they stop excreting cytokines completely. The immune system is shut down. You introduce a galectin-3 blocker into the environment, and they start excreting again. So, the cancer cell is using galectin-3 to evade the immune system and shut down the immune system.

So, you can imagine not only oncology, there is a new wave in immunotherapy and, uh, and checkpoint inhibitors and, and tumor-infiltrating lymphocytes. The reasons that we are not getting the results we wanted, one of the key reasons, is excessive inflammation and evasion of the immune system.

Galectin-3 is sitting at the helmet of the process. We know it anecdotally from patients who have dramatic responses, and by chance were trialed to take my modified citrus pectin. And now, were already starting a clinical trial with these fancy drugs. So, it's, it's very, it's very exciting.

Dr. Stengler: Mm-hmm.

Dr. Eliaz: It, it, and also the idea that it's such a natural—you can't get much more natural than extracting something straight from the peel of the citrus fruit, and then it is all this very unusual science.

Dr. Stengler: So, that's excellent. Now, I wrote an article on the, um, the PectaSol in the past, and this is how I had a summary of its effects or benefits, and tell me if I'm missing anything. "Prevents tumors from metastasizing, again, blocks galectin-3's ability to stimulate the formation of blood vessels and new tu-tumors, which we call anti-angiogenesis. Induces cancer cell death or apoptosis by interfering with important signaling pathways related to cancer proliferation and survival.

"It aids chemotherapy, helps cancer, um, well, it helps healthy cells survive chemotherapy treatment. Improves immune cell activity." And as you said also, it helps remove toxic metals from the body, which of course, can be carcinogenic or cancerous.

Dr. Eliaz: It's actually a very good summary, and since you wrote, you know, we know more about how it does, it—but it's pretty much—it's pretty much the idea. And that's why when you take modified citrus pectin, it's, it's an adjuvant for so many therapies.

So, when we look at its benefit, and we found something that is—effect the conductor of the orchestra, you can see why it's really, like, one of the first, if the first, supplement everyone needs to take. Because there is something that really affects the aging process and prevents that chronic inflammatory damage—which is a driving force of why we have a shorter life and we are sick. There is a way to really address it and then—and because it's an adjuvant, patients often feel better when they take it. When you, when you look at Lyme patients, you know, and, and patients with infections, uh patients with chronic inflammation, you actually—patient tell you, "I feel better," which, you know, Mark, initially, we didn't expect it.

Dr. Stengler: Hmm.

Dr. Eliaz: It was really cancer-targeted, and uh, they discovered the inflama- anti-inflammatory, anti-fibrotic effect. And I did the discovery because we were getting feedback from people who said, "You know, my memory is getting better." Well, there is ten times more galectin-3 in the Alzheimer plaque than in the normal tissue.

Dr. Stengler: Mm-hmm.

Dr. Eliaz: They say, "My joints are getting better." Well, it really affects joint damage in, in rheumatoid arthritis and in osteoarthritis, and we just, as we are—I am being interviewed, we just finished the—enrollment for a double blind clinical trial of our modified citrus pectin in osteoarthritis with Harvard.

Dr. Stengler: Hmm.

Dr. Eliaz: I mean, *[unintelligible]* a major multi-center trial. This is really—it's not only the power of the substance, but it's also what's needed for holistic methods to be accepted.

Dr. Stengler:	Mm-hmm.

Dr. Eliaz: You know, we have—we are doing our work. We also—we are really doing our work from the point of view of research, and we also showed now—we developed an antibody that is, that has a marker.

And we showed that our modified citrus pectin gets absorbed into the bloodstream through the *[unintelligible]*, which was never proven clearly before. So, a lot of progress in this field, a lot of progress.

Dr. Stengler: Well, I used the product with my patients. Um, what are your dosage recommendations? People with cancer, you recommend 5 grams 3 times a day, maybe 5 grams for healthy people wanting to use it preventively? What, what do you typically recommend?

Dr. Eliaz: You are right on the spot.

Dr. Stengler: Okay.

Dr. Eliaz: So, for cancer patients, it's 15 grams a day, either 5 grams 3 times a day, or you can go with either 7.5 twice a day.

Dr. Stengler: Okay.

Dr. Eliaz: Because we know now that the half-life is, is longer than we thought. It's 11, 12 hours. So, it stays a long time with a great benefit. So, if you take it regularly or even twice a day, you get a steady state of, of MCP in the blood. And for people who are really healthy, 5 grams a day. People with inflammatory issue, probably 5 grams twice a day.

Dr. Stengler: Okay, and of course, people can use it in powder or capsule form.

Dr. Eliaz: Right.

Dr. Stengler: I know side effects are not very common. Anything people should be aware of? Um...

Dr. Eliaz: If they take it close to food, maybe 15 minutes before, an hour after. The only, the only thing that people sometime experience, which his transient—it goes away—is sometimes because it's buffered with potassium and sodium,

	people can get a little bit of loose stool and some bloating, but once they get used to it, it goes away. So, it's, it's kind of a side effect-free—it's, it's really GRAS, generally regarded as safe.
Dr. Stengler:	Right.
Dr. Eliaz:	The food, you know, it's a smart, it's a smart food.
Dr. Stengler:	Yeah.
Dr. Eliaz:	It's really—I see it as a gift from nature, and it's kind of an unusual story. I was, I was 12 years old in Israel and, uh, I took a walk to our neighbors, Dr. Ruth and Leo Cohen, which were Ph.D.s in organic chemistries and pioneers in the citrus industry.
	Israel was very famous in the citrus industry in the 20th Century. Now it's famous for other things, and there are no more—very few orchards now. And out of the blue, Ruth turns to me and says, tells me, "Isaac, one day they will find a cure for cancer from the pit of the citrus fruit." Twenty-four years later, when the first study by Azraham Raz came out, I called her from San Francisco. I told her, "Ruth, you wouldn't expect at 12 years old, this 12-years-old kid remembered what you told him. I need your help."
	And she put me together with a key scientist for manufacturing of sophisticated pectins, and from then on, wow, it has really become a journey beyond, uh, what I ever expected. It's much bigger than me. It's multiple centers and NIH-sponsored. I have just been part of the movement, you know, in the beginning.
Dr. Stengler:	Yeah.
Dr. Eliaz:	And the guy who kind of discovers new, new uses and clinically. I'm definitely the most experienced clinically in using modified citrus pectin.
	And I really came to appreciate it as a gift we got from nature, you know? It's really a gift from nature.
Dr. Stengler:	Yeah, I mean, it's, it's amazing the things that our Creator has, you know, put into nature through his design and has

healing benefits in the body. Um, how about all the people out there, the viewers watching who are undergoing chemotherapy and radiation? Um, I use modified citrus pectin, sometimes known as MCP or the PectaSol, as you said. Um, no problems using it during chemotherapy and radiation.

Dr. Eliaz: Modified citrus pectin has shown to be synergistic with multiple kind of chemotherapy. Modified citrus pectin was shown to enhance radiation therapy. When we actually took prostate cancer cell, and we literally radiated them, and we added MCP, our MCP, it killed them at a lower level of radiation or killed more of them.

And radiation produces chronic inflammation and fibrosis.

Dr. Stengler: Right.

Dr. Eliaz: And modified citrus pectin will prevent it. So, it's not about can you use it? It's—you have to use it. And we know—and now, you know, we, we are now starting multiple new clinical trials on different synergistic effects of different protocols in different cancers, and this is all based on all these multiple studies that we are doing.

Dr. Stengler: Mm-hmm. Well, great. Well, you know, thank you for all the years you've done this research. Uh, people don't realize how difficult it is both in time, energy, expense to conduct this type of research. It's not simple. You don't have the backing of big drug companies and all that. So, you've really taken us to a high level, made it very credible, and of course, most importantly, you're gonna help people, uh—

Dr. Eliaz: Right.

Dr. Stengler: —you know, prevent and treat, you know, these serious chronic inflammatory diseases. So, thank you for that.

Dr. Eliaz: Oh, thank, thank you for being aware of it. You know, they say, "First they ridicule you; then they fight you; and then they say it's self-evident."

Dr. Stengler: *[Laughs]*

Dr. Eliaz: Now, now we are in the self-evident phase where, you know, multiple centers are publishing and just using my material.

Dr. Stengler:	Mm-hmm.
Dr. Eliaz:	And NIH is interested and NCI is interested, but it—I liked to call it, it's a 22-year, it's a 23-years overnight success, you know? *[Laughs]*
Dr. Stengler:	*[Laughs]* Well, again, thank you, and thank you for taking this time to share this information with our viewers.
Dr. Eliaz:	Great, thank you, Mark. Thank you.

THE TOP FOODS TO GIVE YOUR BODY ITS BEST DEFENSE

— DR. PAUL ANDERSON —

Dr. Stengler: Hi, everyone. Dr. Mark Stengler here with my colleague, Dr. Paul Anderson. Dr. Anderson, good to see you again.

Dr. Anderson: Good to see you.

Dr. Stengler: And Dr. Anderson and I co-wrote a book called, *Outside the Box Cancer Therapies,* and today, we're gonna get into some very useful information on common cancers and integrative cancer approaches. And so, people are always asking us, friends, colleagues, family members, of course, and especially patients, what are the typical things we recommend to our patients who have cancer? What do we generally recommend for diet, what do we recommend for supplements?

Now, Dr. Anderson, in our book, of course, different cancers do require different strategies, but we have found there are some commonalities quite often with the different cancers, especially the most common ones. So, what I'd like to do in this segment, let's go over some of the common dietary approaches we take, and some of the more well-studied supplements that we commonly use.

Dr. Anderson: Right.

Dr. Stengler: So, let's start with diet. Um—

A lot of information on diet. In our book, we talk about

studies done on huge populations around the world. There are some commonalities, but as I said, there are some differences, too, depending on the type of cancer. But in general, tell the viewers a bit about, um, some of the commonalities with the dietary approaches we take.

Dr. Anderson: Yes, I think that, um, as, as the book elaborates a lot on, and we've spoken a bit about earlier, whatever dietary change works out being the best in a person with cancer winds up being one of the most fundamental and most crucial things that they can do, um, and in a sense, a lot of the supplements and a lot of the nutritional additives, and all these other things, um, can't outrun a, a bad diet.

So, if, if you don't start with the diet, it-it's not that you can't do something. It's just you're not gonna get very far—

Because if you think about it, you know, we're not only taking a lot of our nutrition in that way, as we've spoken about. We also are potentially either stimulating or maybe inhibiting tumor cells, based on what we eat. Um, and the other thing is, is that the digestive system, eh, is a huge part of our immune system.

So, if it's being assaulted by foods that we shouldn't be eating or maybe foods that are full of toxins and chemicals, uh, or just foods that are very out of balance nutritionally, the—none of that's helping us. So, I think that, you know, one of the things you'll see in, and of course in the chapter where we go into, uh, many, many different types of cancers, you'll see many commonalities.

To go more towards a metabolic approach, where you're really restricting glucose sources and sugar sources, and uh, producing ketones, or, or or that end of the spectrum, or whether you're going for, um, you know, you're doing, uh, maybe a secondary prevention with a whole food approach, or, or whatever you're doing, one of the things, I think, that becomes important, and people get a little confused about is there are certain groups of vegetables that are very well known for having, uh, not only a lot of nutrients, but a lot of anti-cancer effect.

So, the, uh, cruciferous type of vegetables, for example.

And because we do so much work with people who are trying to restrict the amount of, say, sugars that they take in, they'll be concerned that, well, any vegetable I eat might be bad for me, right? You know, ketone vegetables have a lot of carbohydrate in them and all that.

And thankfully, now, it's become such a, a wide, uh, a widely known type of therapy, there's a lot more information you can get online. Um, we counsel them to look at the confirmation and the groupings of vegetables, and what you'll find is a lot of the ones that we recommend in the book have a lot of fiber, which is a carbohydrate, but it's not, it's not a fueling carbohydrate.

So, what they're going for is they're getting all of the chemical benefits of the polyphenols and the flavonoids, and all of the nutrients that are in the cruciferous and then some of the other vegetables we talk about. They're also getting a lot of fiber, which is good for digestive health, and they really don't wind up with a lot of sugar for, you know, fueling, uh, the cancer, che—mechanisms, etcetera, so—

Dr. Stengler: Right.

Dr. Anderson: Um, the other thing is, uh, cleanliness of the food, and, and that's not just washing it, but, you know, we talk in the, in the book a lot about, you know, clean protein sources, or clean fat. The last thing that you wanna do under any circumstances, but especially if you have cancer is to go out and get, you know, let, let's say you're gonna use meat, uh, for some protein, or you're gonna get a fat that you're gonna use, uh, within your diet.

You don't want it to have a bunch, you know, of pesticides in it, or other chemicals, because, you know, why bring more damage in with the food that you're trying to bring in? And it's the same with the vegetables. You wanna get them organic and as clean as possible, too.

Dr. Stengler: Right. And have you had a general recommendation for your patients in terms of purified water intake? Just in a general sense?

Dr. Anderson: Yes. We, we try and recommend, and, and somewhat, it depends on what they have available, as far as the ability to get water purifiers, etcetera, but—

We recommend that, uh, any drinking and cooking water that they do, uh, is, is not just filtered like a lot of home systems have, uh, what would be, say, salt filters, or something, you know, for big stuff. Uh, there are filters that can actually remove many or most of the toxic, heavy metals, and a number of other things.

Um, so, we do try to have people be very careful about not just what comes in on the food, but what comes in on the water and the other liquids.

Um, because if you think about it, you know, we're consuming not just, you know, what we might drink, say, from water, or whatever we're mixing the water in, but we're often using the water for cooking or for washing, etcetera, so, again no point putting toxins back in.

Dr. Stengler: Absolutely. And then we have the whole big category of supplements, and we've got a whole chapter on that in the book. Um, some of the more well-researched ones, certainly, are the medicinal mushrooms, as we call them. Why don't you tell the viewers about certain ones, like coriolus versicolor, also known as turkey's tail, or say, mitaki.

Um, well researched, actually considered to be cancer drugs, parts of Asia. Over here, it can be used as dietary supplements, but well, let's start with the, uh, coriolus versicolor, also known commonly as turkey's tail.

Dr. Anderson: Yep, yeah, and, and that's because it actually looks sort of like a turkey's tail when you see it out in the woods. Um, yes—

Coriolus versicolor, uh, is, um, or turkey tail, is a really interesting mushroom, and there, it's really—I think it's one of those things where it's gotten a lot of research here in the West, where, whereas, it's gotten research for a long time in Asia.

Dr. Stengler: Yeah.

Dr. Anderson: So, what has come from that is in the, in the treatment phase, where the person is battling with an active cancer, we often will use a single supplement that would be, say, a coriolus turkey tail supplement, and in the book, we give doses, etcetera. Because we at least have more data that shows, okay, this, this one has—packs a punch in this area of the immune system.

When we get to, say, prevention, etcetera, sometimes what we'll do is use more of a mixed mushroom—

Dr. Stengler: Right.

Dr. Anderson: Because, you know, just like plants, uh, in the rest of the plant kingdom, the different mushrooms—

Might do different immunologic things, and so, sometimes, when you have a big problem like a-aggressive cancer, you do a lot of one, and then you might move to more than one in the, you know, in a more balanced mix later. Um, such as, uh, the—like mitaki and the shitakis, and it's as many, many other medicinal mushrooms that are available to be used.

But you'll find, uh, in the book we recommend turkey tail on many of the cancers—

Dr. Stengler: Right.

Dr. Anderson: Because it's just so well referenced that it's, it's good to start with the ones that have the best data.

Dr. Stengler: Um, the nice thing you get about turkey's tail and mitaki, we do have human studies where patients have used—

These while undergoing conventional treatments, like chemotherapy, radiation, and not only do they not interfere with those treatments, uh, but they reduce the side effects, those treatments, so besides getting the immune-enhancement, the anti-cancer properties, you can actually improve the quality of life while people are undergoing these treatments, which is, you know, nice to see we've got the human research on that.

Which most oncologists just aren't aware of.

Dr. Anderson: Yes, I—I think that's a good distinction to bring up, too, that um, when uh, we were putting that particular chapter together, one of our goals was to try and focus on things that had the most human research. You know, we talked in other areas about more experimental things, you know, sometimes, you have to go and look, and say, "Well, there's no—or there's one human study, but there's a bunch of animal ones, and maybe we'll go there in an experiment."

But for broad use, it's really the best to start with the things that have the best data.

In, in humans, and so we can see, because we, we aren't mice, and we—you know, uh, and uh, we're not whatever else. Um, and I think that uh, one of the other ones that, that we almost universally recommend through most of the cancer types is, uh, curcumin.

Dr. Stengler: Yes.

Dr. Anderson: From the turmeric spice, and most people have heard—I mean, tur—curcumin, as far as a cancer and immune agent has been very popularized in the West. Of course, it's been known about forever, uh, in the East.

And the probably one of the herb/spice medicines that has the most human studies is curcumin. Uh, and exactly like what you said, uh, with say, turkey tail, it has probably the most studies in conjunction with, uh, with chemotherapy and, and sometimes in radiation, where you get a double benefit of not only is it—

Immunologically helping the immune system stay focused, but it also decreases the side effects of many of the standard therapies. And you know, that becomes a, a very, uh, important and sometimes tenuous discussion with, uh, with the other oncology team, because they—you know, of course, their focus is, okay, you know, if I'm a medical oncologist, I do chemotherapy primarily. That's my *[unintelligible]* radiation oncologist, I do radiation therapy.

Dr. Stengler: Right.

Dr. Anderson: Uh, and so, for them, you know, the last thing they want is some patient taking something that's going to interfere with whatever they're doing. And so, um, that's another reason why the specific, uh, supplements that we put in, we, we like to have human data, because then, you know, a patient can go, and they, their physician can look at the references, and say, "Oh, it actually was used with, you know, this chemotherapy or that."

Dr. Stengler: Right, and all these, all these, uh, medicinal supplements we're talking about often do have different, uh, mechanisms of action, like curcumin has many different effects in a helpful way. But one of 'em is it does interfere with chemicals in the body, if you will, that lead to inflammation. And so, that's why curcumin is not only good at helping maybe with joint pain or muscle pain you're experiencing from cancer or from your chemotherapy or radiation treatments, but you know, helping to, uh, affect one of the initiating factors of cancer to begin with.

Dr. Anderson: Yes, it, um, it—curcumin specifically, and, and not unlike some of the mushrooms, um, has this—which, which you see with plants, and you don't see often with single agent drugs, because they work on multiple plains, and multiple inputs into the system, they may look from the outside as, "Oh, well, it's anti-inflammatory—

"And I'm giving you an inflammatory chemotherapy drug, maybe they're gonna cancel each other out." In almost every case, where they've put them together, there's actually synergy where there—you know, they've not only protect against the side effects, but they appear to either have neutral or a positive effect on the standard cancer therapy.

And that, uh, and that's something that's very, like, that is a very new idea for a lot of the oncology world to, to kind of wrap its head around, because if you think of it from mostly the pharmacology point of view, and you've got a drug that's, you know, one chemical, and it's gonna do one thing, and you have another drug that's one chemical that does the opposite, of course they're gonna cancel each other out.

In the case of something like curcumin, often it's working on so many different levels, it doesn't even bother the other therapy, and it not only protects from the side effects, but uh—

Potentiates some of the other therapies. And uh, this is something that we actually worked with a bit in our, our research, as well. Um, and this is something that's, at this point, just a research item, but, um, in-in people getting chemotherapy, and then we would give them large dose infusions of curcumin, so an intravenous curcumin.

Dr. Stengler: Yes.

Dr. Anderson: Uh, and this again was in people where things weren't working. We would often see synergy, uh, with a chemo that had stopped working would start working again. So, um, there's a lot of promise with curcumin. We saw similar things with some of the mushrooms, as well. Yeah.

Dr. Stengler: Absolutely. Here's something a little bit different for the viewers. They may have read in recent years the anti-cancer effects of the common diabetes drug, metformin, also known as glucofage. It appears to have some cancer protective effects. Now, um, in the natural realm, we often use an herb known as berberine—

Uh, which also has blood sugar lowering effects, uh, which then also helps to lower insulin levels, which can be carcinogenic. Why don't you explain that a bit more?

Dr. Anderson: Yeah, so, it's, it's one of those things where the more, um, and metformin's a very old drug, and, and again, I think it's one of those where we, it was developed, and we kind of knew a little about how it worked when we developed it, and then as time went on, we've learned it does lots of other things, other than, you know, just a little bit of glucose manipulation.

Um, probably, and if you look at—you know, there's, there's, there's positive and negative studies. Most of the negative studies around metformin have to do with it does deplete certain nutrients. And you know, there's some things like that that you have to make sure you work on, if you're giving to people—

Dr. Stengler: Possibly could be issues, too, so *[unintelligible]*.

Dr. Anderson: Yeah, so if you're, you're working with metformin, you gotta watch people, etcetera. Um, but that being said, if you look at—

Uh, your likelihood of dying or not, if metformin is part of what you're doing as a therapy, you're less likely to die in-in the cancer setting at the very least. Um, berberine, which, uh, probably back, you know, when you and I first learned about it a long time ago, which we more thought of as an anti-infective kind of an herb, you know, and, and all of that, and there was a little written about it does this and that, um, but no one was really studying it.

Uh, it kinda made a resurgence when people started to look and say, "Well, we've got people on berberine for other reasons in their blood sugar control improved." Then they started looking into, well, would that happen if we just used it, say, instead of metformin, or something of that nature.

So, the way that, uh, and you'll see that berberine figures into many, many of the protocols, um, the way that we see berberine is—

It, and, and again, this is an area where there's definitely human studies on both metformin and berberine. Uh, there's a little bit on them together, or in opposition to one another, but not a whole lot. So, you, you can't say this 100 percent for sure, but what we believe we see is that when—especially if people have reactions to metformin, which some people do. They can't take it digestive-wise, or whatever—

Dr. Stengler: Right.

Dr. Anderson: The berberine seems to have the same effect on muting the insulin surges, which are procarcinogenic. It definitely has benefits on blood sugar control, which again, is much in, in the favor. Uh, but also, because of its, um, structure, um, possibly somewhat like metformin, uh, it actually probably has other anti-cancer effects that are—either we partially or really don't understand. So, we will often with patients—

If they come in, and they say, you know, "I can do everything, but don't give me metformin. I—" They've tried that—

Dr. Stengler: Yeah.

Dr. Anderson: And "I threw up." Or I did whatever.

Dr. Stengler:	Right.
Dr. Anderson:	Uh, we'll say, "Well, you know, berberine almost never has any of those side effects. We can give it with food, uh, and we, we can't say it's the same as metformin, but it's at least in the same ballpark." And, uh, and it has a number of other benefits that are, that are very useful.
	So you'll see berberine in many of the, the protocols, as well.
Dr. Stengler:	Excellent. Uh, another area which has really had a lot of research in recent years, and I know an area you've done a lot of research in, and that's the whole idea of these cannabis extracts, or cannabinoids, and THC. Why don't you give the viewers just a brief overview of what kinda compounds we're talking about, and um, interesting point we talk about in the book, how the human body actually has these cannabinoid receptors and systems, so—yeah, go ahead and talk about that.
Dr. Anderson:	Yeah. Yeah, it's, it's, it's an interesting, um, dichotomy that, um, for—you know, there's a lot of, obviously, legal and political, uh, discussions a-around cannabis, cannabinoids. But if you, you kinda take those away, uh, and you look at the biology of humans and the way we're put together, we actually have what's known as an endocannabinoid system built into us, uh, to help with neural regulation in the brain and the spinal cord, etcetera, help with pain, help with many things.
	Um, so, we're, we're kinda wired with that chemistry already there. Now, what we have noticed, and this is something where definitely there's more and more human studies, but really, in the US, human studies with cancer and cannabinoids are a very, very new thing—
	Be-because of legal issues around the use of cannabis, and, and they're up—up until recently, the only way you could study it was with, with one source for your cannabinoids, and it, it was very difficult, so people pretty much just said, "I—it's just too much for me."
Dr. Stengler:	Yeah.

Dr. Anderson:	And then, what, what happened is you know, certain states started to have waivers where they would allow doctors to, uh, recommend, uh, cannabis, and so then that started at least some observational studies of, well I got these people on cannabis, and these not, and is there a difference, right?
Dr. Stengler:	Mm-hmm.
Dr. Anderson:	So, a couple of things. There's many, many cannabinoids, and that's, that's the broad group of chemistry that's in, uh, cannabis, or in the hemp plant, which are relatives. Um, the two that we normally talk about when it comes to cancer are either the CBD, the cannabidiol or the THC, the tetrahydrocannabinol.
	Um, and they have different effects. So, the THC, for example, has more of a neuron, neural inhibitory effect. It's often used in, uh, seizure and pain, and that sort of thing. Uh, the CBD can have some of those effect at higher doses, but CBD actually, if they're together, like you would have in a whole plant, uh, the CBD actually cuts down on some of the neurological effects of the THC.
	So, the evolution that, that I got to witness as I was practicing in, and I still do in the state of Washington where we had a medical, uh, cannabis waiver act, uh, for quite a long time, uh, going on ten years, I believe. And because we were doing research with cancer patients, that was one of the things you could have a waiver for, so we started to, uh, really, e-experiment, because there was no standardization or anything back then. And as I said, US studies—
	Just didn't even exist, hardly, and the European ones were just starting to be done, 'cause it was just—it's—it's a plant medicine that got, you know, because of its other use, got a bad name—
Dr. Stengler:	Right.
Dr. Anderson:	So, didn't want to be associated with it. But in cancer, what we noticed was we started using it more as, uh, a palliative drug, to try and get people off of, uh, m-many cancer patients, obviously, are on pain medicine, but also, maybe on anti-anxiety medicine, and sleep medications, and all kinds

of other things. And they just don't like feeling that, you know, drugged.

And so, what we started to do was to do a mixture of giving them CBD during the day, which doesn't have a real neurological effect at normal doses, uh, but was starting to show that maybe would have a potential anti-cancer effect, so again, it was maybe it would work, can't hurt.

And then in the evening, uh, we would give them, uh, a liquid extract—

That would have a percent, uh, THC in it. And so, what we do is we'd say, "Well, okay, when you're kinda done with your day, you're winding down, between after dinner and bedtime," we'd start with just drops of this in tea, drop doses of the THC in the tea. "And just see if eventually you can maybe go off some of your anxiety medicine or your sleep medication, or maybe even your pain medicine."

And what we started to notice was over time, some people completely eliminated their sleep medication and their anxiety meds, and a lot of people were able to decrease opiate pain meds. Some people even totally went off. So, that again, you know, in research, things get your attention, and you start to say, "Well, is anyone now looking? This is kind of amazing, really."

So, then, uh, there was sort of an upswing in availability when, um, uh, and this is still a contentious issue with the federal government—

Because the states were kinda driving all of this. But, um, the use of a non-um—uh, non-cannabis-based CBD, so from say a hemp plant, which is legal. Uh, was—started to be distributed and used around the country, and they started to look, and you're getting more research and that. And it—

And uh, so you got a lot—suddenly, a lot wider group of people using at least CBD who had cancer, and starting to see some effect. Now, one thing I will say is because the research is still very much in its infancy, where, where humans go, and we—especially when you move away from pain and anxiety, and those sort of things.

When you get to cancer, it's, it's very early sort of research, but what it, what it appears is that that the mixture is better than them separate, so THC and CBD—

When it comes to actually fighting cancer, there is a ratio of CBD to THC that probably works best. We have people guessing what that is right now, but right now, that's sort of in, you know, everyone's got their own idea, but there, there appears to be a ratio that probably is best.

Um, and we already know that both THC and CBD have some very positive effects when it comes to at least tumor cell lines that they have checked, and that sort of thing. So, what we've done in the book, because we, obviously, don't want anyone to break any laws, or any of that, uh, we, we usually put CBD in as, as a common recommendation, because you can get, in most places, a hemp-based, uh, legal version.

Dr. Anderson: And so, um, my personal opinion is, uh, let's say you're in a state where all you can get is the hemp-based CBD, it's the same, uh, same chemical as the one made from, uh, cannabis, it's just that would be legal, and it's better to do that than nothing. And, uh, and we've seen, you know, again, I, I really hope sometime we get more data from humans with cancer using higher doses, and more appropriate doses—

Dr. Stengler: Right.

Dr. Anderson: But what we've seen so far, um, it can be incredibly helpful in definitely quality of life, definitely reducing other medication use, and probably as an adjunct to some of the other natural therapies for the cancer.

Dr. Stengler: So a lot of people are surprised to find out the sleep hormone, melatonin actually has a lot of good data on it for its anti-cancer properties. Dr. Anderson, what do you—talk to viewers more about that, and why is that?

Dr. Anderson: Yeah. You know, um, I think of everything that we recommend that people take when they have cancer, melatonin is probably the most misunderstood one, because people—they, they know that it, they use it maybe to go to sleep—

Dr. Stengler: Right.

Dr. Anderson:	Or, uh, you know, if recently they've seen, you know, there've been some, uh, of the daytime doctor shows, where, "Oh, you shouldn't take it, or you should take more, or you should take less." You know, there's a lot of confusion—
Dr. Stengler:	Right.
Dr. Anderson:	Around it, right? What you'll find in, in the book is that, um, the doses that we're using in cancer are much higher than sleep doses. Now, there are actually scientists studying melatonin in, uh—

Neuroscience who would say these doses that we use for cancer are appropriate for cancer, but are, are even low for what they're looking at for other purposes. So, where, you know, you might see a 5 to 20 milligram dose range, and think, "Wow, that's a lot of melatonin," um, there's actually applications being looked at for much higher doses.

So, when you think of melatonin, um, yes, it is part of the machinery in your central nervous system that, that starts to tell you, "Okay, it's getting towards the end of the day, it's getting dark, it's time to go to sleep," and it's kind of— it doesn't keep you asleep, but it induces the sleep cycle.

That's one little thing melatonin does, but when you add it, uh, as a supplement, and in many of the cancers, you'll see we write about, we, we do, at the higher doses, it also has, um, much like we talked about with curcumin, multiple effects, and so—

It's not just, "Yes, you, you might feel a bit tired when you take it," uh, but it does a whole number of other things. One is it actually shifts some of your immunology around to make the, uh, uh, to make the cancer setting, uh, less amenable to cancer cells, and it does that through a number of different ways.

It's one of these things that can change the oxidation status, but it, it can actually change it in two different directions, depending on what's needed at the time, hence, a little bit bigger doses. And there's even some human studies just looking at, you know, long-term, uh, if, if we already know they have, you know, this sort of cancer, and there's a group that takes melatonin at these higher doses, and then there's a group that doesn't, that the group that takes the melatonin actually has longer lifespan.

So, so there's, again, like we talked about with the turkey tail, etcetera, there's at least some good, human data on it—

Dr. Stengler: Right.

Dr. Anderson: And it's one of those where, um, you know, I-I would say this would be one where most of the oncologists have run across it, because it's, it's actually, you know, it's, it's sort of found its way into their literature enough that they're at least reading about it. Um, which makes it a little bit easier.

Um, the other nice thing is that there's almost no studied or recorded inhibition from melatonin with other cancer drugs, which is always, you know, we—I mean, if someone that needs to be on a cancer drug, we certainly don't need to be interfering with it, and that's something we're careful about.

So, that's um, uh, but, but often, if we don't have that discussion, that, "Look, this is not about sleep, this is—

Dr. Stengler: Right.

Dr. Anderson: "About your immune system," uh, the, the patient will be confused, and think, "Oh, then he must just want me to sleep more or something," and—

Dr. Stengler: Yeah.

Dr. Anderson: Then they'll get confused and stop taking it, is my experience. So, so, the higher doses, those are immunologic doses, yeah.

Dr. Stengler: Yeah, that's good information. Uh, here's probably a new one for a lot of the viewers. It's actually a medication used in a holistic fashion called low dose naltrexone, or LDN. Let's, uh, review, uh, what that's all about.

Dr. Anderson: Yes. So this is a really interesting, um, use of a, a fairly old medication that is used completely not for cancer. Um, so naltrexone, and uh, it has a cousin named naloxone, uh, are, uh, opiate blockers, and so, these are normally used in emergency medicine if somebody overdoses on an opiate drug.

And so, in North America, you hear about, uh, narcan, or naloxone, is, is usually the one they have on the ambulance, and that, so someone's overdosed, it actually will stop the overdose, and you won't die of respiratory distress. So, then you start thinking, "Okay, what does that have to do with cancer?"

Dr. Stengler: Yeah.

Dr. Anderson: That, you know, that seems like an odd thing. Um, well, number one, what they noticed, and this is a number of years, uh, ago, um, over ten, at, at least, but what they noticed was that because hu—what we'll call high dose naltrexone, will block an opiate overdose, obviously, it's gonna go to opiate receptors, and do something.

Well, some very, uh, smart, astute scientists, uh, in different parts of the world, said, "Well, we know that some of those receptors are also on the triggering activity of either a cancer cell, or a, uh, cancer triggering cell. So, what if we, we obviously can't give people these big, high doses, 'cause they haven't taken opiates, and that would make them sick. What if we give them very, very tiny doses of this, and would that work? Would it do anything?"

And so, the two areas of research that—

Were looked into, really, were cancer and autoimmunity. And the, the shortest version of the story is that, um, when you go in a tiny amount, and kind of calm these receptor sites that the naltrexone goes to, again, kinda like the curcumin story, the immune system doesn't either shut off or overregulate. It kind of mellows out and kind of levels out.

And that's actually the—one of the most anti-cancer things you can do long-term, is to level the immune system. So, sometimes we do, you know, increase it, like with mistletoe. Sometimes, you know, we, we might calm it way down for other reasons. But leveling it is actually what homeostasis, that's what our normal body is supposed to do during, uh, keeping cancer away.

Dr. Stengler: Right.

Dr. Anderson:	So, it's sort of morphed from, uh, autoimmune things—
	Like using it in multiple sclerosis and other things, and then them noticing, "Well, it's kind of a similar effect to what we could do with cancer." And uh, just kinda shorten the story up, um, there, there was a, uh, a landmark study done in England, looking at it with not only with cancer cells, and cell viability, meaning if we put it in the petri dish, do the cancer cells die faster, etcetera?
	Which it turned out they did, if you dose it appropriately. But the other thing was they took three of the most common chemotherapy drugs, and they put the naltrexone in the chemotherapy drugs together, and the chemotherapy drugs worked better, which was another pushback we would always get as well. Is it gonna stop the chemo and all that?
Dr. Stengler:	Yeah.
Dr. Anderson:	So, you'll see LDN, low dose naltrexone, recommended. It is something you'll need to find an integrative physician to prescribe, because it is a medication. Uh—
	It is used at low dose, so it's not the anti-opiate, you know, sort of dose. Um, but we are more universally recommending it, because again, it's one of those things like curcumin, where in the background, it's, it's not going to harm anything. And if anything, it's gonna push your immune system in a direction that makes cancer harder to propagate.
Dr. Stengler:	Excellent. And then we have good old vitamin D. Let's end on the vitamin D. Uh, it's certainly one of the nutrients, the least in conventional medicine. They're aware, there's a number of studies showing that vitamin D deficiency is a risk factor for a variety of different types of cancer. So, talk about that, and its mechanism, if you would.
Dr. Anderson:	Yeah. So, vitamin D, um, what—I think one of the things to start with that's probably the most important is there are certain vitamins that, that really shouldn't have been named vitamins—
Dr. Stengler:	Right.
Dr. Anderson:	And vitamin D is one of those. Uh, vitamin D is actually a—

Uh, a hormone, and it is made in the same cascade that your steroid hormones are made in. So, its structure, it's a, a fat-based molecule. Its structure is, is similar to other steroids. One of the things that we see, whether, uh, whether it's just a natural, uh, steroids produced in the body, or if we give someone overdose of steroids, it changes immune function, okay.

Well, because vitamin D is, although it binds to different receptors, it works very similarly, same thing. If we don't have enough vitamin D around, we wind up with a change, not only, we think of vitamin D for our bones, let's make our bones strong. Let's get enough vitamin D, and that's true.

Uh, but vitamin D actually has crossover receptors with some of the places that trigger, um, things like breast cancer cells to, to grow, and certain prostate cancer cells, and other hormone receptive type, uh, tumors.

And then just in general, kind of like we've alluded to before, where you know, people will say, "Well, on the list of triggers of cancer is stress," well, stress isn't just some mythical thing. It's actually chemistry in your body, a lot of it being steroid hormones. Well, the same reasons that steroid hormones, if they're going way too high or way too low, will be a trigger for cancer cells. Same thing with vitamin D being too low.

There's not enough support, um, for the, um, for the receptor sites that are, uh, are supposed to be kind of on guard for, uh, not turning cancer on. So, just like we see with, you know, if you imbalance estrogen and progesterone too long, or cortisol too long, or whatever, vitamin D is a, is a steroid hormone, right?

Dr. Stengler: Right.

Dr. Anderson: In there, whether you keep it too low too long, it's not, it's not going to be protective like it ought to. So, what, what we, uh—

Recommend are some dose ranges, and then of course, having it—your levels checked—

Dr. Stengler:	Right.
Dr. Anderson:	Because that's, that's critical, too.
Dr. Stengler:	It looks like most studies are, are finding a blood level around 45 to 50 in general, seems to have the best cancer protection. I mean, studies vary, but that seems to be about in the ballpark.
Dr. Stengler:	At a minimum, you know—
Dr. Anderson:	Where you'd see a cutoff, uh, and um, of course, if you're listening in the UK or Canada, those will be slightly different numbers. But the, the punchline to me with the blood level seems to be if you look at the normal range as, you know, 0 to 100 percent, we usually tell our patients, you want to be in the upper third, so, uh—
Dr. Stengler:	Right.
Dr. Anderson:	You know, uh, and, and that's pretty easy to see. And you don't—there's very few times you need to be higher, but you, you don't want to be lower.
Dr. Stengler:	Right, right.
Dr. Anderson:	And so, 40, you know, 40 to 50 in our, in our American units, uh, is right kinda at the bottom of that third—
Dr. Stengler:	Yeah.
Dr. Anderson:	You know, which would make sense.
Dr. Stengler:	So, in summary, it seems that vitamin D is anti-inflammatory, helps with normal cell division, immune activation, uh, and probably many other mechanisms—
Dr. Anderson:	I think a lot of other, um—
Dr. Stengler:	Which haven't even been, uh, discovered—
Dr. Anderson:	A lot of other things, yeah.
Dr. Stengler:	Yeah, so yeah, but it's a great anti-cancer nutrient. More for prevention, but certainly should be part of our protocol, as well, just because of all the mechanisms—
Dr. Anderson:	Yeah.

Dr. Stengler:	Involved with it.
Dr. Anderson:	Yeah. And we see many of our cancer patients when they screen in the beginning, their vitamin D levels really aren't very high, and so—
Dr. Stengler:	Right.
Dr. Anderson:	You, you know, even for just general health, they need to be brought up.
Dr. Stengler:	Right. Well, there's many supplements we talk about in the book. There's many supplements that could be used, theoretically, in a preventative and treatment, uh, protocol for cancer. We can't go over all of them tonight, but they are in the book, and that was a great review for the viewers, so thank you for that.
Dr. Anderson:	Yes, thank you.
Dr. Stengler:	And if you've been watching this, which I'm sure you have been, um, look into these supplements we're talking about. Again, these are the ones which have good data on 'em. Very good research, very scientific, and so, you don't need to be fearful for a lack of information, and, and good science behind them. Take care, and we'll see you on the next, uh, video.

EPISODE 5: YOUR CUSTOM CANCER PROTOCOL

How to Treat—and Cure—
Your Specific Diagnosis with a
Fully Customized Plan that's
Tailored to Your Needs

THE CΛPLESS METHOD TO TREATING PROSTATE CANCER

— DR. GEO ESPINOSA —

Dr. Stengler: Welcome to *Outside the Box Cancer Therapies*. Now, I wanna welcome Dr. Geo Espinosa; he is a naturopathic doctor and certified functional medicine practitioner, recognized as an authority in urology and male health. Dr. Geo is clinical assistant professor at New York University Langone Medical Center, Department of Urology, and lectures internationally on holistic therapies for urological conditions. As an avid researcher and writer, he has authored numerous books, textbook chapters, and scientific papers, and wrote the popular prostate cancer book, *Thrive—Don't Only Survive!* On his time off from work, he enjoys writing on his popular blog, drgeo.com, spending time with his wife and three kids, and practicing martial arts. Welcome, Dr. Geo.

Dr. Espinosa: Thank you so much, Dr. Stengler. It is a pleasure, a pleasure to be here.

Dr. Stengler: Well, everyone in our industry knows about you; you really are probably the leading expert in men's health, prostate health for sure, and, um, you've got a very interesting background. Why don't you tell the viewers how you got interested in men's health, and, you know, how you got all this expertise in, in prostate health?

Dr. Espinosa: Well, that's *[laughter]*, uh, that's, uh, you know, that's, uh, that's a phenomenal question, because why would anyone wanna be an expert in prostates and penises, right?

Dr. Stengler: *[Laughs]*

Dr. Espinosa: Um, that, that's probably a reflection of my quirky personality, or at least, uh, to some degree. Um, but it turned out, when I was in school, in naturopathic medical school, uh, *[unintelligible]* long time ago, let's just say *[laughter]*, um, you know, I started seeing, clinically, uh, as a student, I, I started seeing a lot of men, and men were asking for me.

Then one day, um, uh, I live here in New York, so we lived, uh, at the time, I lived in an apartment building, like most of us here, so we pay a lot of money for very little. Uh *[laughter]*, um, uh, so, I'm taking the, uh—so, it, I had, I remember, so in order for me to go from where I lived to University of Bridgeport, which is where I got my degree, it took me roughly about an hour to get there.

If I left—and that's if I left at 6:30 AM, for my 8:00 class, *[unintelligible]*, so, roughly, I got there at 7:30. If I left at 6:45, then I, I, I would hit traffic and I would be late for my 8:00. It, it was, I had it down to a science. One day I go up to, so, one day I'm, you know, I'm, uh, so, I'm, you know—and the joke was, for my 8:00 class, "You know, Geo is always late."

Dr. Stengler: Yeah.

Dr. Espinosa: So, one day I'm actually early, 6:30, got my books, you know, you know, I, I, I have a, kind of a stroll with me, like, "Hey, the joke is on them." And then I open up my *[unintelligible]*, I was, like, "God, I forgot my, the book that I needed for the class." So I have to go up—I live in the 16th floor, and I was, like, that was it, then, once I had to do that, I knew I was gonna be late, "God—" I go up, come back down; on the way down, I, a friend that, you know, we played volleyball together, he didn't know what I did, I didn't know what he—he says, "Geo, where are you going? It's early." I said, "Well, I'm a student, naturopathic medicine." I said, "Where are you going so early?" well, he says, "I'm a urologist."

Dr. Stengler:	Hm—
Dr. Espinosa:	So, "Tell me about naturopathic medicine. I don't know what that—" "Well, it's natural medicine," I explained. He says, "Wow, fantastic. How, how can I get you to work with me? I mean, all my patients are asking me about *[unintelligible]*, and I don't wanna—" you know.
Dr. Stengler:	Yeah.
Dr. Espinosa:	So, then, you gotta pay attention, right? That is, like, if you believe in whatever, the universe or God, something is hitting you in the head and saying, "Hey, idiot, this is where you need to go."
Dr. Stengler:	*[Laughs]*
Dr. Espinosa:	And that's what I did. So, you know, the, the, the rest is history; then I worked with, uh, Dr. Aaron Katz, at the Holistic Center of Urology. Then I became absolutely obsessed with men's health and urology: I bought every book, naturopathic, conventional. I wanted to know everything, uh, every naturopathic approach for every urological and male problem. I wanted to know every conventional approach, even though I didn't practice conventional medicine, but I wanted to see, you know, I wanted to see how that type of medicine worked. Long story short, uh, you know, years, maybe 13, 14 years later, now I'm at NYU heading the, uh, Integrative Function *[unintelligible]* Urology Center, here in New York.
	And, you know, it is the best decision I've ever made, besides marrying my wife.
Dr. Stengler:	Mm, nice, well, you're a, you're a unique character, for sure. *[Laughter]*
Dr. Stengler:	—I don't know of any other holistic doctors, certainly naturopathic medical doctors, who are working at a conventional medical center in urology. You were at Columbia; now you're at, what, Langone, right?
Dr. Espinosa:	Yeah, NYU-Langone, yes.
Dr. Stengler:	Yes, so, I, I don't know anyone else, in, in the history of naturopathic medicine, who's done what you have done, do you?

Dr. Espinosa:	Uh, I, I appreciate that. I'm just humbled, you know, with the opportunities. I couldn't be happier being at a very, very conventional, uh, orthodox medical setting, quite frankly.
Dr. Stengler:	Yeah, well, you're making us look good—we thank you for that.
Dr. Espinosa:	My pleasure—thank you.
Dr. Stengler:	Now, as you know, more than two-and-a-half million men in the United States have prostate cancer, over a billion men worldwide.
Dr. Espinosa:	Right.
Dr. Stengler:	And, thankfully, we've got guys like you out there helping people, helping to prevent prostate cancer, helping men get through the treatment with prostate cancer, using the best of both worlds, integrative medicine, integrative oncology.
Dr. Espinosa:	Right.
Dr. Stengler:	So, Dr. Geo, as you may know, I've got a book, here: *Thrive—Don't Only Survive!*, and it happens to say "Dr. Geo's Guide to Living Your Best Life Before and After Prostate Cancer."
Dr. Espinosa:	That's right.
Dr. Stengler:	So, a great book—this really is, is an excellent reference book to, to help families, to help men, help practitioners walk through the world of integrative oncology, and to, to give the best information on how to help men prevent and treat prostate cancer. So we're gonna go through some of the, we're gonna go through some of the main sections, and get your, um, comments on it, okay?
Dr. Espinosa:	Absolutely.
Dr. Stengler:	Now, let me start about the prostate gland itself. You start, as you know, we first see the patients with prostate problems, the men, they don't really understand what is this prostate gland all about. So, maybe give us a little bit of a primer on the prostate gland.
Dr. Espinosa:	So, yeah.

So, the prostate gland, um, it's, uh, roughly a walnut-shaped gland; it's a gland and it, it's a muscular gland, meaning, there's muscles around these glands that secrete different things, including this marker that provokes anxiety, called PSA, right?

Dr. Stengler: Right.

Dr. Espinosa: So, so, um, so it's about the size of a walnut, if, that's if it's a normal size. That, that prostate, that "size of a walnut," can get bigger, and bigger, and bigger. And what, and, and, the, *[unintelligible]* only one purpose for the prostate gland, which is interesting consider that it causes so much trouble as a man gets older. *[Laughs]* You know, you would think it has multiple functions *[unintelligible]* if you're gonna go through all the hardship as you get older, it should have, you know, multiple life, life longing, uh, functions. It has one function, *[laughs]* and that's for conception, right?

Dr. Stengler: Right.

Dr. Espinosa: It's to conceive, um, because it's, it's, it plays a major role in the production of semen, and the expulsion of semen, uh, out of the penis.

And that's its only role, uh, you don't wanna undermine it, I mean, there's no life without the prostate, right? So you don't wanna undermine that role, but still, you know, it causes, uh, a significant amount of problems for men as they, as they get older, and sometimes even in men, uh, that are younger. when you look at a whole walnut that's encapsulated with a shell, um, roughly, that's, that's a prostate. And actually, I've had the opportunity of going to the OR multiple times with the surgeon, and really looking at the prostate and touching a prostate, and, wow, it is so, I, so similar to a walnut, And it really is, in terms of size and everything.

Dr. Stengler: That's a good description. Now, in your book, you talk about the warning flags of prostate cancer, and, of course, a lot of these are similar to just enlarged prostate, which most men are gonna deal with over the age of 50.

Uh, warning flags could be dribbling urine, trouble urinating or an inability to urinate, frequent urge to urinate, burning or painful urination, pain in the urine or semen, painful ejaculation, difficulty having an erection, frequent pain in the lower back, hips, or upper thighs. So, a lot of crossover from large prostate; I guess that's what makes it a little bit tricky in the diagnosis.

Dr. Espinosa: A lot of, yeah, a lot crossover with, uh, uh, BPH, or benign prostatic hypoplasia *[unintelligible]* enlargement of the prostate *[unintelligible]* crosses over with prostatitis, which typically occurs in, uh, younger men. The reality is that, um, most men with prostate cancer have absolutely no signs and no symptoms, so, there's no way of them knowing, so, it oftentimes is just found, uh, by just routine visit to the doctor, they get a PSA test, PSA is elevated, they get a biopsy, biopsy, biopsy comes out negative, uh, or positive in this case. Um, and, and that's pretty much it.

If there is any of these symptoms that are associated with prostate cancer, *[unintelligible]* some of the ones that you mentioned—painful ejaculation, even erectile dysfunction, uh, difficult time urinating—that might mean that there are tumor cells—not just enlargement of the prostate or inflammation—tumor cells that's actually squeezing the tube, the urethra, that brings *[unintelligible]* the urine and the ejaculate. So, that may be, uh, one of the, uh, early signs; more often than not, those signs are related to, as you mentioned, to an enlarged prostate and prostatitis, not prostate cancer. Again, I wanna, for your listening audience, um, I wanna let, make sure they know that there are, typically, no signs, no symptoms, related to prostate cancer.

Dr. Stengler: *[Crosstalk]*

Dr. Espinosa: *[Crosstalk]* the time they have lower back pain, hip pain, and things like that, again, that could be muscular, of course, but if it is associated with prostate cancer, that might mean, already, metastasis, uh, prostate cancer spreading to the bone.

Uh, typically, when we see a patient and we're gonna rule out prostate cancer, maybe take us through kind of the, the typical things *[unintelligible]* get into more detail: the prostate exam, um, the PSA blood test, that's maybe getting some of the other tests you talk about in the book that people may not know about. Uh, of course, people wanna know about the PSA—it's always, it's been a controversy for a number of years, and for doctors like you and I that see patients on a daily basis, we know it has some value. Um, it's obviously far from a perfect test, but let's get your expertise on, walk us through the, the exam of a prostate, the palpation, uh, the bloodwork, starting with PSA, and maybe some of the other tests which you, you like to use.

Dr. Espinosa: The bottom line is this: the reason why the controversy with PSA, should we use it to screen or not, is because many clinicians, urologists, have used PSA, uh, wrongly, in terms of getting a PSA. PSA is low, but low normal or low abnormal, in some cases, and ordering a biopsy than then they or, then the biopsy comes up positive for prostate cancer. Meanwhile, it's low-grade prostate cancer, which the treatment doesn't really improve their, uh, longevity, uh, from prostate cancer. And then, it's just downhill from there in terms of side effects from the prostate treatment, and then, of course, increase in healthcare costs. And then, the—

So, the United States Preventative Taskforce, around four or five years ago, say, "Hey, stop screening with PSA." That's not necessarily a good thing. And the reason I'm going, I'm giving the audience, uh, uh, this background is because, you know, you go to any urologist or any doctor, they may have a different approach to how they screen for prostate cancer, right?

Dr. Stengler: Right.

Dr. Espinosa: Typically, of course, the guys that are coming to see you and I, Mark, they want—less is more: they're trying to avoid a biopsy, right? So, so, so that I can answer your question *[unintelligible]* what's your process, I have to say, this is my protocol as to how I help men, um, find prostate cancer when necessary, okay? Um, so, because, uh, and why is that the case? Why? Because, yeah, who wants their, you know, no, there's no men, that I know, wakes up in the morning and they say, "Hey, man, woo, I can't wait to get that biopsy, today," right? Big nice probe in your rectum, and poking and clicking going on, blood coming out of your urine and semen for a week.

"I can't wait for that," possible infections, "I can't wait for that." Well, and, and, so then we have to be more responsible, I think, with even, way before we even send them to a biopsy—I think we have that opportunity. And in urology, I mean, look, medicine is big business—no one should undermine that—and, you know, there is an incentive, a financial incentive, to do biopsies and to treat, all in all. I'm not saying every doctor does it for that reason, but there is some sort of an incentive. All right, let's get right to it. New patient comes in, 55 years old, PSA 4.5, should you—what's the process to determine if they have prostate cancer or not? There are about, there are several things that I look at way before even a biopsy, okay?

Dr. Stengler: Okay.

Dr. Espinosa: I look at PSA history, and PSA velocity, meaning, how, you know, how has this PSA changed within the last one to two years?

So, this guy, 55 years old, PSA of 4.5, I'm not alarmed, particularly if he's giving me or showing me signs of an enlarged prostate, okay?

Dr. Stengler: Right.

Dr. Espinosa: So there's this, there's this questionnaire of, uh, um, called the "IPSS questionnaire," based on that questionnaire, you can, um, quantity their urinary symptoms that might be associated with prostate enlargement. So, if their IPSS, for argument's sake, is—normal that's one indication, in my head, to me, that says, "Hey, maybe the, his prostate being 4.5 is just from an enlarged prostate, not related to cancer." Then we look again at the PSA velocity, within the last two years or so. So, just that number by itself doesn't scare me, but let's say that number went—he's always had a PSA of—you know, within the last two years been, it was 5, uh, two years ago, then 6 months after that it was 3.5, uh, 6 months after that it was 4.2, uh, 6 months after that it was 3.8, and then now it's 4.5. Cyclically, that's not concerning to me, right? When it's, it's more concerning when, when it, when it, when the velocity is continuously upward, okay?

Dr. Stengler: Yeah.

Dr. Espinosa: So that's the other thing, right, that I look at. Then, so then, the third thing is, the, the, the, the prostate exam—it's very important, 'cause you're looking nodules, or the absence of nodules. Nodules can signify—not always—prostate cancer.

So, if the, if the, if the prostate feels a little like an enlarge prostate—and there's certain things—I don't' wanna get into the weeds—uh, there's certain things that you're looking for, and it feels like an enlarged prostate, there again, PSA 4.5 might be related to, uh, uh, an enlarged prostate. So that's number three. The fourth thing you look at is a PSA density, what is that? Well, if, if we have to value the, the, the weight of the, or the size of the prostate, from either an ultrasound, or even better, from an MRI, then you could make a calculation. And then, which is, um, you, you, you divide PSA score over PSA, uh, size, and anything above 0.15 is associated—not caused—or related, uh, strongly related, to prostate cancer. So, so, anything above, uh, .15 is more associated with prostate cancer. We look at that.

Dr. Stengler: Mm-hmm.

Dr. Espinosa: Still concerned—maybe he has a family history of prostate, "Hey, my father had prostate cancer." "Okay, let's do a 4Kscore." The 4Kscore is actually a blood test that's much more specific, uh, and sensitive to prostate cancer, more so than PSA. Anything much higher than 7.5 percent might indicate, yeah, that it's not only prostate cancer, but the, the type of cancer that you might wanna pay attention to, right, the type of cancer that might be deadly.

Dr. Stengler: Right.

Dr. Espinosa: If the PSA is, uh, if the 4Kscore is 11—I had a patient this morning, his PS, his 4Kscore was 11—just because it's higher than 7.5 doesn't mean, "Oh, my god, we need to biopsy right away." If it's a 25 percent, different story, okay?

Dr. Stengler:	Right.
Dr. Espinosa:	So, that's that, we, we do, so—and then, lastly, so, if all these, these five things that we're looking at, if they indicate, "Yeah, you know what, family history, uh, let's just say—" Well, in this case scenario, the thing, it's not too alarming, to me, if their—if their 4Kscore is 11, uh, cyclical PSA within the last two years, uh, it, enlarged prostate, IPSS high, that's not too alarming. I'd say, "Hey, hold off on a biopsy. Let's continue to monitor." In a different case scenario, where it's, like, all these, uh, many of these things are, uh, high—4Kscore is high, uh, continuous rise in velocity of PSA, uh, abnormalities in the, on the prostate exam—the next step is, "Hey, let's get an MRI of the prostate." The, the modern, the, the new technology with, um, what's called T3 Tesla, or T, 3T, or 3 Tesla MRIs, are, um, is, is, is really good. It's not perfect; it's not that they can see actual tumors there, but it's very good, it's very good, and you can see suspicious lesions. And they rate that in a, in a, what's called a PI-RAD score, in a scale of 1 to 5—higher up on that score, more significant to something incredibly suspicious.
	Now we have all this data—we have a 3T MRI; now we could do what's called the, a targeted, um, focused biopsy. And in that case, in the latter, uh, case that we spoke about, where everything kinda seem, seems, uh, seems a little bit abnormal, now, yeah, a biopsy should be performed. And then, it should be the right biopsy, which is a, a, a, a MRI-guided, uh, or what's called a fusion biopsy: MRI, ultrasound, fused biopsy, where the areas of interest are, is, they're more, they're more pronounced, and you can target that area a lot better. Than doing what most people are still doing, a blind biopsy, ultrasound-guided, which is really a blind biopsy. All you can see in an ultrasound is where the prostate is, not for, that, you can't really see anything that's that suspicious; maybe some calcification or something, and then *[unintelligible]* you're just shooting 12, 15 times, blindly. So this, this former form of biopsing is much better, if one needs to go there.
Dr. Stengler:	Now, what percent, what percent of biopsies would you say are the targeted, the better kind, as you're saying?

	What percent, in America, do you think are being done the best way?
Dr. Espinosa:	Still low, still low. Why? Because this M, MRI technology is very expensiveSo, big centers, and sometimes, you know, big cities, even private places, have one, too, in, in, in big cities. So, yeah, they're not widely available; the machine is very expensive. And I'll say this, it, which is actually also important: you could have the machine, that's great.
	Who's reading the, the, the images? So, what's happening is that some people have the machine, but the radiologist who's reading it and interpreting it is not that experienced in just prostate. They might be experienced in, uh, uh, suspicious tumors, and breasts, and other areas, and then they start doing prostate. So the interpretation of those images become as important, and perhaps even more important, than having that technology
Dr. Stengler:	Okay. Now, what about for the viewers out there, across America and around the world, seeing this series, here, what would you recommend if they don't have the option of getting, you know, the best MRIs?
	What I would say is this: You know, if, if, if your, if your car breaks down, you're gonna do some research online, so you can have a conversation with the mechanic as to what needs to happen, so you don't get screwed, right? *[Laughs]*
Dr. Espinosa:	Like, you're gonna have, you're gonna have some idea, so, you're gonna learn the language a little bit, right? I gotta say, people have to be proactive.
Dr. Stengler:	So I think that, um, I think that the layperson, the lay male, has an opportunity to really educate themselves about this process, be proactive, be well-informed, right, and ask good questions.
Dr. Stengler:	Mm-hmm.
Dr. Espinosa:	You're forcing the person, the, the, the physician, to answer your good—so, the better the question, the better the answer. So I think that—and, and the reason why I say that

is because some men will, probably will not need a biopsy, even if it's, uh, ultrasound-guided. Okay, so let's just say that they do need a biopsy, and there's no MRI available, no target, what do they do? So then they get what, what's available. *[Laughs]*

I wanna get to the, you know, some of the expertise you have in integrative treatment.

Dr. Espinosa: Okay.

Dr. Stengler: Now, let's get into your CaPLESS method—why don't you define what the CaPLESS method is, let's go through that and kind of define that, okay?

Dr. Espinosa: So, you know, within the last, uh, decade, I've, I've intensely looked at research on what is the proper lifestyle. You know, not the proper lifestyle, not the proper diet, for cancer. What's the proper lifestyle, what's the proper diet for prostate cancer? So I kind of got very specific, very granular, and, more importantly, whatever the research says, how can that be implemented, right? 'Cause research is good, it's great, wonderful, right? Uh, you know, studies show that plant-based is good. Okay, how do I apply that? Oh, studies shows that exercise is good. What kind of exercise? What—right?

So, research, research doesn't work, is not good, unless people are able to implement. So, that's exactly what the CaPLESS method is, is an acronym, so, C, capital C, lower-case A, capital P, stands for carcinoma of the prostate. Uh, L stands for "lifestyle," E stands for "exercise and, and, and eating," uh, and "SS" stands for "selected supplements." So, the CaPLESS method, so, it's a, it's a, it's a focused program on helping men that have been diagnosed, how to create a microenvironment that's hostile to cancer cells, and at the same time, prolong their life from all cause, uh, uh, of mortality. You know, we, we still know that most men with prostate cancer die from heart attacks, not prostate cancer, right?

Dr. Stengler: Right, so, your, your program, it can be used by men who are under active surveillance, *[unintelligible]* being monitored by their doctors, seeing if there's changes or not, integrating holistic techniques. Or men who are getting treatment for prostate cancer, you'd still wanna incorporate the things we're talking about, like the CaPLESS method.

Dr. Espinosa: The guy in active surveillance is different than a guy with advanced disease, slightly, uh, who have, uh, metastatic bone disease, let's just say, guy undergoing radiation—I just gave a talk to a group, a group of radiation oncologists, so I went right into the wolves, so I had my, uh, boxing gloves on, right?

Dr. Stengler: [Laughs]

Dr. Espinosa: I'm, like, "All right, I'm, I'm ready for you guys, uh, you know, I do martial arts, be careful."

Dr. Stengler: Yeah.

Dr. Espinosa: Um, and, really, my point is: "Why are you guys taking your, your, your patients off of supplements when they're undergoing radiation? What's the basis of that? This horrible theory that the cancer cells are protected from a little, like, 15 milligrams of selenium, or, or 200 micrograms of selenium? Is that the—" uh, it just, so we're, so—

So, part of that, uh, the CaPLESS method is, yeah, the 80-20 rule, 80 percent, you're gonna do better by following. There's a, there's a little bit of a nuance, here and there, depending on, on what, what's the patient's, you know, uh, sick personal situation.

Dr. Stengler: Sure, well, [unintelligible] give us the highlights—so let's go through each one—give us the highlights of lifestyle, first, [crosstalk].

Dr. Espinosa: So when you, yeah, so, when we talk about lifestyle, we talk about, uh, we talk about eating, we talk about exercise, we talk about managing stress, and sleeping properly, right?

Dr. Stengler: Mm-hmm.

Dr. Espinosa: So, obviously, we can get into, um, into details with each part of those, uh, each one of those categories. But with, so, with, um, so with eating, let's say, what do you, what do I eat, right?

Dr. Stengler:	Right.
Dr. Espinosa:	I, I think what's interesting, lately, is not only what do I eat but when, when should I eat, okay? So I have become a big fan of this intermittent fasting thing—something that I really started doing 20 years ago, um, and there was no science.
Dr. Stengler:	Yeah.
Dr. Espinosa:	And now, like, everybody's into *[laughs]* fasting and intermittent fasting. So, I think it's a matter of, you know, you know, when not to—and, and there's exceptions to that rule. Metastatic prostate cancer, when the patient is kinda becoming cachectic or losing a lot of weight, I would not do intermittent fasting *[crosstalk]*.
Dr. Stengler:	Right.
Dr. Espinosa:	But, but for most men who have had prostate cancer, or had it treated, here's the thing—very important, maybe this is the most important—I like to think that everything I've said so far is very important.
Dr. Stengler:	*[Laughs]*
Dr. Espinosa:	Here's one good takeaway: The, the, once a man is diagnosed with prostate cancer, you own prostate cancer, forever. I don't care what the treatment is, right? The, the recurrence rate, in men, after treatment of prostate cancer, within ten years, is up to 40 to 50 percent, depending on what you read.
	That's significant. What does that mean? Cancer coming back, based on PSA rising after treatment, whether it was radiation or, or surgery. So, you never, and, and it's very important for men to understand that, they owe it—so how do you manage it? Always through the CaPLESS method. So the eating part *[unintelligible]* when not to eat; you don't eat, you know, 12 to 16 hours, uh, I, in the book, I think I talk about 12 hours of, you know, of time-restricted eating. Um, now I'm kind of pushing more towards 16, between 12 and 16, based on certain researched that I've read.
Dr. Stengler:	Mm-hmm.

Dr. Espinosa:	Uh, and then, when you do eat, what do you eat? There's a food rating system that I have online, uh, where I, I, I, I help rate foods on a scale of 1 to 5—foods that are higher up on the scale are more protective. So, the more protective foods are actually, uh, the cruciferous vegetables, things like broccoli, Brussels sprouts, cauliflower—cauliflower is one of the main white foods that I recommend.

I don't recommend too many white foods. |
Dr. Stengler:	Right.
Dr. Espinosa:	So, so that's that—kale, very, you know, very—they have *[unintelligible]*, different, um, phytochemicals that are, are in these vegetables, that actually have not only, uh, antioxidants and *[unintelligible]* good minerals, good—they have anticancer properties specific to prostate cancer. So you wanna eat more of those, right?
Dr. Stengler:	Right.
Dr. Espinosa:	So, there's more foods you should eat, more 4s and 5, uh, and less 1 and 2s. One and 2s are the flours, uh, the simple carbohydrates; the well-done meats are one, right?
Dr. Stengler:	Mm-hmm.
Dr. Espinosa:	Uh, for example, slow-cooked meats that are not too brown on the outside are a 3, neutral, right? Fish is actually very interesting, and I'll—you know, let's, we'll move on quickly, uh, but I'll say this about fish, uh, fish actually—here's the story with fish. Based on research, fish is this: colored fish much better than white fish, okay?
Dr. Stengler:	Okay.
Dr. Espinosa:	From a, from a prostate cancer protective, uh, uh, uh, uh, effect, colored fish—salmon, sardines—better than things like codfish.
Dr. Stengler:	Mm-hmm.
Dr. Espinosa:	Okay? Then, slow-cooked colored fish is a 5, right?
Dr. Stengler:	Okay.
Dr. Espinosa:	Uh, or, or fish, fish that's, colored fish that's cooked in low

temperature is a 5. Colored fish that's grilled or broiled is a 4—still somewhat protective; not as much. White fish that's, uh, heavily cooked is a 1, actually promotes more hydro cyclic, uh, uh, amines, and nothing else to counteract that, right? Hydro cyclic, hi, hi, hydro cyclic, cyclic amines are these—I know you know, but, you know, just, your audience—are these things that are created when you expose, uh, muscle meats to, to high heat, uh, that browning and stuff, it—and so, hydro cyclic amines are, uh, uh, a potential, if not just outright a carcinogen.

Dr. Stengler: Yeah.

Dr. Espinosa: So, uh, so white fish—and white fish that's fried is, is a 1, and so forth.

So, it actually can get very specific and granular—uh, again, all, this is all based on research; this is not my opinion.

Dr. Stengler: Yeah.

Dr. Espinosa: Um, exercise, exercising, with moderate to, uh, high intensity, four hours a week—okay? Four hours a week, that's based on science. So, guys that, so, research shows that guys who have had prostate cancer, who exercise—actually, three hours a week; I just think four is better, uh, based on my experience—three, three to four hours a week, with moderate to high intensity, have a lesser risk of dying from prostate cancer after they are diagnosed.

Dr. Stengler: Yeah, and that's quite significant—you put it in your book, there, [unintelligible] that study, uh: "Three hours or more of vigorous physical activity, per week, these men with localized prostate cancer had a 49 percent lower risk of death from all causes, and a 61 percent reduced risk of dying from prostate cancer, compared with men, compared with men who got less than 1 hour of vigorous activity per week."

So, that, I mean, there's no drug supplement diet that can compare to that.

Dr. Stengler: And here's an interesting question—and, and, and there's, of course, no poll, I don't think, that's ever been done, but—what percent of urologists, in America, do you think, give that very specific, uh, information out to patients, to encourage them to get that three hours or more of vigorous exercise, which is so significant? *[unintelligible]* what percentage, if you had to estimate, guesstimate?

This is my plight: How can you not make those kind of recommendations? Well, I'll tell you how you can't: the system is such, is such where you only have ten minutes with each patient. Right now, as we speak, many of my colleagues out there, you know, they're seeing 40 patients, today, in one day.

Dr. Stengler: Right.

Dr. Espinosa: Do you think you're gonna talk about exercise? No way, that's another five- to ten-minute conversation *[crosstalk]*—

You know, a lot of these doc, doctors I work with are actually healthy and health-conscious, but most are not. I tell you, the amount of times that I see diet Cokes and pretzels all over the—and that's a good diet, diet Coke and pretzels.

Dr. Stengler: Mm—

Dr. Espinosa: Right? So, there's a lot of come, and some, many of them just don't exercise—they don't have the time, they are very busy, all these things. So, if you don't do it, why would you recommend it? You have to do it and live it, to sell it. *[Crosstalk]*

Dr. Espinosa: Now, according to your average urologist—'cause I hear it all the time in my office, when patients come in—there is no science behind supplements for prostate cancer.

Dr. Stengler: So, comment on and take us through some of the key ones you commonly use, and why.

Dr. Espinosa: Let's, let, let me say this. I was on Dr Radio Show, the other day, you know, it's hosted here at NYU *[crosstalk]*—

Dr. Stengler: I'm there quite a bit, and the other day a caller comes in, "Hey, do you know that you're, what you are saying is evidence-based?" And, actually, I was, like, caught off-guard, and I said, "Well, listen—" and right before I was about to answer, uh, the, the other medical doctor said, "Hey, let, let, hold on, I'll answer. Let me say this: What we do is likely less than ten percent of evidence-based." And he, he was honest.

Dr. Stengler: Mm, wow, yeah.

Dr. Espinosa: So, let's just say that it's very—let's start with the premise of, when you look at what's great research, it's very expensive, very arduous to do, very complicated, and, and, and, and nothing is patented, at least with regard to a dietary supplement.

Dr. Stengler: Right.

Dr. Espinosa: Now, having said that, there is absolutely great research, or good enough research, so, for us to at least to act on the proper use and the selected use of dietary supplements.

When you look at things like, um, when you look at selenium, for example, which a lot of men are deficient in it, ironically, when you look at Isomineral, when you look at curcumin—tons of research on curcumin—who's gonna deny that curcumin has benefits, um, if not for, you know, prostate cancer, for all cancers, for, you know, prevention of Alzheimer's, and things like that. Uh, other, like [unintelligible], for example, excellent herb; Vitamin D, Vitamin D3, "Oh, well, listen, I'm outside a lot. Do I need Vitamin D3?" Yeah, you're outside a lot, but you're, you're fully covered, so you're not making, you know, the, the, the, the, the sunrays are not really stimulating enough Vitamin D in your body for it to be, uh, effective and preventative, and, and help your body prevent, um, diseases and prostate cancer. Uh, zinc, another, uh, very important mineral that is actually concentrated in the prostate, uh, and the thymus gland, of course.

Um, so they're just different but modified [unintelligible], in fact, there's a lot of different botanicals, that come from nature, that once we have'em, uh, in a pill form, um, can, can, can enhance the therapeutic effect or the, this idea of creating this microenvironment hostile to prostate cancer. Look, I don't think [unintelligible] I have, I have to say—thank goodness, knock on wood, there's some case reports in the book—I don't think I cure prostate cancer. I never say, "Hey, you know, Dr. Geo cures prostate cancer," I never say that. I help people—I help Mr. Jones, who's walking in with prostate cancer. And by doing so, you are interfering with all the different pathways that, that, uh, that are involved in the development and progression of prostate cancer. I deal with the pathways, right? So what are the path? Reduce inflammation, stimulate the immune system, uh, control blood sugar and insulin production, um—

—prevent against oxidative stress, promote detoxification, Phase 1, particularly Phase 2 detoxification, right? So when the crap comes in, the potential carcinogen that you may not know about, your body should be good enough and strong enough to eliminate it.

Dr. Stengler: Absolutely, that's true, it's multifactorial. And one of the nice things in your book you really stress is that prostate cancer is not a localized cancer. You've gotta look at the body as a whole, because there's a breakdown in the whole body, the whole immune system, or oxidative stress, uh, many other, you know, mechanisms, as mentioned. And so, that's why you have to address the diet, the supplements, the stress, the exercise.

Dr. Espinosa: *[Crosstalk]*

Dr. Stengler: And maybe in that last little segment here, maybe talk about the importance of hormone balance and prostate health. You know, as holistic doctors, we know the hormones are very influential in the prostate, and *[unintelligible]* great things through diet, supplements, help reduce that hormone stimulation of this very hormone-dependent gland.

Dr. Espinosa: —here's the deal: for 60 years it was thought that, "Hey, high testosterone, uh, that ignites prostate cancer, and even makes it worse. So keep your testosterone actually low, particularly as you get older," right? Within the last 10 to 15 years, thanks to, uh, uh, uh, Morgan Tyler from Harvard, and his book, and his work, and his scientific research, thank goodness, we know that, hey, not only is testosterone not a causative effect for prostate cancer, low testosterone actually is involved in, in men getting high-grade or probably deadly prostate cancer. So, low testosterone is not, is not a problem; low testosterone is a problem in terms of men getting or being diagnosed with high-grade disease, right?

So, we have to look at that a little bit differently. Then the other thing is, the testosterone-estrogen ratio. We know that there are receptors for estrogen in the, around the prostate, and much research shows that it's not—forget about high testosterone. Perhaps the imbalance between testosterone and estrogen, where estrogen is so high, that is stimulating the progression, uh, and development of prostate cancer itself. Then we could look at cortisol, right? High cortisol, what does that do? And of course, high cortisol is most, comes from mostly stress. High cortisol, uh, weakness your immune system. A weak immune system is a party for cancer cells in your body, right? It's a party, they have a party.

Dr. Stengler: *[Laughs]*

Dr. Espinosa: Why? There's no police officer going in, and arresting people, and putting people in jail, and killing people, right? So all these hormones, um, testosterone, estrogen, cortisol, they're all involved—in, in many ways, and sometimes not even ways that we think, uh, with regards to the development and progression of prostate cancer.

Dr. Stengler: Excellent. So, *[unintelligible]* in closing, why don't you, given all your years of experience in this field, give the viewers maybe a summary. Uh, and we know you're a truthful guy—a summary of what you see when patients, men with prostate cancer or a history of prostate cancer, incorporate the things you talk about in your book: the diet, the stress reduction, the lifestyle changes, the supplements, all these good types, good types of things. What difference overall do you think it really makes? Is it really obvious to you, in all the men you've seen throughout the years, versus men who just do the old mainstream conventional therapy?

Dr. Espinosa: It's a gamechanger.

Dr. Stengler:	Mm-hmm.
Dr. Espinosa:	It is a gamechanger. Okay, let's say I'm biased. Let's say, "Hey, of course you would say that—this is what you do. Of course." Go into the literature, go into PubMed and say, "Hey, exercise and prostate cancer, uh, diet and prostate cancer, the effects of a low-inflammatory diet and prostate cancer, the effects of a low-glycemic diet and prostate cancer."
	You do that yourself, and once—and here's where the magic is. Because, of course, when you look at the research, it's, "Oh, diet and prostate cancer, oh, exercise and prostate cancer, oh, meditation and prostate cancer." The magic is where you combine all of these things together, and apply it, right?
Dr. Stengler:	Right, synergistic *[crosstalk]*.
Dr. Espinosa:	So, synergistic, that's a gamechanger. What happens is— numerous things. I guess the main thing that—uh, it's just so many things going in my head—the main thing happens is that now the patient is saying this: "Man, thank god for my diagnosis of prostate cancer," and you're looking at them, like, "You're crazy." I'm not, but most people would, "*[unintelligible]* what do you mean? *[unintelligible]* cancer." Well, because of this diagnosis, I'm actually living a healthier life, I'm stronger than ever, I feel sharper than ever, I'm more energetic, I lost 20 pounds, and, you know, and I'm off my cholesterol drugs.
	Because of the diagnosis of prostate cancer, right?
Dr. Stengler:	Mm-hmm.
Dr. Espinosa:	Something that I would've never changed, I would've never made these changes, unless I was diagnosed with this disease.
Dr. Stengler:	A blessing in disguise *[crosstalk]* look at it that way.
Dr. Espinosa:	A blessing *[unintelligible]*, uh, an opportunity to live a much better or your best life. And that's why the subtitle of the book—it wasn't just something that can sell, you know, it was, like, "Hey, no, how can you live your best life, as a result of your diagnosis?" So, that, I think that's the, that's where, uh, certainly where I get my, um, uh,

	where I feel the best is when I—and I see these patients coming back, and not only is their PSA under control, and all these things, but they're saying, "Hey, I, I am, I am living a great life. I mean, I, I'll, I, I tell you, I'm 60 now, I, I'm in better shape than when I was 50."
Dr. Stengler:	Yeah.
Dr. Espinosa:	And that's, that's rewarding.
Dr. Stengler:	Well, this has been phenomenal information, Dr. Geo. And to the viewers out there, the key is: get educated. That's what this series is about. Dr. Espinosa, he's given you great information, Again, his book, which is on the screen, *Thrive—Don't Only Survive! Dr. Geo's Diet to Living Your Best Life Before and After Prostate Cancer.* And, uh, Geo, just before we end, you've got a few different websites—why don't you give those out, and we'll put'em on the screen as well. Again, so, education, people *[unintelligible]* educated, here.
Dr. Espinosa:	Yeah, thank you. So, the main website where you could get anything you want is drgeo.com—that's "geo" with an E, so it's D-R-G-E-O .com.
Dr. Stengler:	Okay, and thank you again—this has been great.
Dr. Espinosa:	My pleasure—anytime, Mark.

HOW ONE DOCTOR CURED HER OWN BREAST CANCER – NATURALLY!

— DR. LISE ALSCHULER —

Dr. Stengler: Hi, everyone. We've got a great interview today. We've got Lise Alschuler. She's a naturopathic doctor with board certification in naturopathic oncology, so that's quite an interesting specialty. She graduated from Brown University with an undergraduate degree in medical anthropology and received a doctoral degree in naturopathic medicine from Bastyr University. She's the past president of the American Association of Naturopathic Physicians and a founding board member and current president of the Oncology Association of Naturopathic physicians. She's also an independent consultant in the area of practitioner and consumer health education. She speaks a lot to lay audiences, to healthcare professionals, doctors all the time.

Dr. Alschuler is also the coauthor of *The Definitive Guide to Cancer*. She cocreated and cohosts a radio show Five to Thrive Life on the—Cancer Support Network about living more healthily in the face of cancer. And she has a very interesting background we're gonna talk about today. She herself is a breast cancer survivor and that what makes her an expert in the integrative treatment of oncology combined with her training of course. And so, Lise, so great to have you today.

Dr. Alschuler:	Yeah, my pleasure. Happy to be here.
Dr. Stengler:	Well you certainly have the credentials to be talking on the subject today, and tell us a bit more about your background. You have extensive training in medicine and naturopathic medicine, but being a breast cancer survivor maybe take us through that, and I presume that had some impact on you getting into this field.
Dr. Alschuler:	Yeah, for sure. I think as you know our training is very comprehensive and we learn how to help people from a very educated place. But that's a whole different thing than going through an experience of an illness yourself. And so even though I had been working with people diagnosed with cancer, as that was my 100-percent focus before I was diagnosed, I had the experience—first of my father being diagnosed with pancreatic cancer and had really the honor of being able to be both his daughter but also his sort of unofficial doctor during his experience and really was able to witness even in that very aggressive cancer how powerful combining natural therapies with integrative therapies when that's done safely can be. He outlived his prognosis of three months. He actually lived 17 months. What was most remarkable about that though was about a year or so into that survivorship we were sitting on a porch in some nice afternoon ray of sun having a cup of green tea and he said, "I just want to thank you because I have felt healthier over this past year than I've felt in the last 20." And he had advanced pancreatic cancer, so that was really powerful to me. And of course, I had more to learn, because then two years after he passed, I was diagnosed with breast cancer.

And because of the kind of cancer it was, I *[laughs]* got to experience surgery and chemotherapy and radiation and tamoxifen. But of course, concurrent with all of that really utilized of course all the things I recommend for my patients from a lifestyle and supplement perspective. And throughout that entire sequence of events, even though I did have some side effects they were covered really well, I always felt like a healthy person with breast cancer, a health person getting radiation, etcetera. So I think that really helped me to understand and experience the power |

of integration, and then of course having had that experience and patients say to me that they can just relate to me a little bit differently because they feel that I know what they're going through.

Dr. Stengler: Right, yeah. Well that's a powerful story. I think it was 2008 you had the breast cancer, was it?

Dr. Alschuler: Yep, so nine years out. Yeah.

Dr. Stengler: Well that brings us into our topic for this segment, and that's breast cancer.

Now obviously it's a huge subject and that's why you've written books on it and have articles and see patients in person. But for our viewers out there, can you maybe walk them through what you think are the most powerful integrative treatments with diet, some of the key supplements, other things you recommend? You know in this series it's all about integrative oncology.

Dr. Alschuler: Mm-hmm.

Dr. Stengler: You know we presume the average person is under the care of an oncologist and has a medical team, and we're trying to provide information on credible things which can enhance their health, help them with the side effects, help their immune system, help with quality of life and of course better outcomes. So maybe take us through that if you would.

Dr. Alschuler: Sure. So I guess let's start with sort of the fundamentals. I think most people come in to me and they say, "What should I eat?" is their first question. And the good news is the answer is very simple and that is to eat a diet that approximates the Mediterranean style of diet, by far the most evidence-based diet for the reduction of risk in association with breast cancer and most cancers actually.

And the Mediterranean diet is not difficult for people to do. It's essentially a plant-based diet. It's unique in that there is minimal meat, although meat is allowed; it's more like a side dish. In the traditional Mediterranean diet, people ate meat from animals grazing on the hillside, so it's really grass-fed meat that's included, lots of fish, lots of olive oil; there's a very important component of the Mediterranean diet. And no processed foods, so it's really a whole plant-based food. If you look across all the diets that have had some studies or some indication of benefit, so we're looking at the Mediterranean diet. We're looking at what's called in the research the prudent diet, which is kind of a proximation of the Mediterranean diet. There's been some studies on low-carb diets, low-fat diets, all that stuff. The only diets that show up in the literature as having any benefit are ones that are plant based, so that's the common denominator.

So I think that is the most important and it makes a lot of sense. When we think about plants, we think about lots of natural colors. Those colors represent flavonoids, and flavonoids are a unique group of compounds that are only found in plant foods and they are very powerful. And they're powerful in terms of cancer because flavonoids reduce the risk of cancer, specifically by being anti-inflammatory. They stimulate cell repair. They support the ability of the immune system to target cancer cells, so they do all the things we need to do to lower the risk of cancer growth. So I think you know if there's nothing else, that's the message from diet.

Dr. Stengler: Yeah, that's great. Like you said, that's something the average person can follow, and I agree with you. I've written about it for years too. I mean just you know put in Google or put in Pub Med and put in Mediterranean diet and you know it'll take you days and days to go through the studies in regard to cancer and heart disease and many other things, so that's great advice.

Dr. Alschuler: And just if I could say one quick thing on that. It's not something to kind of shake your finger at, because there was a study that actually showed that the Mediterranean diet reduced the risk of breast cancer by 44 percent, so that's pretty significant. So it's you know a powerful stretch I would just add.

Dr. Stengler: Absolutely. One last thing on that. Is there any advice you'd give in terms of grains only in that you know the American breads and pastas and stuff tend to be different than what you find over in you know Mediterranean area or Europe and so forth?

Dr. Alschuler: Right.

Dr. Stengler: Is there any particulars on that you advise?

Dr. Alschuler: Yeah, so specific to breast cancer, there's been several studies now that have shown that women who have high levels of insulin and specifically a condition called insulin resistance increase their risk of breast cancer and breast cancer recurrence. And in fact, women who have insulin resistance who are—going through chemotherapy have a worse outcome than women who do not have insulin resistance. So insulin resistance is really, simplistically put, the outcome of eating a diet that has too many refined carbohydrates and saturated fats and not enough whole grain type of fibers and vegetables. So with that being said, I think particularly in relationship to breast cancer, it's very important to keep the consumption of refined carbohydrates, which would be pastas, desserts, breads at a minimum. I don't think they have to be completely avoided unless somebody has some kind of intolerance to grains, but I do think it's really important to keep that at a minimum. You know one just kind of little tidbit on this. In the Mediterranean diet they eat a lot of pasta, but they eat their pasta al dente, which means it's not overcooked. And there's been research that's shown that when you make pasta al dente it doesn't raise blood glucose—as much, really at all interestingly, compared to overcooked pasta. So there's also little things you can do if you just have to have some pasta every once in a while.

Dr. Stengler: Yeah, that's a great tip. And of course, you know there's been some studies on the olive oil seems to have some powerful effects and the omega-3s, so omega-9s, omega-3s. Maybe just comment briefly on that if you would.

Dr. Alschuler: Yeah, the olive oil both for its fatty acids, as you mentioned, which are anti-inflammatory and help to educate the immune system to better target cancer. Olive oil also contains a unique group of flavonoids; they're referred to often as polyphenols. And these polyphenols are very powerful. If you put some of those olive oil polyphenols in a petri dish with some cancer cells, those cancer cells will die, and that's through a process called apoptosis. So these polyphenols help our cells, the injured, mutated kind of cancerous cells, undergo a process of death.

And so if we eat olive oil on a regular basis, then we are encouraging that kind of cleanup, daily cleanup. And in fact, in the Mediterranean diet, people have a container of olive oil on their dining room table and they're just putting it on like we use salt they use olive oil. They just put it on everything.

Dr. Stengler: Yeah, and it's a fair amount of olive oil on kind of a regular basis, much more than people think in terms of a lot of the you know cancer-preventative properties and cardiovascular properties, isn't that correct?

Dr. Alschuler: Right. Yeah, a couple tablespoons a day is what I recommend.

Dr. Stengler: But you know, Mark, if I had to—if I was on a desert island and I could only take one cancer-prevention tool or anti-cancer tool with me, it actually would not be diet, as important as it is. It would be exercise. And I'm a big, big fan of exercise or movement, if exercise is a scary word for people.

The data on the importance of movement, daily movement, is just incredible and particularly for breast cancer. So there's two cancers that actually are the most sensitive to the benefits of exercise, and those two cancers are breast cancer and colon cancer. In some studies, there is a 60-percent reduction of risk for breast cancer in people who regularly exercise. Now the line where we start to see that benefit is about 30 minutes of a moderately-brisk walk five days a week. So that's kind of where we start to see the benefit. But what we now know in the last couple of years, the data has also indicated that yes you get benefit there, maybe about a 25-percent risk reduction, but if you add both time and intensity to the exercise, the benefit increases in almost a linear fashion. So what I really counsel people about—is wherever they're at in terms of their fitness, they want to stay at that edge and keep moving their fitness forward and so that they build their capacity over time, 'cause as you move and exercise more, you gain fitness so then you can do even more. So exercise should always be fun but it should never be easy is kind of the way that that works. And it's so powerful.

Dr. Stengler: Maybe just for the average viewer out there, how would that translate into say walking, something a lot of people can do?

Dr. Alschuler: Mm-hmm. Yeah. So vigorous in terms of walking would be fast walking, or actually jogging. There is another way to kind of get the same benefits without having to do a jog, and that's to do interval training. So if let's say you're going for a 30-minute walk, you can every five minutes, so for a minute, do one minute of walking as fast as you absolutely can.

So you're just motoring it as fast as you can, and then you go back to your moderate pace for four minutes and then you do another minute of brisk. So that sort of inserting intervals conditions the cardiovascular system in a way that almost mimics doing a 30-minute jog.

Dr. Stengler: Yeah, that's great advice. What would be next? What would be the next category you'd want to talk about in terms of integrative treatment for people?

Dr. Alschuler: Yeah. So I know we want to get to supplements but I have to insert stress management in there first.

Dr. Stengler: Oh, absolutely.

Dr. Alschuler: Good. So this is really particular to breast cancer. There's some data now that has found that women who have a poor social network, and a social network is defined not necessarily with lots of friends but having good quality relationships with others. Women who don't have those good quality relationships that now is an independent—risk factor for recurrence, meaning that it is very impactful for breast cancer risk. So and we know now on sort of a mechanistic perspective we know more and more about how stress can lead to cancer, and there are very clear and direct pathways connecting stress with cancer, and particularly breast cancer. So stress management is so important. I kind of describe stress as a thread that unravels the whole sweater of life, and if you pull on that thread too hard, more stress, not good stress management, everything else collapses.

Dr. Stengler: Right.

Dr. Alschuler: So really getting good, quality. You know first being aware of one's stress and then thinking about how it would make sense to each person to manage that stress. Meditation is a tried and tested method. Doing even you know creative work like artwork or engaging in hobbies, spending time with loved ones.

All those things make such a difference and it really needs to be on a daily basis because the impact of stress is relentless and it's cumulative day to day.

Dr. Stengler: Well it's a great point. I mean people get the exercise in order. They're focusing on their diet. That's all good, but if you're not handling the stress properly, it's you know gonna be a major problem in terms of your risk and recovery, so that's very important.

Dr. Alschuler: Yeah, yeah.

Dr. Stengler: Well people always ask about supplements.

Dr. Alschuler: They do.

Dr. Stengler: And I know as doctors like ourselves here we use them. We try to always emphasize to patients you gotta do the core work first, you know the diet and the exercise and the stress reduction and the detoxification. But nevertheless, we do have some good supplements that can be helpful for people, so what do you generally recommend in terms of breast cancer are some of the main ones you think are credible?

Dr. Alschuler: Well I'm gonna start with one of the best-studied substances, so it's melatonin. Melatonin is a hormone that we produce ourselves when we go to sleep. The production is triggered when we have dark at night, and melatonin at that kind of physiological level is very important to maintaining a lot of our functioning throughout our body, including important things like cell repair, immune restoration. And there was a researcher, gosh, about 20 years ago now named Paulo Lissoni in Italy who started to research using melatonin in a much higher dose than we produce ourselves, and his studies have all used 20 milligrams, 20 milligrams, of melatonin at night. And now there's almost, actually now over, 100 clinical studies specifically on melatonin at that dosage range, sometimes it goes down to 10 milligrams, in the context of cancer.

And what we find is that melatonin improves people's outcomes when they get conventional treatment and reduces side effects kind of across the board. With breast cancer specifically, melatonin has been found to have those risk-reducing effects, and melatonin is a natural estrogen inhibitor, so it blocks estrogen receptors, like the action of tamoxifen, not nearly as strong as tamoxifen so it's not a substitute for tamoxifen in any way. It's more like an adjuvant or something you can use to make tamoxifen to work even better. And for people who have finished their tamoxifen, for example these would be for estrogen-receptor-positive breast cancers, melatonin can extend that anti-growth effect. And then too, it helps people get good rest. Rest is really important 'cause it does people to feel very tired so they have to take it at night, and then you know you get all these immune and cell-repair benefits.

So melatonin I think is probably in my top five for sure.

Dr. Stengler: Yeah, it's amazing how much research is on that. And I don't know about your experience but I don't see patients coming in from their oncologist having been recommended melatonin still to this point.

Dr. Alschuler: Yeah, and I don't know why because there was actually a very nice review about a year-and-a-half ago on Medscape, which is a very well-respected kind of web-collection site of research articles that medical doctors read and really extolling the virtues of melatonin. And the conclusion of that review was hey, we should all be recommending this, so I'm not quite sure why it hasn't made its way in it.

Dr. Stengler: Yeah, okay. What would be another one you like, recommend?

Dr. Alschuler: So another one I like is medicinal mushrooms, so I'm saying medicinal mushrooms because of course there are lots of mushrooms out there but there are some that have very potent abilities to stimulate the activity of a particular part of our immune system.

So our immune system is actually quite complex. It's kind of like an orchestra and we have all different you know types of instruments in there and you know having just a really strong immune system would be in this analogy like asking the orchestra to just play louder, and that's not gonna work. So what we really want to do with cancer is figure out what sections of this orchestra need to come up in their volume and how we can coordinate the section with other sections and really make good immune music. So in that sense, what medicinal mushrooms do is they target two populations of cells in our immune system, what are called cytotoxic T-cells and natural killer cells. So you can tell by these names these are potent cells that directly attack cancer cells. And people who have cancer generally have lower activity of both those cell types, the cytotoxic T-cells and the natural killer cells. So when we ingest mushrooms on a regular basis,—we're supporting those direct anti-cancer or cancer-killing cell types. And we can certainly get some of this benefit by eating cooked mushrooms. Mushrooms if they're in your diet should always be cooked. But there's also supplements that concentrate some of the compounds that have this capacity in mushrooms, and when we take these supplements, typically water-extracted mushroom supplements, we can get more polysaccharides, which are what do this in mushrooms. And then we can accentuate that immune-supportive benefit, and that using mushrooms has been shown to improve long-term survival in people that have a diagnosis of breast cancer.

Dr. Stengler: Right. And within that category I presume you're a big fan, I of course have your books and listen to your webinars, so I presume you're a big fan of the Coriolus versicolor, the maitake, maybe some other ones. Would you say those would be your top two picks, the Coriolus, also known as turkey's tail, and the maitake?

Dr. Alschuler: Yeah, I would have to say those are the two that I go to the most, absolutely.

Dr. Stengler:	Right. Well same as me. and interesting to note that in Japan and China they actually can be used as drugs used by oncologists, both IV injection and orally.
Dr. Alschuler:	Mm-hmm, mm-hmm.
Dr. Stengler:	And of course, here in the U.S. we use them orally as dietary supplements, so very well researched.
Dr. Alschuler:	Right, right.
Dr. Stengler:	What would be third on the list? What's your thoughts maybe on fish oil in terms of—
Dr. Alschuler:	Fish oil. Okay, yeah. So fish oil—what's unique about fish oil are the omega-3 fatty acids, EPA and DHA. And these fatty acids are very potent anti-inflammatory agents. And what we know about breast cancer in particular is that the breast cancer tumor will grow—when the environment, the cellular environment, around the tumor cells is basically inflamed. That is called a tumor microenvironment, to shorthand this. And so with that being said, if we can keep the what we call chronic inflammation in our bodies low or somewhat suppressed, then we're less likely to create these tumor microenvironments, which in turn encourage tumor growth. So omega-3 fatty acids being such potent anti-inflammatories really do that. In addition, they also can modulate the immune system to help create a better targeting of cancer cells. And I'm not a fan of big, big doses. You know the research really seems to indicate that when we approximate a dose with what we would get if we ate fish, then we're kind of in the right range. And that's really only about 1 to 2 grams of omega-3 fatty acids a day.
Dr. Stengler:	Okay. Great, great. I think there's some good research too in terms of—the omega-3s and people aren't going to chemotherapy. I'm not sure if that's breast-cancer specific, but just shows there's some good compatibility there.
Dr. Alschuler:	Absolutely, absolutely.
Dr. Stengler:	Excellent. What else is on your mind in terms of supplements? Maybe just one or two more.
Dr. Alschuler:	Mm-hmm. You know I guess I would have to say that I

think it's important just to think really basically about vitamins and either through a multivitamin or as long as that includes sufficient vitamin D. So vitamin D, as I think many people are now aware, is really emerging as an important vitamin that many of us are deficient in. And with deficient vitamin D, we can't have competent immunity. Our cells are much more prone to develop into cancer cells because our cell-repair processes are somewhat crippled or hampered. We're more likely to be insulin resistant. So for breast cancer, vitamin D is really important. And there actually is some data now that even in aggressive—breast cancers like there's a certain subtype of breast cancer that is HER-2 positive. Even in that subtype, vitamin D having sufficient vitamin D levels improves prognosis. So I think vitamin D is particularly important, but then you know vitamins work best in association with other vitamins. So a good-quality multivitamin covers a lot of bases. You're gonna get your B vitamins, your vitamin D. You're gonna get vitamin A, which has some benefit, some basic minerals. You know the key there is good quality, so just in general if you're taking a One-A-Day tablet you're probably not getting much out of it. It's really hard to—you know those tablets are made by compressing everything so tight it's really hard for the body to break it up and to get those vitamins out. So a good-quality multivitamin generally, not 100 percent, but generally is in a capsule form, usually requires more than one a day, and certainly something that you consult with an integrative practitioner to get some guidance on.

But I think that you can get a lot of mileage from just a good-quality vitamin.

Dr. Stengler: Yeah, that's great. Now on the vitamin D, are you—with your patients, are you shooting to get a blood level above 44? A lot of people are starting to get their vitamin D levels tested.

Dr. Alschuler: Right.

Dr. Stengler: You know for the viewers out there, general range is 30 to a certain unit of measurement.

Dr. Alschuler: Yep.

Dr. Stengler: I've seen some good research. Seems to be about 44, 45

	seems to be like the most preventative range, but you're an expert in this area, what do you recommend?
Dr. Alschuler:	Yeah. So you know it's interesting because I think we're still learning a lot about this. Most of the data is actually just when you get sufficient, so when you get above 30, or it used to be 20 then you start to see benefit. There are a few studies that, like you say, indicate there may be a more optimal range, and I try to get my patients to at least 40, and I don't like to see them above 80. I think that there's also some indication now that when you have too much vitamin D you can create some resistance to it.
	So usually between about 40 and 80, and I think your target of 44 is right on the mark.
Dr. Stengler:	Oh okay. Great, great. Well good. Any other comments you have then?
Dr. Alschuler:	I think we've covered a lot. You know I guess I would just say that I think for women with breast cancer and men with breast cancer that there are a lot of options from an integrative perspective available and we've just scratched the surface. And so the main I guess thing I would say about this is this is a really good opportunity for people to avail themselves of an integrative approach not only to help them recover from treatment but to maximize their probability of having a post-cancer-free life.
Dr. Stengler:	Yeah. I think one of the main points, which you've done a great job on with your writings and lectures, this isn't theoretical. We have just a tremendous amount of data, very good scientific data, showing these are powerful integrative therapies.
	And really if someone's just doing conventional treatment only, obviously it can be beneficial, but to not incorporate the kind of things you're talking about with diet and exercise and stress reduction and some of the more well-studied supplements, you're just not getting a comprehensive approach and you're limiting the likelihood of better quality of life and better outcome.
Dr. Alschuler:	Right, exactly. Well said.

Dr. Stengler:	Now, I know you have like a unique website or app we could give to the viewers that could be helpful for them.
Dr. Alschuler:	Yeah. I've written books, as you said, with my coauthor Karolyn Gazella, and together we've created an app called I Thrive, or the I Thrive Plan and it's available at ithriveplan.com. And really what this is about is takes—there's a survey and then with that survey we individualize lifestyle-based recommendations. And all of it is evidence based, so it's based on clinical research. It's matched to each person. It evolves with usage over time.
	And it's really our attempt to make this kind of widely available to people. So yeah, that's ithriveplan.com.
Dr. Stengler:	Wow, that's a great resource. Well, Dr. Alschuler, great information, very credible information, a lot of experience, your own personal you know testimony of how these things can be very powerful and effective. And so we want to thank you for your time and also let the viewers know we have a different video segment with you where we talk about what does science show how we can best manage the aftereffects of conventional treatments like chemotherapy and radiation, surgery. And so we definitely would recommend you know the viewers watch that segment as well. But again, thank you for your time today.
Dr. Alschuler:	Thank you.

KNOWING YOUR CANCER PROFILE

— DR. LEIGH ERIN CONNEALY —

Dr. Stengler: Well, hi, everyone. Welcome back to Outside the Box Cancer Therapies. In this series, we're interviewing, as you know, the experts around the country in integrative oncology, and today is no exception. We have a powerhouse with us, Dr. Connealy, who's got a beautiful practice here in Irvine, California. And, uh, Dr. Connealy, great to have you with us.

Dr. Connealy: Well, thank you, it's a pleasure.

Dr. Stengler: Uh, you've been in medicine how long, now?

Dr. Connealy: Thirty-one years—a long time.

Dr. Stengler: Okay—31 years and going strong.

Dr. Connealy: Yeah, and we're at 42,000 patients, now.

Dr. Stengler: And you have a passion for integrative oncology. Your book, I think it came out a year ago, *The Cancer Revolution: A Groundbreaking Program to Reverse and Prevent Cancer*.

Dr. Connealy: That's right.

Dr. Stengler: But you go through, what I like is you go through all the things people need to do to prevent cancer, to treat cancer. But more than that, uh, there's a lot of books out on this now, but yours gets into the cutting-edge therapies, which really give the, uh, the stronger therapeutic effects, not in a negative way but in a positive way. So, you're a researcher, I mean, you're practicing but you're, you're a researcher, for sure.

Dr. Connealy: Researcher and teacher.

So, I do lecture to doctors and groups, because pa, there are lots of patients that are interested in this. But I also want other doctors to know—there are too many patients, I can't take care of them all, and I want other doctors to know all of their options and all the things they can do. And all the things you gotta think of, and, you know, the body is a tapestry: you gotta, you gotta be addressing every single thing all the time. And so, I want patient, I want, I want, truly want doctors to know—and other practitioners, because I teach health coaches, chiropractors, everything—everybody can add their little bit, and also help someone that might not have been helped from somebody not knowing the knowledge.

Dr. Stengler: Now, of course, conditions, you know, or diseases like cancer, obviously, we do have very specific targeted therapies we only use for cancer.

Dr. Connealy: Absolutely.

Dr. Stengler: But they won't work that well unless you're doing all the other things we're talking about, the foundational things, right?

Dr. Connealy: That's right, yes, you must do all the foundational things. There's no way, even if you go see a conventional oncologist, even if you go see a conventional surgeon—so, if I have a patient who's *[unintelligible]* surgery, I prepare their body for two to four weeks, Mark, before they even have the surgery.

Dr. Stengler: Mm-hmm.

Dr. Connealy: Because why? They're gonna recover immediately if I do that.

Dr. Stengler: Yeah, absolutely.

Dr. Connealy: And I'm gonna be taking care of the cancer before, 'cause what does cancer do to—what does the surgery do to the cancer? It makes the cancer spread and grow. Because the doctor can't see microscopic cells, so he's doing the best job. So, if we're covering the patient with health, and healing, and fighting cancer before they even have surgery, think of all the outcomes we are gonna have.

Dr. Stengler: Well, I tell people there's always a place for integrative medicine, no matter what kind of treatments you're getting, what kind of providers, what kind of illness you have, there's always a place for it. Would you agree with that?

Dr. Connealy: Oh, abs, well, no, that should be your starting place, Mark.

Dr. Stengler: Hm—

Dr. Connealy: Okay, every doctor today should be doing integrative functional medicine. If they're gonna care for the patient, every single doctor.

Dr. Connealy: And why does it take a death sentence like cancer, heart disease, heart attack, why does it take that to wake all of us up?

Dr. Stengler: Right.

Dr. Connealy: Why can't we start early and say health is the most precious asset we have, and we have the information, the tools, the testing, the information, to prevent most diseases that people have.

And we can't listen to journalists who have never seen a patient. What I know is not from medical school; what I know is 31 years, 42,000 patients later. And so, what we now have, but nothing on the news, nothing in *People* magazine, nothing in newspapers, is telling patients that prevention is priceless. We would save lots of hassles. I tell my children, I go, "Look, you need to listen what I tell you to do and what I'd like you to do, because your life directly affects me. And if you become ill, then, not only you're affected, but your entire family system, your employment." So, this is a rippling effect that affects many, many different people—stress, financially, time, energy.

But if we try to preserve the human frame, think of the world we could have.

Dr. Stengler: Well, you know, it's still a small percent of doctors who are thinking like that. Um, are you seeing that changing at all?

Dr. Connealy:	Yes, it's interesting, because I've been practicing 31 years.
Dr. Connealy:	And I've been practicing five or six days a week, a long time—I don't take a lot of vacations, because my hobby is working. I don't knit; I don't shop. *[Laughter]* I like to, I like to work, I love to research.
Dr. Stengler:	Yeah, yeah.
Dr. Connealy:	And I love seeing patients, because I learn so much from the patients.
Dr. Stengler:	Mm-hmm.
Dr. Connealy:	I do see that change, and I'll tell you, if I would've told a patient, "What is the first thing you've changed since your diagnosis of cancer?" they would look at me like, "Well, what do you mean?" But now, every single person, hands-down, now, for about five years, Mark, you know what the first they've done?
Dr. Stengler:	Mm-mm.
Dr. Connealy:	Radically changed their eating, got rid of sugar, got rid of carbs, got rid of dead food, and are eating a plant-based diet and juicing—every single patient.
Dr. Stengler:	One, one of the things we have found, as you would, would hope, as a commonality in interviewing the experts in this series, is if patients don't change their diet—of course, there's many other things that need to be focused on—it's, it's a, it's a major problem; you just can't get the results. Has, has that been your experience?
Dr. Connealy:	Yes, absolutely: you've gotta change your mind, and you have to change what you are putting in your mouth.
Dr. Stengler:	Now, tell us more about the mind, because you—a lot of holistic doctors, obviously, focus on the mind and spirit, or at least, you know, they have it on their website. But you actually, talking to your staff, put a big emphasis on that. Tell us more about that.
Dr. Connealy:	Right, well, what I have learned, also—and this isn't something I started out at all doing in the beginning of my practice—uh, but I realized—I was listening to Thich

Nhat Hanh—on a cassette tape, so that was a long time ago—and he is Vietnam—you probably know him. He's a Vietnamese Buddhist who is, uh, phenomenal at teaching love and compassion.

Dr. Stengler: Mm.

Dr. Connealy: And I was listening to his cassette tape, and he talks about how to turn negative seeds into positive seeds. Because we know, first of all, from the diagnosis alone, that we have seen, now, positive, I mean, PET imaging of the brain, that it's changed from when the patient's diagnosed and when they have resolution of their cancer, that the brain has changed back to its positive state.

Dr. Stengler: Wow.

So, the first thing I have every patient do, Mark—it's mandatory; it's not negotiable—is, they see me.

Dr. Stengler: Mm-hmm.

Dr. Connealy: At the end of the visit, I ask them how do they perceive the stress level in their life. And some of them, most of them cry, and most of them will tell you, "This, this, this, and this. It's my—I'm taking care of my 85-year-old mother. My husband had an affair," or, you know, a multitude of situations. And, and I said, "Well, that emotional stress is just as important as the cancer stress." So, all of my patients see the nutritionist and, to learn the science of food, to really understand the science of food. Not just how to eat, but really understand how every molecule is going to change the cells and how they function. Then, they will see the emotional, because a lot of times, their, patients have the diagnosis; they have outrageous fear.

And fear, you know, is False Evidence Appearing Real. And so, we wanna reframe their diagnosis, and the word "crisis" is danger and opportunity.

Dr. Stengler: Mm-hmm.

Dr. Connealy: This is an opportunity, get the microscope of your life, and say, "Why, where, when, and how did this happen?" We must understand the origin of any diagnosis, which is just a, a label. And I tell patients, "Don't become your label. Do not own your diagnosis. This is a time of health opportunity, for you to learn and master the human mind and body and spirit, and we're going to walk you through this journey." Health is a skill—I can't teach you in a visit, and my team can't teach you in a visit.

Dr. Stengler: And so, that's what I tell the people, 'cause they, uh, they think they need to fix everything today, and I'm, like, "No, from one cancer cell to tumor formation is about 10 or 12 years, depending upon the size."

Dr. Stengler: Mm-hmm.

Dr. Connealy: "And so, this just didn't happen, so we've got to stop the runaway train, turn it around," and I said, "That will take some time." So, uh—

Dr. Stengler: Well, sure, 'cause, like, like you said, you have to address all the different aspects of what's affecting someone's health, like you said, the diet, and the toxins, and the emotions, and the spiritual factors.

Dr. Connealy: The emotions, the hormones.

Dr. Stengler: Uh, your clinic, I mean—let's go over some of the things you have in this clinic.

Dr. Connealy: So, yeah, so, anyways, I know it's a lot, but maybe just walk us through a bit, you know, what makes this place so unique?

Dr. Connealy: Yes, well, yeah, oh, this is unique, first of all, we have an amazing team that is passionate about increasing the health of humanity, one patient at a time. That's number-one.

Dr. Stengler: Mm-hmm.

Dr. Connealy: Number-two, you have to have different modalities, because there is, like we said, no one pill, one modality, one IV, one injection, one vitamin, one herb, one structural judgment.

It's not. It's the body has trillions of cells, influenced daily by everything that we think, eat, drink, do, and put in our body. We don't live in a bubble; we live in the world. So every, when you walk out of here, there's a whole series of bombardments, good and bad, that are happening to you.

Dr. Stengler:	Mm-hmm.
Dr. Connealy:	So, when a patient comes in, we always do a head-to-toe assessment, okay? And so, that will include their entire history, and we do a very, very—because we wanna know what's the status of their mouth, what is, how many surgeries have they had, how many medications are they on. All of that influences how we are properly gonna take care of the patient. And then we or, all of us doctors order a complete panoramic view of your blood, not just a chemistry and a CBC. A chemistry checks liver, kidney function, electrolytes, but I tell people, "That's a snapshot in time."
	Your blood count shows if you're anemic or infection, but it doesn't show cancer. Then you've gotta check people's sugar levels, you gotta make sure they're not prediabetic or diabetic.
Dr. Stengler:	Mm-hmm.
Dr. Connealy:	Then you gotta check their hormones.
Dr. Stengler:	Mm-hmm.
Dr. Connealy:	Then you have to check their adrenals. Then you have to check their Vitamin D levels, you gotta check their inflammatory markers. Then we do a nutrient assessment testing, that checks every vitamin, every mineral, checks your gut, checks your toxins, checks your *[unintelligible]* enzymes, check your heavy metals, checks your antioxidants, checks Omega-3—everything that makes you work. So I tell people, "Today, we don't have to guess. We test and we have the information we need to specifically fix you. If you came in to see me, 'Oh, Mark, just take these vitamins,' 'Well, do I need them?'" No, we specifically ascertain what you to, totally need or don't need.
Dr. Stengler:	We have the technology to do that.
Dr. Connealy:	Yes.
Dr. Stengler:	Why wouldn't you use it? A lot of doctors don't, but—
Dr. Connealy:	Right. And then, I will decide what treatment. So, one treatment, uh, might be ONDAMED.

So, ONDAMED is a device that was designed in Germany, and I got the machine probably 15 years ago. And what it does, you wear a receptor site, uh, uh, around the neck, and then the practitioner feels the pulse and runs through all the electro frequencies and hurts of the patient's body. We know what every electrical frequency is, right? We know everything—everything is dialed in to a, you know, your heart is this, your liver this, your lung this, et cetera, et cetera, et cetera, et cetera.

Dr. Stengler: And, and just, and just for the viewers, I mean, a lot of people just aren't aware our cells communicate by electrical frequencies.

Dr. Connealy: Yes, thank you. Anyway, and so, I will say—so, for example, you may tell me, "Oh, I feel terrible, terrible," and I go, "Well, your bloodwork doesn't show that much, and you need a few little vitamins," "But, Dr. Connealy, I still feel right." So, I will say, "Okay, let's do, let's, uh, do an electrical biochemical assessment of the body, and it will tell me—" and then it corrects the frequencies and balances out the imbalances that you had.

Um, then, I may patient, I may have, have a patient do hyperbaric oxygen. So, hyperbaric oxygen, what is the first thing we need? We need oxygen. We need oxygen to live. We, we, we'll all die without oxygen, right? Within a couple of minutes.

Dr. Stengler: Mm-hmm, mm-hmm.

Dr. Connealy: And so, when patients, the characteristic features of a cancer patient are low oxygen, acidity, and sugary environment. And so, hyperbaric oxygen helps heal wounds, if you have diabetes, it helps cancer patients, 'cause *[unintelligible]* oxygen-rich environment suppresses the activity of a cancer cell.

Dr. Stengler: Mm-hmm.

Dr. Connealy: Uh, it, it, it's very, uh, helpful with people with any kind of infection, because it enriches the oxygen environment so microorganisms don't live.

Dr. Stengler: Mm-hmm.

Dr. Connealy:	Then, um, I may have the patient do PMF, pulsed electromagnetic field. So, that has about 1,000 PubMed studies on it.
	But specifically, here, we use it for pain, or we use it for, to enhance the delivery of IVs, because it actually changes the, the cellular membrane receptivity of every IV that we do.
Dr. Stengler:	Yeah, so, all of a sudden your patient's getting IV and getting that treatment at the same time, yeah.
Dr. Connealy:	Same time. So, all the patients do that either before, during, or after their IV. But also, a lot of'em have pain, and also, a, a cancer cell is a very low energy frequency. So, we are raising the energy frequency of the entire body, when we do the pulsed electromagnetic field. Then we have the nano bath. The nano bath was given to me, uh, by the inventor, and it is basically nano bubbles of oxygen that go through and seep in through the skin—'cause your skin is your largest or, organ in your body, and absorbs it the most, more, absorbs more than your mouth—people don't even realize that. And so, you have this nano bubbles of oxygen going through, and it basically kinda does an oxygen dialysis of your entire body.
	So, it, so, when people have pain, there's decreased oxygen, right? When cancer cells have, uh, uh, patients have cancer, they have low oxygen. So this makes the patients feel significantly better, because of the oxygen, but it's a different delivery system than hyperbaric. Then we have, as you mentioned earlier, we have the chiropractor that does many different things. So, we have chiropractor who does, uh, you know, body adjustments, okay, which is very important. Then, we use a device called the Scenar—S-C-E-N-A-R—and I found that in a United Kingdom publication, and I thought, "Oh, this sounds really interesting." Well, it was designed by the Russians, about 40 years ago, and it's obviously become, uh, you know, more advanced.
Dr. Stengler:	Yeah.
Dr. Connealy:	But it is the most unbelievable little TV remote thing, that basically helps the nervous system, helps the immune sys-

tem, helps restore adrenal gland function, phenomenal for pain, uh, phenomenal for just recalibrating the entire body.

I mean, I've used it on sinus infections; I've used it for many, many, many modalities. And we've only been using that, really, for maybe only ten months, and we're still even learning more about that. Because there's, the, the, the capacity of that is just unbelievable, and a lot of times our patients bring'em home to use at home. Then we have our tranquility room. Our tranquility room has the Biosound, so, a lot of us have never learned how to meditate. And one of the best ways, the easiest way—we talk about popping a pill—there's no better way to meditate than to put some Bose headphones, listen to meditative music—which, that has been studied that shows changes the frequencies of the brain to be like a Zen monk. So, I tell people, "No, you don't have to go, 'Ommm,'" you know?

So, talk about getting the body in the most relaxed peaceful state—it's amazing. Then we have the healing mat that I got from Russia, and what it does—you've heard of orgone energy, right?

Dr. Stengler: Mm-hmm, mm-hmm.

Dr. Connealy: So, all of our [unintelligible], but we are depleted every day, because of the new electrical signals called EMFs. So, the EMFs, from the cell towers to the cell, uh, cell phones, to the iPad, everything, and the light—

Dr. Stengler: The Wi-Fi, all that, yeah.

Dr. Connealy: Everything. So, as you mentioned earlier, we are, as Nikola Tesla said, we are, above all, an electrical being—electrical energetic being.

And so, that is first and foremost, because we know that all of our cells have photonic energy with them—every single cell [crosstalk]—

Dr. Stengler: Couldn't survive without it.

Dr. Connealy: You can't survive without it. So people always have a hard time understanding energy, but it's energy. I always tell people, "When you hug your child, did you feel different?

Yes, you felt different, because there was an energy exchange." And so, um, so, energy, just like I tell people, EKG is energy; it's assessing the electrical energy of our heart. If you do a quantitative EEG, that's a energy quantitative analysis of the brain.

Dr. Connealy: So, this puts, it directs all that energy that's been spattered all about, and puts it, all of the orgone energy, back into the body. And when you go in there, you'll see, when you go in the, you immediately get energy, the, your, your pain your body is gone, and you are very, very, very, very calm, cool, and relaxed.

So, then we have the infrared sauna; the infrared sauna we've had in our clinic for 17 years. Infrared sauna is amazing. We know that sweating is powerful medicine.

Dr. Stengler: Mm-hmm.

Dr. Connealy: People don't understand your fat tissues are a depot for chemicals, and so, even though you might do liver cleansing or some kind of cleansing, even fasting, you're still not getting it out of your fatty tissues.

Dr. Stengler: I tell patients that, you know, they do a three-day cleanse from the health food store, a seven-day cleanse, and I say, "Well, that's great, but you know what, you cannot cleanse all the toxins out of the deep fat tissue in three to seven days."

Dr. Connealy: Correct. So, you need to do—sweating is great. Infrared, people say, "Well, what about just a *[unintelligible]* sauna?" I go, "Well, any kind of sweating is gonna be great— exercise, sauna, dry, wet sauna—but there is nothing like the power of infrared."

Dr. Connealy: We've got lots of IV therapies. I have, well, we've been doing IVs for about 25 years, and, of course, I started out with a very simple little menu, and now I know—so, why would we even do IV? Do you know, if you were really sick and you went to the emergency room, I'd say, "Mark, we have to go on IV, because it's 100 percent to get to your body," right?

Dr. Stengler: Mm-hmm, yeah.

Dr. Connealy: Medicine or no medicine.

Dr. Stengler:	Right.
Dr. Connealy:	But what do they do? They start a line of IV fluids, of salt fluid. Why? Because what is the, what is the liquid that all of our cells bathe in?
	Salt.
Dr. Stengler:	Yeah.
Dr. Connealy:	It's salt fluid, like the ocean.
Dr. Stengler:	Mm-hmm.
Dr. Connealy:	And so, we start that, so because we know that we have 100 percent introduction of something that we want to help you and enhance you. So, we do IV Vitamin C—there's many, many studies about IV Vitamin C killing cancer. Um, there, we do, also, vitamins and minerals, because we all usually need other vitamins and minerals, especially when we're sick. And, and the different thing of taking it orally, when you take an IV, it goes straight to the cell, immediately; it, it bypasses the gastrointestinal tract.
Dr. Stengler:	Mm-hmm.
Dr. Connealy:	So, it is phenomenal at, at a, at immediately making someone feel better.
Dr. Stengler:	Mm-hmm.
Dr. Connealy:	Now, we do IV glutathione, which is your master ant, antioxidant; we do IV phosphatidylcholine. Phosphatidylcholine is the ingredient, each one of your cell membranes, along with the essential fatty acids.
Dr. Stengler:	So, with the cancer, with the patients who have cancer, the IV therapy—uh, as I explain it to patients, it's just, we can get a therapeutic effect in a much shorter period of time. Um, you know, supplements are good—we both use'em—but the IVs just are such a—
Dr. Connealy:	They're powerful.
Dr. Stengler:	—a much stronger therapeutic effect. I mean, with cancer, you've got to get on top of it, I mean, you can't be—

Dr. Connealy:	Right, you've gotta get in front of it.
Dr. Stengler:	I like that term even better.
Dr. Connealy:	Yeah, you have to get in front of the cancer, immediately, and a lot of the patients don't understand that, because when they go to their doctor, their oncologist, or their surgeon, the doctor just says, "Oh, well, just cut it off and get your chemo, and you're gonna be fine." Well, no, that is not how you fix a cancer patient. You don't fix any kind of patient like that, because you must do an integrated approach to any chronic condition, because the patient is so multi-faceted, like we mentioned earlier, that many things—did you change the condition that the patient originally got the cancer? If you didn't change their—the World Health Organization publishes—what is the cause? Lifestyle and diet.
Dr. Stengler:	Right.
Dr. Connealy:	What doctor talks to patients about lifestyle and eating?
Dr. Stengler:	Well, they do, they just say, "Eat healthier," and then, and then your visit's over. *[Laughs]*
Dr. Connealy:	No, no, no, no, they tell you you can eat anything you want, Mark.
Dr. Stengler:	Well, a lot of the oncologists, uh, have said that, that is true.
Dr. Connealy:	Yes, my patients always tell me that their doctor says you can anything. I say, "Well, does that make sense to you?" Does that make sense to anybody? No, it does not make sense. But also, you have to do an examination analysis of their lifestyle: if they work 80 hours a week, that cancer's not gonna, gonna go away. They have got to stop, look, listen, examine how they got there in the first place. So, um, and then, um, one of our doctors talked about IV Salicinium—
Dr. Stengler:	Yes, we talked about that, yeah.
Dr. Connealy:	And we talked about IPT—IPT, we do low-dose chemo, uh, and the only reason we usually use low-dose chemo is because, if we need to shrink tumor burden, chemo helps. But let me make one very important point about that, because chemotherapy, people think, "Okay, we gotta do

chemotherapy, and you're gonna kill the cancer."

Well, people don't understand, from the beginning, that the genetics of every cell, of every cancer cell that you have in your body, is unique—every single one—and they're constantly mutating. Then, when you do chemo testing and chemo sensitivity testing, even if you don't do chemo sensitivity testing—which is not typically done by the doctors of today—there are a few doctors, but not a lot.

Dr. Stengler: Mm-hmm.

Dr. Connealy: But they don't understand that 50 percent of the cancer population is chemo-sensitive and chemo-resistant. So, you are going to miss 50 percent; when you give the chemo, 50 percent of those cancer cells are not gonna be killed because they're resistant. And then, if you look at the efficacy of cancer, the agents, let's say you have three great agents, what are they? Eighty, 81, 82 percent. Nothing is 100 percent.

So that means you can't just rely on chemo, because you have something called chemo, I mean, uh, cancer cell sinensis: they're sleeping, they're, they're, they're in their own, they're, they're silent there. And then, when the chemo's gone, *[snaps]* they grow exponentially and become more virulent, and the cancer stem cells grow more, more virulent. And people don't understand that you, what is the definition of remission and/or cure? The definition, in oncology books today, is your circulating tumor cells are zero. Who is checking circulating tumor cells.

Dr. Stengler: I haven't had any patients come in where they've had that data.

Dr. Connealy: No, it is done in all over, literally, it's done all over the world, even the United States. The laboratories in the United States are not very accurate, yet, but it's being done all over the world. And when the patients tell the, their doctors, "Oh, have you thought about checking—" "Oh, that's all experimental." No, it's not experimental. First of all, there's laboratories all over the world that do it.

And we know what exterminates, terminates, circulating tumor cells: surgery, chemo, and radiation does not kill circulating tumor cells, which is responsible for 95 percent of metastasis. So, if you wanna make sure that cancer is not gonna come back, you've got to measure the circulating tumor cells, assess what natural things, rotate those natural things, because you're playing chess all the time with the cancer cell.

Dr. Stengler: Mm-hmm.

Dr. Connealy: So, you, and remember, these cells are immortal; these are cells that are immortal. So you have got to constantly be negotiating with these guys and outsmarting'em all the time, and like I said, you have to get in front of the cancer, immediately. And that's what I love, is early detection and prevention, which we'll talk about in a minute.

Dr. Stengler: Yeah.

Dr. Connealy: But, but that's why chemo is just one—can, oh, can only be, for any patient, whether you, uh, see a conventional doctor or me, it can only be one facet of the treatment, because you must be addressing the whole body and targeting the cancer cell in many other ways.

Dr. Stengler: You wanna get the best results, so, yeah.

Dr. Connealy: Yes, we're getting the best results, and our patients, as you know, most, a lot of our patients, I'd say 50 percent of our patients, come to us after they've exhausted every avenue in conventional medicine. Which is surgery, chemo, and radiation, and maybe a couple of times.

Dr. Connealy: And I tell them that every single modality that we provide here will not hurt you, only enhance your health and wellbeing.

Dr. Stengler: Mm-hmm.

Dr. Connealy: There are no negative side effects; it's only health enhancement.

Dr. Stengler: And it seems, just in recent years, you're seeing published data from the conventional oncology community on "quality of life" questionnaires and scores. Um, but of course, to us as holistic doctors, I mean, that's of prime importance, yeah.

Dr. Connealy: That is the number-one importance. For example, if a patient has breast cancer, and they're estrogen receptor-positive, there's theoretically given an estrogen blocker. They're

	given tamoxifen if they're premenopausal; they're given Anastrazole postmenopausal.
Dr. Stengler:	Mm-hmm.
Dr. Connealy:	Many patients, I've put it on, put them on it, okay, or their doctor has put them on it, and they tell me, "Dr. Connealy, this is terrible way to live. I ache all over my body, I'm very moody, I'm very anxious, I feel horrible, and I have no energy." So, and I tell them, "Okay, if you feel that bad, it's not worth it."
	Because if you, we know if you're depressed you're more likely to be sick.
Dr. Stengler:	Right.
Dr. Connealy:	So, I find—there are natural estrogen blockers, believe it or not, like Estraderm, like broccoli, like, uh, I use an herb, uh, called myomin. So there are other things that we can do to—again, it's all about learning the entire spectrum. There are some patients that are, can handle Anastrozole, and so, we pick and choose. And I tell people, "We must treat the patient, not the disease."
Dr. Stengler:	Now, were you surprised, coming from the conventional community, originally, then getting into holistic and integrative medicine—
Dr. Connealy:	Yes, integrative.
Dr. Stengler:	—were you, were you somewhat surprised how much more research, in publications and studies, there were on diet and all these natural agents? Of course, we have a lot more, especially the last 10 to 15 years, but were you somewhat shocked? Because obviously, in conventional medical school, you don't get any exposure to that.
Dr. Connealy:	You don't [crosstalk] you have no exposure, whatsoever— that sulfurane, um, helps inhibit cancer cells, or corsatun inhibits cancer cells, or ardemesent, okay?
Dr. Stengler:	Yeah.
Dr. Connealy:	This is all—and like you said, the scientific validation of all of these agents is enormous—enormous—sometimes,

in most ca, a lot of cases, more than in conventional pharmacology. And so, but the, at, the most important thing is, what, what is the good, bad, and the ugly of what we're doing? To each patient.

Dr. Stengler: Mm-hmm.

Dr. Connealy: And natural substances, natural nutrient medicine, does not give you the bad deleterious injurious side effects, like pharmacological intervention.

Dr. Stengler: Right, I always explain to people, at least in, in my view, um, you know, there's a design behind the human body. And so, you have a certain fit between what you find in nature and how it interacts with our cells, kinda like a lock and key, so to speak.

Dr. Connealy: Exactly, exactly. So, so, uh, that is a, a very—but, but the most, the most important thing is people aren't dying because of natural plant interventions, whether it be vitamins, nutrients, or herbs.

And people don't realize, in herbs, there's so much pharmacology in herbs. So, why wouldn't we even try that first, to preserve the quality of the patient? That's our job, right?

Dr. Stengler: Now, you do a great job on testing. Now, of course, that's a whole big field, but let's talk a bit about other ways to assess, uh, people with cancer in terms of tests. Um, of course, you talked about some testing, already—very important.

Dr. Connealy: Right.

Dr. Stengler: Take us a bit through that—I know it, it's a big field, but take us through some of the more important things, if you would.

Dr. Connealy: Right. Okay, so, my whole, uh, mission, now—besides what I said earlier about increasing the health of, of humanity— is, cancer rates, now, are 1 in 2 men and 41 percent of females. It's the largest killer 1 to 85; over 1,600 people die a day, and you never hear about it. How is that possible?

Dr. Connealy: Uh, because they don't want people to know how serious it is, and then, it would create panic and fear.

Dr. Stengler:	Mm-hmm.
Dr. Connealy:	And then, *[unintelligible]* unfortunately, pharmaceuticals control most of the news stations, uh, if not all.
Dr. Stengler:	Yeah, they spend a lot of money and they have a lot of influence.
Dr. Connealy:	And they have a lot of influence. And so, um—
Dr. Stengler:	It would show it's a failure, in a lot of ways, with those kind of stats being out there on a regular basis.
Dr. Connealy:	Yes, well—right.
	Well, conventional medicine has reached its point of no return in chronic illnesses. If there's an emergency, there is the, we have the best.
Dr. Stengler:	Can't beat it, you can't beat it, right, right.
Dr. Connealy:	We can't beat it, okay? The emergency room doctors and the care they provide, it's, uh, phenomenal, best in the world.
Dr. Stengler:	Yeah.
Dr. Connealy:	But the care for chronic illnesses, like cancer, like heart disease, autoimmune disease, Alzheimer's, et cetera, conventional medicine doesn't work, okay? So we must be on the search for finding the best options available, all over the world, not just in the United States, because the world is our oyster. So, now that cancer rates are so high, and now I, we believe that cancer now is going to surpass heart disease, but we can completely, I would say, with over 95 percent, we can prevent cancer, and have early detection, and do something about it.
	But there is no money in that, okay? Because then, because the money is in the diagnosis and treatment.
Dr. Stengler:	Right.
Dr. Connealy:	And so, and nobody really, really, really is talking about this.
Dr. Stengler:	There's kinda lip service to it, but not in reality, it's not—
Dr. Connealy:	And so, of course my whole mission is how not to get cancer.

Dr. Stengler:	Yeah.
Dr. Connealy:	And so, that's, I have researched every single thing how, uh, about that, whether it's in the blood. So, some of the, perfect little indices you can do in your blood, that any doctor can do, whether they're, they're integrative or conventional. There's three tests they can do. Check your Vitamin D, because Vitamin D is a, is a hormone and a vitamin, and it's critical for GcMAF, which is your macrophage activating factor, which plays a very important role in your immune system and prevention of cancer.
	You check your hemoglobin A1C—your hemoglobin A1C is a reflection of your blood sugar over 90 days, but we know the higher your sugar, the higher incidence of cancer. Not only the higher incidence of cancer, but higher incidence and prevalence of aging.
Dr. Stengler:	Yeah, and so many diseases, yeah.
Dr. Connealy:	It's aging, aging, aging—correct.
	[Crosstalk]
Dr. Connealy:	So, every disease, what? Is involved with aging.
Dr. Stengler:	Mm-hmm.
Dr. Connealy:	Then, the CRP—the CRP is the C-reactive protein. Even slight elevations are critical importance. I tell patients, even if it's 1.2, 1.5, I have found cancer. And so, so, people, on the lab it says it's, looks like it's normal; some of the laboratories say 0 to 3.
Dr. Stengler:	Yeah, they have wide ranges, yeah.
Dr. Connealy:	Yeah, wide range. Well, it's, ours says less than 1, okay?
Dr. Stengler:	Right, right.
Dr. Connealy:	And yours probably says less than 1.
Dr. Stengler:	Yeah.
Dr. Connealy:	So, anyway, but the CRP is a nonspecific marker of inflammation.
Dr. Stengler:	Mm-hmm.

Dr. Connealy:	So, that tells me there's a red light on the engine frame, on the frame of your car, okay? And we know we can't put duct tape over that red light. We usually go—we may drive a little bit, but we don't drive too far without, with an engine alert on, light on, right?
Dr. Stengler:	Right.
Dr. Connealy:	We go in to the car dealership, or the car mechanic, to see what is wrong. And what do they do? They run—
Dr. Stengler:	Diagnostics.
Dr. Connealy:	They diagnostics, they do all this testing—they have very sophisticated testing, now, and they go, "Oh, it's this, this, and this."
Dr. Stengler:	Oftentimes, much more expensive than our, our lab tests we do for people.

[Laughter]

Dr. Connealy:	You're right, you're right, very, very good point. But anyway, and so, those three tests anyone can do anywhere, on their own, with a doctor, without a doctor, you can do that. Now, three are some more sophisticated testing that I do; one is called the cancer profile. The cancer profile is a blood test developed by Dr. Schandl, at American Metabolic Laboratories. It checks HCG. HCG is the hormone of pregnancy and the hormone of malignancy.
	So, he does a blood and urine; along with that panel is a blood test called the PHI. The PHI is the enzyme of hypoxia. What is hypoxia? Low oxygen. That exists in all diseases. Then it checks your DHEA, which is your hormone of stress *[unintelligible]* longevity. It checks TSA, which is your thyroid assessment. It checks CEA, which is a nonspecific marker for many cancers. And it checks GGT, which is the most sensitive testing for liver function.
Dr. Stengler:	Mm-hmm.
Dr. Connealy:	So, those give us a picture of maybe there's something maybe not right, not balanced. So, we, we've learned how to interpret that and what the next step is. Now, there used

to be a blood test called the ONCOblot. Now, the ONCO-blot is no longer around—it checked the ENOX2 protein on the cancer cells, and it told what organ. So, that was, I would say it's a pretty good test, probably somewhere between 90, 90 and 95 percent accuracy.

So, now they have something called the IBGENE. The IBGENE is a new test that checks tumor DNA stem cell markers, okay? And so, it's a blood test, very inexpensive; uh, I think it's a couple hundred dollars.

Dr. Stengler: Mm-hmm.

Dr. Connealy: And, and, I never just use one test; I always triple-check everything. Then there's the blood test from Greece, called the circulating tumor cells—the lab is RGCC, which I'm sure you've hear of it—and that will check your circulating tumor cells. So, a person without cancer should not have circulating tumor cells. And they go, "Well, no, everybody gets cancer." Yes, we all have cancer, every single day; that's why we have this amazing immune system that is killing it, uh, second by second.

Dr. Stengler: Yeah.

Dr. Connealy: But circulating tumor cells means there is something going on.

Dr. Stengler: Beyond that, yeah.

Dr. Connealy: So, it appears when something is about a millimeter in size—a millimeter is like a pencil line—it's already releasing circulating tumor cells. And so, that is responsible for 95 percent of metastasis, but that's also used as early detection that there's something going on in the system.

So then, I will put their picture together, right?

Dr. Stengler: Mm-hmm, mm-hmm.

Dr. Connealy: I use ultrasound, MRIs, all kind—

Dr. Stengler: Yeah, [crosstalk] and the standard things, too, sure.

Dr. Connealy: I use the standard of care, too, because I wanna make sure that I'm not missing, so we do all kind of imaging, whether it's breast, abdomen, CTs, MRIs. I do, even do PET scans on my patients; I have to do PET scan all the time. So, and then I do the bioenergetic testing, I've done that for 19 years. So I put this picture together, and then I tell each patient what they need to do. Or sometimes people have nothing, and that's awesome and that's great, and then they know that.

Dr. Stengler: And plus, with all that information, especially preventatively, I'm sure it's a great motivator for the patient, to make the lifestyle changes, and the, the stress and stuff, 'cause they can see objectively there's imbalances going on, and take care of it now or you'll pay for it later.

Dr. Connealy: Right, exactly, you do.

I tell people, "You, you know, there's old, there's a saying that we spend all of our, all of our years acquiring wealth, and then we spend all of our money to get health, when we get sick."

Dr. Stengler: Yeah, a lot of Americans do do that, that is true.

Dr. Connealy: Yeah, and so, we, we have to change that, we, we need to [unintelligible] that our true asset in our life, for themselves and for the world, is true health.

Dr. Stengler: I want people to know, I want people to be given the knowledge. That's why these webinars are so amazing,

But what I do is, I look at the tapestry of the entire system, and say, "Okay, this patient needs this, this, this, this, and this," and we slowly accomplish it. And the patient and I are partners, right?

Dr. Stengler: Yeah.

Dr. Connealy: These patients are coming in with last resort situations, and so, we have to find answers now.

Dr. Stengler: Yeah. Well, in this last part, uh, you, you know, in this series, we're, we're giving people the best truth that we can. So, what I'd like you to do is tell the viewers, just given your background in conventional medicine—and now in integrative medicine, and includes integrative oncology—how effective are these treatments overall? The diet, and the supplements, and the IVs, and the other things, I mean, how do you assess that? Is it a gamechanger, compared to just doing conventional alone? I mean, how would you, what would you tell the viewers out there, uh, as someone who gives, like, uh, an honest assessment? I mean, is this something every person with cancer should be, you know, getting into, assessing? Um—

Dr. Connealy: Every single patient—let's say you don't have cancer. If you don't have cancer, today especially, because 50 percent of our children—about—some people say 25, some people say 35, some people say 50—say that our children suffer from a chronic illness.

So, if they have a chronic illness now, what are they gonna be at 30? So, now, everybody needs to be addressed, correct?

Dr. Stengler: Yeah.

Dr. Connealy: Then, you have the patient who's just 30, or 40, but I have 30-year-old patients with cancer, Mark; I have 40-year-old patients with cancer.

Dr. Stengler: Yeah, we're seeing more of those.

Dr. Connealy: Yes, and so—a lot of them, unfortunately. So that means, really, everyone needs what they call a once-over, once a year, go to a doctor who looks at the broad spectrum of the patient, talks to the patient, makes sure you understand their stresses. If they need somebody to help them with stress, they do that; make sure their blood and their nutritional status is great.

Dr. Stengler: Yeah.

Dr. Connealy: There's, there, the basic rules, they're sleeping—about 50 percent of the population doesn't sleep; sleep causes cancer and heart disease, top two killers. Water—people don't drink water; water: solution to pollution is dilution.

Dr. Stengler: Mm—

Dr. Connealy: Then, they don't move—we have 800 muscles; we need to move. We moved 100 years ago; we don't move now. We've gotta move.

We've gotta teach them how to move, and they're at the computer every day, well, get up every five, every hour, and walk five minutes.

Dr. Stengler: Mm-hmm.

Dr. Connealy: We have to teach the patient how to eat and understand the science of food. Most of the supermarket is dead toxic food, so we can't eat like that. We can't nourish, strengthen, and heal our bodies with dead, toxic food. Then, we have to understand what nuances in the blood that need to be tweaked. Then, if you're over 40, you most likely are going to have a hormonal imbalance. So, what are the hormone problems? Thyroid, pancreas with blood sugar, adrenals in male and females, and then, men testicles, women ovaries. So, we have to make sure all these hormones are working; they work in a orchestra, so—and if your hormones, if you don't have hormones, then, you can't work and function and think everyday.

Dr. Stengler: Right.

Dr. Connealy: So, it's not that difficult, and you could easily create a little assessment—I was listening to the guy who wrote *Abundance*, and I was, like, "Okay, how can we really make healthcare efficient and wonderful?"

And I go, "You know what, I'm gonna create the plan." *[Laughs]* So, because I feel like I, I'm good, after 7 kids, and 31 years, and 42,000 patients, I'm, like, "I know how to streamline. I know, I get that, I'm a multitasker, I know how to, you know, make this a system that can work, that can be affordable." Like you said, it's more expensive to go to your car mechanic than get your body assessed and fixed. And to find out if you have cancer, it's very inexpensive.

Dr. Stengler: So, like you said, it's gotta start with the prevention, at the youngest age you can; prenatal care, even, we're showing, with, um, um—

Dr. Connealy: Exactly, that's—yes.

Dr. Stengler: Yeah, that's, yeah, so, epigenetics, prenatal care can influence for your health the rest of your life, so, absolutely. How about the people that have cancer, though? I mean—

Dr. Connealy:	Okay, so, the people that have cancer, then, I tell patients, "If you have cancer, you must see an integrative practitioner." Whether it's a naturopath, whether it's an acupuncturist, whether it's a medical doctor who schooled— you have to go to school for all this.
Dr. Stengler:	And everyone thinks it's so scientific, and these holistic therapies aren't, but it's, it's a, it's a myth.
Dr. Connealy:	Exactly—it's a myth, exactly, just like the BRCA1 and BRCA2 genes. Okay, that gets so much publication—it is probably a tenth of one percent of the population; over 50 percent of the patients who have BRCA1 and BRCA2 don't even get cancer. And if you'd just eat right, you wouldn't trigger BRCA1 or BRCA2. But it gets so much, and then, people, if it's a breast cancer patient, they just take off the breast. Well, the, the *Lancet* published, said if you do a mastectomy or a lumpectomy, the survivor rate is the same. So, why would you be biologically, anatomically hacking someone's body?
Dr. Stengler:	They don't have the information.
Dr. Stengler:	Mm-hmm. Well, you know, this has been phenomenal information, and I know our viewers will greatly appreciate it. And, of course, you're here in Irvine, California; you've got your center here, which, um, as we've said at the beginning is, wow, it's, um, there's no center like it here in the United States, for sure. So, again, thank you for your time and all you do for all your patients, and the education, and your books, and your newsletters, and your website—and so, we greatly appreciate it.
Dr. Connealy:	Oh, well, thank you, Mark. I appreciate you advancing all of the mission for all of us.

THE IMPORTANCE OF TESTING

— MOLLY FINI —

Dr. Stengler: Hi everyone. I'm here with Molly Fini here at the Cancer Center for Healing, and she's gonna share an interest—interesting perspective on what we call bioenergetic testing. So Molly, good to meet you.

Fini: Nice to meet you too.

Dr. Stengler: And so you work with a lot of cancer patients obviously here at the center.

Fini: Yes. Yes.

Dr. Stengler: And so tell us more about what you do. This is—technology has been around for a while. I've been familiar with it. A lot of colleagues that use it really like it.

Fini: Yes.

Dr. Stengler: Uh, tell us how you're utilizing this technology to help people, you know, preventing and treating cancer.

Fini: Okay. Okay, well we—our idea here is to try to find the underlying reasons of why people maybe have cancer or, you know, the toxins that are in their body—you know, it can be chemicals, parasites, viruses, funguses, pollutions, emotions—that's a big thing, emotions and stress. And so what I do is the biomeridian testing which is a bio, you know, um, energy testing.

Dr. Stengler: Mm-hmm.

Fini:	A patient comes in and I test them. I test the meridians which, um, correlate with all the tissues and organs of their body.
	So I—the first part of the test is I get a baseline. I find out where they're in balance and out of balance. The second part of the test is I explain the bioimmune survey. We call it a bioimmune survey because what we're trying to find out is how strong your immune system is, and I explain to them how important it is to have, you know, a strong immune system because that correlates with wellness, as you know.
Dr. Stengler:	Right.
Fini:	And so, um, you know, I give them the explanation on how important it is that it—their immune system is strong and how cancer or any disease doesn't just like—it's not like one day you just wake up and you have cancer. There's— you know, in theory, there's a—it's a 12-year process, so conventional medicine usually can't pick it up or identify it till it's 8 years in. So we have this invisible area from year zero to year eight that a lot can be going on in your body, and a lot is going on in your body whether it's emotional, whether it's, you know, emotional stress, chemicals, toxins; you know, whatever it could be.
Dr. Stengler:	Right.
Fini:	Whatever suppresses your immune system is gonna effect your body in many ways, and then at that point it gets to be where it might be too late. And it's not that it's too late to correct it, but it's a lot harder when it gets in year 8 through 12 than year 0 through 8.
Dr. Stengler:	Right.
Fini:	And that's why prevention and early detection is so important, and with the bio meridian testing or the bio energetic testing, we're able to see like kind of the invisible, things that the conventional medicine really cannot pick up. And so that's mainly what we do, and that's how I do it, and then I'll find like whatever toxins are in their body, or something— you know, is it a nutrition deficiency? Are they eating foods that's hurting their body? Um, and I test them on, uh, Chinese

herbs to find out—and they're very effective to, um, reverse whatever's going on in their body. And so the first part of the test is the biomeridian to find out where they're in and out of balance, and the second part of the test is testing them on these Chinese herbs that we call *[unintelligible]* to just find out what's going on in their body and if they test positive.

And I don't test for cancer. I test for an overgrowth of abnormal cells. So that's what I'm looking for.

Dr. Stengler: Right, so good point. So I always explain to patients "It's— It's like a more subtle type of testing, like on blood tests and urine tests, these types of things."

Fini: Yes. Yes.

Dr. Stengler: It's like you said, often you can only pick up things when they're already advanced.

Fini: Yes, that's very true, and it is subtle. So it's like if we have, um—you know, we all have like 75 million cancer cells, give or take, and if our immune system's been—is strong, it keeps those into check. But when something that's very subtle—like let's say that everything starts at an emotional or energetic level. That information travels to the meridians, and then that information travels to the nervous system, and then to the cells. So all of that time from the emotional energetic level to the meridians to the nervous system to the cells is a lot of years. The calls are where conventional medicine can start picking things up. So that is the invisible.

Dr. Stengler: Right.

Fini: Okay, so that's what we look at. Does this person have candida? Does this person have fungus, parasites, toxin— you know, are there chemicals in their body? I find things that—chemicals that they got in their body 20 or 30 years ago that's affecting them. So that's the good thing about biomeridian or bio—bioenergetic testing, is we can find these things and then give them—whether it's homeopathics or whatever they need, um—do they need to—a drainage, a purification cleanse, a, you know, detoxifier to get that out of their body and start healing and going through the layers of their body to heal their body.

Dr. Stengler:	Right, so you're using nontoxic therapies to balance the system out so it can work better on its own.
Fini:	Exactly.
Dr. Stengler:	Right.
Fini:	Exactly.
Dr. Stengler:	Now of course here at the center, you guys do the—the regular testing too. You guys do blood tests and conventional tests, and this integrated in with it. That's why it's integrative oncology; not just using one system or the other, but using the two together.
Fini:	Exactly. Right.
Dr. Stengler:	So it's done very responsibly, and it just helps the patients at a deeper level. Is that what you'd say?
Fini:	Yes, I would say, and I see these patients over and over again, and a lot of these patients have gone to just an oncologist, which a lot of these patients do want both, and that's the neat thing about what we do here is we offer everything, and that's what patients love. And so I see these patients over and over, and they get better and better and better because the reports that I give—um, I don't know if you're familiar with homotoxicology, but I can see in their report like from the first time they came to the second to the third time that if they're taking these homeopathics or the—these detoxifiers or cleaning their body out that they're getting better and better, and their scores are going down. You know, so—
Dr. Stengler:	Yeah, you have—you have objective standards to see—
Fini:	We have—we—and we have the—the stats to see it, and the patients get very excited because they look at it and they're like "Oh, all this hard work is paying off. I'm glad that I'm doing this because it doesn't matter what we're doing if I can see on paper that I'm showing that—I mean, I do feel better, but am I really better? But I can see on the results that I am better." And that gets the patients excited.
Dr. Stengler:	Yeah, usually what happens is like with the biomeridian testing—you're telling me this is what you find, you can

see on the testing you do things are improving. Then at some point later on you will see the changes in the regular bloodwork and urine work as well.

Fini: Oh, definitely.

Dr. Stengler: So it goes up a line, so to speak. Yeah.

Fini: It matches. It pretty much matches. Like somebody can come in—even though I'm seeing something before maybe it would show in blood, it pretty much matches how they feel, and when—you're right, after they've come for a few times and we're really healing their body and going down the layers and getting everything out, they'll go to their—and get their bloodwork, and it's like "Oh gosh, the parasites are gone. The candida's gone. All of these things match with the blood."

Dr. Stengler: Yeah, so it seems like you got the subjective symptoms, what the patient feels, which is important, of course.

Fini: Yes, of course.

Dr. Stengler: And then what, uh, your testing shows, which is objective, and that at some point then kinda the regular conventional testing will show the improvements as well, so you can see it down the line.

Dr. Stengler: Yeah, these oncologists see the improvements.

Fini: Uh-huh.

Dr. Stengler: Are you starting to see some of them telling other patients to come into your center to get this benefit because they're seeing it in the patients that are showing up already?

Fini: I see the ones that are open-minded.

Dr. Stengler: Okay.

Fini: Yes, I do.

Dr. Stengler: Yeah, that's the key, right?

Fini: Yes. That's the—that's the key, because if they're willing to be open-minded and seeing "This patient is benefiting from this center and whatever treatment that they're getting" and will be open-minded to it—yes I do see the recommendations, and I do have some patients that have very good relationships with these doctors that they'll listen to them and like "Okay, we'll admit that whatever you're doing there is working because look at your numbers. This is like incredible." So I do see that.

Dr. Stengler: That's great. Do you think we're getting beyond the point where—in years past, I'd often—[unintelligible] patients tell me—you know, they'd speak to an oncologist—

—they're getting improvements with what they're doing with—you know, with natural holistic treatments, and often their oncologists would say "Well, yes, you are doing better. That's good. But you know what, I really don't wanna hear much about it. But you can keep doing what you're doing."

Fini: Yes.

Dr. Stengler: Do you think we're starting to get beyond that point?

Fini: Um, I think—um, I don't know if it's 50/50 yet, but like we're seeing the open-minded ones.

Dr. Stengler: Mm-hmm. Right.

Fini: I do hear that a lot, but I think a few more are starting to say "Whatever you're doing is working. Keep doing it."

Dr. Stengler: Right.

Fini: Because you have to realize that sometimes they're in practices that they have to be careful what they say too.

Dr. Stengler: Right.

Fini: But I think that some of them are becoming more open-minded.

Dr. Stengler: Well, this has been great information. Thank you so much.

Fini: Yes. You're so welcome. It was nice to be and talk—here and talk to you.

Dr. Stengler: Great, thanks.

Fini: You're welcome

PATIENT STORY

— GLENNA G. —

Dr. Stengler: Well, we're here with our popular and friendly patient, Glenna, so good to be with you.

Glenna: Thank you.

Dr. Stengler: And, um, we just want to tell the viewers your story. You know, cancer, unfortunately, is just so common now days.

Glenna: Mm-hmm.

Dr. Stengler: I mean, last 10 years my practice the amount of people coming in just wanting nutritional and holistic supports have sky rocketed.

Glenna: Mm-hmm.

Dr. Stengler: So it's good we can help these people, but, you know, it's sad that almost 50 percent of the population at some point in their lifetime are going to have cancer.

So why don't you, um, walk the viewers through your story. What, what, what you encountered and what you experienced.

Glenna: Mm, well it was, uh, February of 2015 I was diagnosed with Stage III breast cancer.

I had four positive lymph nodes. I had a 5.6 centimeter tumor, so it was quite large. Um, I—the treatment that they recommended was six rounds of chemotherapy followed by surgery and then 33 radiation treatments.

Dr. Stengler:	Wow. Pretty intense, huh?
Glenna:	Pretty intense.
Dr. Stengler:	So at what point did we meet up in that course of treatment?
Glenna:	It was, uh, just after my diagnosis actually. Uh I hadn't had a first treatment yet. Um, so it was in between my diagnosis and my first chemo treatment, which was in March.
Dr. Stengler:	And did a, a friend refer you in, or...?
Glenna:	I did.
Dr. Stengler:	Okay.
Glenna:	You know, actually, it was interesting I had several people that I ran into had referred me.
Dr. Stengler:	Okay, okay. So you came in you already just started treatments and, uh, tell the viewers the kind of things we were, you know, recommending for you.
Glenna:	Well, so when I first came in—
Dr. Stengler:	Mm-hmm.
Glenna:	Um, started with the high dose Vitamin C IV's and I started those. Um, and I proceeded with my second treatment.
	And I, I had minimal side effects of the chemo and it was, it was hard chemo.
Dr. Stengler:	Mm-hmm.
Glenna:	It was some pretty aggressive chemo. Um, I had minimal side effects. After my second chemo treatment, um, I forgot to take the anti-nausea pills and I didn't actually need them, um, after my second chemo treatment all throughout.
Dr. Stengler:	And your, uh, oncology doctors were pretty surprised were they?
Glenna:	They were very surprised.
Dr. Stengler:	Mm-hmm.
Glenna:	And they did ask me—
Dr. Stengler:	Mm-hmm.

Glenna:	You know, what I was doing.
Dr. Stengler:	Mm-hmm.
Glenna:	And I did tell them.
Dr. Stengler:	Mm-hmm.
Glenna:	Um, and, uh, they were very surprised. Very surprised.
Dr. Stengler:	And did you find them supportive, or not really saying one thing or another depending on what you were doing with this integrative treatment?
Glenna:	You know, the—my radiology oncologist was very supportive.
Dr. Stengler:	Mm-hmm.
Glenna:	Uh, my oncologist was supportive, um, asked me to do, uh, the high dose vitamin C maybe three days before and three days after. But otherwise she was more intrigued.
	I have to admit she asked me frequently what I was doing, how I was doing, because I was still working every day. I still exercised every day. And, um, so she was very surprised.
Dr. Stengler:	Yeah. And so you kept going through the courses of treatment.
Glenna:	Mm-hmm.
Dr. Stengler:	You were doing very well and so was the comment just basically not what they typically would see if their patients in terms of side effects?
Glenna:	Oh, absolutely.
Dr. Stengler:	Mm-hmm.
Glenna:	I mean, that was probably the most surprising to them was that I didn't have—with the, with the degree of chemotherapy. Because it was an aggressive cancer I had HER2 positive.
Dr. Stengler:	Mm-hmm, mm-hmm.
Glenna:	So, um, that's what, I think, surprised them the most was that I had so minimal side effects and so they, you know, they did—they were very curious. Uh...

Dr. Stengler:	Now of course we did more than just, you know, intravenous vitamin C.
Glenna:	Sure, sure.
Dr. Stengler:	Maybe tell the viewers a bit about what you're doing for diet and supplements and some of the things like that.
Glenna:	Well the diet, of course, I, I, I juiced.
Dr. Stengler:	Mm-hmm.
Glenna:	I eliminated, uh, dairy and, and meat.
Dr. Stengler:	Mm-hmm.
Glenna:	Um, by choice. Um, and, and then I did supplements, a lot of supplements. Um, turmeric.
Dr. Stengler:	Mm-hmm.
Glenna:	Um, vitamin D, magnesium, adrenal, things like that. And I continue to, actually.
Dr. Stengler:	Yeah, yeah. And so how long's it been now since the first—
Glenna:	Three years.
Dr. Stengler:	Three years, yeah.
Glenna:	Three years.
Dr. Stengler:	And you had a follow up just, what was it, today or yesterday?
Glenna:	This morning.
Dr. Stengler:	This morning!
Glenna:	This morning. I had a follow up this morning.
Dr. Stengler:	Your oncologist and how—
Glenna:	Mm-hmm.
Dr. Stengler:	What was the conversation?
Glenna:	She asked me, um, she said, "So I made a list of all of these supplements that I currently take and she, she said, "Why you're still doing this?" And I said, "I am." And she said, "What else are you doing?" And I said, "I continue to do, uh, Vitamin C IV's monthly and ozone therapy monthly."

	She said, "Whatever it is you're doing I want you to continue to do."
Dr. Stengler:	Yeah, that's great.
Glenna:	So she was very—she's very supportive of it now. Very much so.
Dr. Stengler:	And how is your quality of life? I mean, how would you rate your health now compared to, you know, say three to five years ago?
Glenna:	You know, I feel great.
Dr. Stengler:	Mm-hmm.
Glenna:	I mean, I feel great. I have—I, I listen to people who have gone through chemo and some of their residual side effects continue.
Dr. Stengler:	Mm-hmm.
Glenna:	I have none. I don't have—I, I just have none. And I feel very blessed by that.
Dr. Stengler:	Yeah and you're very active; you work very hard, you work fulltime—
Glenna:	Correct, mm-hmm.
Dr. Stengler:	and you travel, um...
Glenna:	Yeah.
Dr. Stengler:	You're just very busy. Right?
Glenna:	Very busy; run every day. Yeah, very busy.
Dr. Stengler:	Mm-hmm.
Glenna:	And, I just, I feel great!
Dr. Stengler:	That's great, yeah.
Glenna:	I feel great.
Dr. Stengler:	Yeah. Well thank you for sharing your story to everybody.
Glenna:	Absolutely. Yeah, thank you.

PATIENT STORY

— TOM C. —

Dr. Stengler: Well hi everyone. You know, prostate cancer is just so common in men and we're lucky enough to have Tom here, uh, a patient at the clinic, uh, gracious enough to share his story and to give the viewers an idea of what it's like to be involved in, uh, natural cancer therapies.

And, Tom, thank you for coming in.

Tom: You're very welcome.

Dr. Stengler: So maybe tell us the origins. I mean, you got little bit of a story. It's been a number of years before you first had cancer. But take us through kind of the first type of cancer you had and what happened after that.

Tom: Okay. When I was about—about the year 2000 I was in my early '50s and I noticed a lesion in my groin area and, uh, went and had it excised and they didn't think much of it, but then it came back and said that it was a pretty rare form of sarcoma.

And so the surgery that followed there was—actually had four surgeries. Uh—

Dr. Stengler: Mm.

Tom: They said it was not where they gave me chemotherapy or radiation it was just, uh, surgical procedures. And I got through that pretty well and then the oncologist handed me off—this is the typical, uh, natural, uh, medical system that I was following.

Went to a general practitioner and I gave me—he gave me yearly exams and part of the exam, at my age, was a PSA.

Dr. Stengler: Mm-hmm.

Tom: PSA came in and he noticed it started rising and so then he handed me off to a, uh, urologist. I went to the urologist. Uh, he watched it for a while and he says, "Well, why don't we go in and, and do a biopsy on it?

He went in, it was a—my recollection 8-point test.

Dr. Stengler: Mm-hmm.

Tom: Came back one of them, uh, had some, uh, malignancy and it was, um, scored as a Gleason Score of six.

Dr. Stengler: Mm-hmm.

Tom: From there, um, I sort of stumbled. I, honestly, I felt as though the doctor didn't give me a lot of hope and they wanted me to go in immediately and have a, a surgery, have my prostate removed.

I wasn't comfortable with that. A lot of it was because I had had four surgeries. I was pretty gun shy from the scalpel.

Dr. Stengler: Mm-hmm.

Tom: And so I decided to go a different route and I started investigating some things and, uh, going into—I went into a process of cleansing. Uh, and, and et cetera, et cetera, and the—it's been nine years now.

And then recently I saw that you had been working on some things and I contacted you and came down, we set down together, and you've said, "We're going to go on a procedure." And I'm very comfortable with it and that's why I'm here.

Dr. Stengler: Yeah. Yes so you do the intravenous vitamin C, right, and some—?

Tom: Right.

Dr. Stengler: Um, what all—what other treatments are you all doing?

Tom:	I'm doing the, uh, uh, IV—
	Uh, Vitamin C, the glutathione.
Dr. Stengler:	Mm-hmm, mm-hmm.
Tom:	Uh, every other time I'm doing the blood ozone.
Dr. Stengler:	Ozone, yeah.
Tom:	And those are primary the treatments I'm doing. Uh, you also have me on a procedure for the mercury. I don't know if that—
Dr. Stengler:	Oh, yes, the he talks *[unintelligible]* he texted me in *[unintelligible]* and—
Tom:	Right and that was part of the overall testing procedure.
	So that's pretty good. I mean, I feel great.
Dr. Stengler:	Yeah.
Tom:	Uh...
Dr. Stengler:	What kind of, uh, diet or supplements do you incorporate into your regimen?
Tom:	I try to follow—you have me on a, a new procedure. Um, new diet. Uh, I try to avoid, you know, sugars.
Dr. Stengler:	Mm-hmm.
Tom:	Grains, uh, eat a healthy diet. I exercise, I work out with a trainer a couple times a week. Uh, I practice yoga. I meditate. I—we go into systematic, um, cleansing procedures.
Dr. Stengler:	Mm-hmm.
Tom:	And that's primarily it is, is keeping the system clean and healthy and it's—I have no symptoms at all.
	I never had symptoms.
Dr. Stengler:	Yeah. And it's great you got a wife who's very much into natural health too, right?
Tom:	Very much so. Yes, she is.
Dr. Stengler:	So, yeah. And then, so how's your PSA been doing and how are your...?

Tom:	It's been stabilized. It has, it has been stabilized. I'm—I have not gone and had another biopsy or anything like that.
Dr. Stengler:	Right, right. It all seems stable and you're doing well.
Tom:	Everything seems stable. I, I have no symptoms at all.
Dr. Stengler:	So we're about, what, 9, 10 years *[unintelligible]* for diagnosis? So...
Tom:	Almost 10 years, yeah.
Dr. Stengler:	It's great. Well, any, uh, any other advice you'd recommend to the viewers? Just to be proactive, or what would be your recommendation for them?
Tom:	I think that what got me into this procedure here is—and I don't want to knock on anyone, but I felt before I wasn't really given any hope.
Dr. Stengler:	Mm-hmm.
Tom:	I felt that I was put into a system and said that you have to do this, this, this and if you don't your irresponsible. And I just wasn't comfortable with that. And what I really like about this procedure is, uh, uh, you have—you give us hope.
Dr. Stengler:	Mm-hmm.
Tom:	And I know it's my responsibility. I'm not an irresponsible person.
Dr. Stengler:	Mm-hmm.
Tom:	I'm not going to do something that I'm going to jeopardize my health in, in, uh—
Dr. Stengler:	And you still do the labs and make sure you're *[unintelligible]* good in all that, so you're very responsible in that way, so yeah.
Tom:	Oh, absolutely. Very responsible. I do the, do the—uh, systematic lab tests, uh, and, you know, again, uh, I really believe that part of it—I'm going to get out on a limb here, but part of it is, uh, the emotions.

Dr. Stengler:	Mm-hmm.
Tom:	There was a time in my life I had a lot of repressed emotions.
Dr. Stengler:	Mm-hmm.
Tom:	And I do believe that contributed to some of the problems that I had.
Dr. Stengler:	Yeah.
Tom:	And so I been working just systematically getting—healing those things.
Dr. Stengler:	Yeah, mm-hmm.
Tom:	Healing those past wounds and that along with the just keeping cleansing and the, the natural approach I'm very comfortable with it.
Dr. Stengler:	So you just, like, have a kind of a comprehensive, holistic approach. You're addressing the many different factors which influence cellular health and your immune system and all of that. Perfect, yeah.
Tom:	Absolutely. From the—from mental health to emotional health.
Dr. Stengler:	Mm-hmm.
Tom:	Gets—especially getting rid of the blockages.
Dr. Stengler:	Mm-hmm.
Tom:	Uh, so that the systems regular, regular added— In the, you know. Colon regularity.
Dr. Stengler:	Mm-hmm.
Tom:	Uh, just emotional cleansing, et cetera.
Dr. Stengler:	Yeah. Well great. Well you're doing a great job and, uh, thank you for sharing your story to viewers here!
Tom:	Oh, well thank you.
Dr. Stengler:	Yeah, thank you.

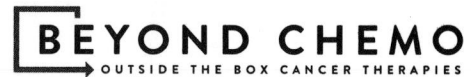

EPISODE 6: HOW TO PREVENT THE CANCER COMEBACK

Your Step-by-Step Guide to Overcoming the Side Effects of Chemo, Avoiding a Recurrence, and Living Cancer-Free for the Rest of Your Life

THE SUPPLEMENT GUIDE TO ELIMINATING CHEMO BRAIN

— DR. LISE ALSCHULER —

Dr. Stengler: Well, hi everyone. We have a very important video segment today, and we're gonna be with, uh, integrative oncology expert, Dr. Lise Alschuler. And she's gonna talk about managing the after-effects of conventional treatments. So, if you're gonna be undergoing, let's say, chemotherapy or radiation, um, and you've already—or you've already had these treatments, what can you do naturally, based on good science, to help heal from these treatments? A lot of people suffer side effects. So, we've got Dr. Alschuler with us again. Great to have you back.

Dr. Alschuler: Thank you. Great to be here.

Dr. Stengler: Of course, you've got great credentials in this, you know, category. Um, you've got board certification in naturopathic oncology. You've been practicing since 1994. As you told us in a different segment, you had cancer yourself.

Dr. Alschuler: Mm-hmm.

Dr. Stengler: And so, you're well-versed with what people go through, which is, you know, very powerful for people. They can resonate with that. Uh, you're still practicing today out of Naturopathic Specialists in Scottsdale, Arizona. You've written some great books on the subject.

Uh, one I wanna recommend to the viewers is the, is *The*

Definitive Guide to Thriving After Cancer, which is exactly what we're talking about today. And, um, you know, the vast majority of people with cancer are getting conventional treatment. And so, in this series, you know, we're just trying to support people to get better outcomes and reduce the side effects. So, um, you've done webinars for doctors on this and public lectures, and so, it's very important to help people to get through these treatments.

Dr. Alschuler: Mm-hmm.

Dr. Stengler: Um, you know, emotional after-effects. Depression and anxiety very common going through these treatments and afterwards. What are some of the more well-studied or credible naturopathic approaches to help people, say, with anxiety and depression as a result of, say, chemotherapy or radiation?

Dr. Alschuler: Yeah, good question, and you're right, very common, uh, for lots of reasons. So, when people have anxiety, uh, after treatment, you know, the first thing I would say is to—if it's serious to get help, of course.

And I think that there's a really good role for, uh, engaging in a therapeutic counseling relationship. Uh, from a naturopathic perspective, in addition to that, there are some ways that we can help, uh, physiologically or biochemically to get peoples' mood kind of back to more stable, uh, a stable place. So, some of the things that, uh, I've found to rely on quite a bit—I'm gonna highlight maybe two of them for—

Dr. Stengler: Okay.

Dr. Alschuler: —particularly, anxiety. So, one is a compound that's extracted from green tea. Unfortunately, you'd have to drink so much green tea to get enough of this compound; you really have to take it as a supplement. But it's called L-theanine, and L-theanine has a unique ability to relieve anxiety and to create what's, uh, often referred to as a relaxed state of mental alertness. So, if you have ever meditated, after meditation, that's exactly how you feel. You're relaxed, you're calm, but you're also very aware and present.

And that's what L-theanine does, and they've actually done

studies to show that when people take L-theanine, their brainwave pattern looks just like the brainwave pattern of somebody who's meditated. So, it definitely affects the brain in that way. Um, you don't need a lot of L-theanine to get this effect. You know, usually, the, the L-theanine supplements are in 200 milligram capsules.

Dr. Stengler: Mm-hmm.

Dr. Alschuler: And I find that, uh, if people take—if they have to take it throughout the day, they can take, like, 200 milligrams in the morning and then another 200 milligrams in the afternoon, and then 400 milligrams at night will help them sleep. That would be a—an example of a regimen. Really, no interactions with medications. A very safe thing for people to take. So, that would be one of my first.

Dr. Stengler: Yep.

Dr. Alschuler: Um, another one that I absolutely love is lavender. Uh, now, lavender essential oil has been long-used in traditional herbalism to relieve anxiety, and it's used in a lot of different ways. So, uh, you can take dried lavender flowers—and put it in a little, uh, sachet, like, made out of thin cloth, and put it in your pillowcase, and so you kind of inhale the aroma as you sleep. And that can really help sleep and anxiety. Uh, people can get this effect from drinking lavender tea, and there's now a dietary supplement available that's been extensively studied in Germany for the most part. It's where it was developed. It's called Silexan WS, and, uh, this is available in this country as an oral—so, it's an oral supplement of lavender essential oil, and over 400 clinical trials, very safe.

No drug interactions, and remarkably effective, even just one or two capsules a day of this lavender extract can be very potent. So, those would be kind of my first from a supplement perspective, go-tos for anxiety.

Dr. Stengler: Excellent. Uh, how about depression? Obviously, that's very, very common. People—

Dr. Alschuler: Mm-hmm.

Dr. Stengler:	You know, diagnosed with cancer or going through the treatments, sometimes that's greatly aggravated just because of the way they feel, you know, emotionally and physically.
Dr. Alschuler:	Yeah, so depression is a little bit more complex because, um, the depression can be the result of an imbalance in neurotransmitters. So, my, my honest answer is that people, from a naturopathic perspective, I think, should get evaluated for—there's some testing we can do—actually, urine testing that we can do to help us see what the neurotransmitter balance is like, and then we can be more specific in our approach.
Dr. Stengler:	Right.
Dr. Alschuler:	Now, having said that, um, you know, it, it, without that, there are some general things. So, the first thing, actually, is exercise. Exercise has been shown to be one of the most effective ways to relieve depression, and so that's foundational.
Dr. Stengler:	Yeah.
Dr. Alschuler:	Um, from a supplement perspective, uh, many people with depression are actually—and especially after treatment—are suffering from amino acid deficiencies, which amino acids are found in proteins. Uh, chemotherapy, radiation are very protein, uh, drawing therapies—so that peoples' amino acid stores can decrease as a result. So, after treatment, sometimes simply repleting good amino acids is, is sufficient. And that can be done pretty easily in a bri- in a, a well-balanced protein powder.
Dr. Stengler:	Hmm.
Dr. Alschuler:	And people can start doing that, um, and that may take care of the issue, actually.
Dr. Stengler:	Absolutely, that's great. Now, one of the big problems people experience, especially with chemotherapy—you know, they call it "chemo brain" so to speak.
Dr. Alschuler:	Mm-hmm.

Dr. Stengler:	Problems with cognitive function, memory, focus, uh—
Dr. Alschuler:	Yep.
Dr. Stengler:	—you've provided some excellent information to doctors about this and in your writings. Uh, please tell the viewers what's going on with that, and some good natural ways to help that.
Dr. Alschuler:	Yeah, this is a big problem and, uh, increasingly recognized as a very clear consequence of both the diagnosis of cancer itself—so, the cancerous process—as well as chemotherapy and radiation therapy can cause this, and even some of the hormonal therapies.
	Um, what we think is happening is that all of these various events are creating inflammation in the brain, which is called neuro-inflammation, and that, uh, neuro-inflammation disrupts the ability of brain cells to work efficiently and communicate with one another. So, there are some, uh, and I should just preface this by saying that, unfortunately, we don't have any good clinical trials for chemo brain, specifically. So, we're translating some of what we know in other, uh, cognitive-deficient issues or, uh, situations and translating it to this, uh, application.
Dr. Stengler:	Right.
Dr. Alschuler:	I would say in my clinical practice, I've seen this to be effective, but that—with that being said—
Dr. Stengler:	Yeah.
Dr. Alschuler:	—um, there are lots of things that we can do to increase something that's call- uh, in the brain called nerve growth factor. Well, when we increase nerve growth factor, we allow or we support the ability of neurons to kind of reorient and re-stretch out and connect with one another. At that same time, we wanna try to reduce the inflammation in the brain.
	And so, we need to do all of that with things that can actually cross into the brain. So, for example, for the—when we go backwards with the inflammation aspect, something as simple as curcumin from turmeric root is a very good way to reduce inflammation in the brain. In fact, going

back to our discussion on depression, there, there's actually been a clinical trial that shows that, uh, curcumin re-reduces depression because depression is another aspect of this neuro-inflammation. Um, so depre- uh, cog- curcumin or turmeric is good.

There's lots of different forms of turmeric. Uh, that can be quite confusing, but generally-speaking, it's important to use a form of turmeric that will get absorbed and go into the brain. So, Theracumin is one branded ingredient that I look for. Uh, another one that will do this nicely is, uh, curcumin in a phytosome form, and that's called Meriva curcumin.

Dr. Stengler: Mm-hmm.

Dr. Alschuler: And then there's another form called BCM-95.

They all work. *[Laughs]*

Dr. Stengler: Yeah.

Dr. Alschuler: Um, and generally, you're looking at of, of those kind of things, you're looking at about—I mean, it's hard to generalize the dose, but, uh, I will anyway.

Dr. Stengler: Yeah.

Dr. Alschuler: So, you're looking for kind of, uh, between a gram and two, uh, two grams a day.

Dr. Stengler: Okay.

Dr. Alschuler: Uh, then the—to stimulate this nerve growth factor, there's some great things we can do. So, uh, just a couple I'll mention. One is, um, a mushroom that's, uh, really a wonderful mushroom called lion's mane mushroom. And this has been studied in people with dementia and—or early dementia, I should say. *[clears throat]* And it's been found to be very helpful in improving their cognition, and uh, this is, uh, two grams of lion's mane mushroom extract, hot water extract.

And I've found this to be very helpful for people with, uh, chemo brain, especially if I use it with another compound called acetylcholine. Acetylcholine is an ingredient that, uh, has—so, it complements, uh, lion's mane because lion mane—lion's mane is gonna increase that nerve growth factor.

And then acetylcholine allows this neurons to communicate better to one another because it raises a necessary—it's a co-factor or it's a building block for some of the chemicals that neurons use to communicate with one another.

Dr. Stengler: Mm-hmm.

Dr. Alschuler: Um, and the nice thing about acetylcholine is that you don't need very much of it, uh, to get a really strong benefit. Even something as little as 400 milligrams is sufficient. So, uh, I really like acetylcholine combined with, uh, lion's mane—

Dr. Stengler: Wow, that's great.

Dr. Alschuler: —as, as a good chemo brain support.

Dr. Alschuler: I missed that dosage. It was 250 milligrams of acetylcholine.

Dr. Stengler: Yeah, great. Yeah, I usually use 250 to 1,000 milligrams depending on the person, and that's—

Dr. Alschuler: Mm-hmm.

Dr. Stengler: —that's a good dose recommendation. And then lastly, peripheral neuropathy, uh, is just a very common side effect.

Dr. Alschuler: Yes.

Dr. Stengler: Uh, what have you found in the research? I know you've written on this clinical path just to be helpful for these people because it's not fun to be having abnormal—

Dr. Alschuler: No.

Dr. Stengler: —nerve sensations in your extremities and numbness and tingling and pain.

So—

Dr. Alschuler: Right.

Dr. Stengler: What are your thoughts on that?

Dr. Alschuler: So, one thing I would say really, honestly, at the beginning is just to go see an integrative practitioner, a naturopathic oncologist who is trained in this because they'll be able to

	go back through your history of treatment and figure out which agent caused that neuropathy and then match that, that sort of history with the best supplement.
Dr. Stengler:	Right.
Dr. Alschuler:	Um, uh, so that being said, generally, across the board, there's some newer data that's found that people who take omega-3 fatty acids from fish oil, uh, have less neuropathy and can heal from neuropathy more, uh, effectively. In addition, actually, people who are deficient in B vitamins, particularly B12, uh, are more likely to have neuropathy. And when their levels are repleted, their neuropathy symptoms can get much less severe, and the same is true for vitamin D. People who are sufficient in vitamin D have less neuropathy.
	So, you know, at a basic level, we're looking at just repleting, uh, or making sufficient omega-3 fatty acids, B vitamins, and vitamin D. And then in addition to that, there are some, uh, sort of more specialized nutrients, which, again, depending on the chemotherapy that was used, can be helpful. So, you know, we could think about L-glutamine if you've had a TAC in chemotherapy, for instance, or, uh, acetyl-L-carnitine if you've had a, a platin chemotherapy. So, you know, we kind of mix and match from there.
Dr. Stengler:	Wow, that's great. So, like you said, you can be very specific, depending what's been causing the problem, the kind of chemotherapy. So, that's taking it to another level. That's really good.
Dr. Alschuler:	Mm-hmm.
Dr. Stengler:	So, in summary, how would you summarize, um, the effectiveness of these integrative treatments, naturopathic treatments in preventing and reducing the side effects of, say, chemotherapy and radiation overall? You find your practice, it's, uh, consistently helpful for people?
Dr. Alschuler:	It, uh, without a doubt.
Dr. Stengler:	Yeah.
Dr. Alschuler:	One hundred percent, yes.

I mean, you know, I, I would go so far as to say that I wish that every single person going through chemotherapy or radiation had the opportunity to utilize integrative natural treatments concurrent with and after those conventional treatments because the recovery is so much more complete. Uh, the risk reduction benefits are there. People actually can regain wellness and even optimize wellness to a level that they didn't even have before the cancer.

So, I mean, it's just so tremendous and, you know, there are, of course, long-term side effects that will take a lot of work to—

Dr. Stengler: Right.

Dr. Alschuler: —to get people back in line. So, I'm not gonna, you know, sort of make this out to be, "Ah, it's easy. Just come in, one treatment; you're done."

Dr. Stengler: Right.

Dr. Alschuler: But, uh, for sure, there's huge, huge benefit from these therapies.

Dr. Stengler: And, of course, you wrote, you wrote a great book on this, *The Definitive Guide to Thriving After Cancer*, where you talked about these types of things. So, that's a great resource for people as well.

Dr. Alschuler: Absolutely. *The Definitive Guide to Thrining-Thriving After Cancer*.

And uh, my co-author, Karolyn Gazella and I who wrote that book, we also developed an app, actually, that's, um, available at iThriveplan.com, which is kind of all of this information individualized. So, uh—

Dr. Stengler: Wow.

Dr. Alschuler: —that's a great resource as well.

Dr. Stengler: Absolutely. Well, thank you again for your time, Dr. Alschuler. I know—

Dr. Alschuler: My pleasure.

Dr. Stengler: —the viewers are gonna be very happy with what they learned today and, um, you know, their knowledge greatly is gonna be increased, and they can work with an integrative doctor, incorporate these therapies and get better.

Dr. Alschuler: Great, absolutely. Well, thanks. It has been my pleasure. Thanks for having me on.

Dr. Stengler: Thank you.

FIGHTING A RECURRENCE

— DR. NASHA WINTERS —

Dr. Stengler: Today, I'll be speaking with Dr. Nasha Winters. She is a visionary and CEO of her own company as well as a best selling author, lecturer, and she has more than 25 years of experience in the healthcare industry. She is a thought leader in personalized precision medicine and Dr. Nasha works to educate clients, doctors, and researchers worldwide in how to apply integrative oncology philosophically and therapeutically. Well welcome, Dr. Winters. Again, it's great to be with you.

Dr. Winters: Thank you so much. This is a joy to be here.

Let me give the, uh, viewers and interesting statistic here. According to the president's cancer panel, only a few hundred of the more than 80,000 chemicals in use in the United States have been tested for safety. They also say many known or suspected carcinogens or cancer causing chemicals are completely unregulated. So you and I both know that in conventional medicine, they just don't address, you know, the concept of detoxification. Um, so let's talk about the carcinogenic effects of, you know, different toxins and why it's just critical in preventing cancer, helping people with cancer, and preventing, you know, relapses in the future.

Dr. Winters: Wonderful. Well, my coauthor, Jess Kelly, does a great presentation when we do our cancer retreats and she basically kind of does a little skit where she shows, "Okay. By the time you get out of bed and through breakfast, you've already pretty much lathered your body with over 20 different—"

You know, ingested or put over 20 different chemicals on your body before you've even left the house for work on average. Okay? So that's coming down to what we're washing our hair with, what we're putting on our skin afterwards, what cosmetics we're putting on, what—what creamer we're putting into our coffee, you know, our—especially if it's like a non-organic or an instant coffee process. Um, what, uh, you know, what room deodorizers we have going on, you know, in the—in the house. You know, just all those things add up. Not to mention the—the fats—what's in our fabric, what's in our furniture, what's in our, um, the new flooring.

You know, I've—I've can't tell you how many times I've seen people have a recurrence or a progression that just did a recent remodel on their house. Um, these chemicals are coming at us every single day and they're invisible. We don't see them. So, you know, I have a perfect example of living in this beautiful place of Durango, Colorado and you look on a map.

People come here, flock to us for the natural outdoor beauty of where we live and yet, a few years ago, our river turned the color of mustard orange when an old gold mining mountain town, uh, 50 miles up North of us basically broke open and flooded millions of gallons of toxic chemicals that were part of the mining process into our river and turned it to this crazy color that made international news. Everyone freaked out even though it had been leaking that, a couple hundred gallons a year for 100 years. But then suddenly when it's, you can see it and there's millions of gallons, now everybody's up in arms and yet, no one wanted to talk about as myself *[unintelligible]* and my colleagues and my community wanted to bring awareness to the water quality for years and when it went orange, we thought, "Okay. It's our chance."

But within a few days as happen, dilution happens, everyone's like back on their rafts. They even had a river parade.

Our governor came and took a drink of water right out of our river. *[Laughs]* You know? We're like, "What?"

We just go into amnesia so quickly when we don't see it. When it's out of sight, it's out of mind.

Dr. Stengler: Yeah.

Dr. Winters: Today, we can't—like she said, those 80,000 chemicals are constantly swarming around us so we have to start taking concerted efforts to lower our exposure to these things every single day. So just like we did a pantry overhaul, you have to start walking around. Open up your—you know, I'm the person who comes to your house and opens up your medicine cabinet and looks under your sinks because I want to be—I wanna feel safe when I'm visiting my family and friends but I want them to have awareness as well.

And so going into your garage, seeing if you've got a—an old bottle of Round Up in there, these are the things that are just—they seem like an—not—like not a big deal but it's the cumulative effect that we're—we're all being crushed under. And we don't know how, let's say, your and my chemistry are very different. We have different fingerprints of who we are. Our threshold is very different. You know? I'm like a canary in the coalmines. Someone smokes a cigarette driving down the road and it makes me immediately nauseous that I smell that.

Other people could just sit in an entire smoke—you know, smoke the cigarette and sit in a nice smoky bar and have no symptoms whatsoever. So we all have our own personal threshold as well as the fact that we're being bathed in it constantly. So we have to start to create some awareness of what we're being exposed to an dhow to mitigate it, how to avoid it, and how to get it out of our bodies.

Dr. Stengler: Right. And you do a great job in your book going through that. Um, it goes back to what you said. If we wanna have healthy mitochondria, healthy inner workings on the cell, we don't want there to be damage occurring, abnormal cell division. These toxins can do it. We know many of them which can and there's many more we don't know about which we'll find out in the future also can create the, um, environment for cancer. But as holistic doctors, one of the beauties we have in our therapies, we have many good tools in helping people to detoxify.

Now, of course, you don't wanna put these things in the first place as you said, um, but when we need to detoxify and there's many different things that can be done—maybe we'll go through some of the basic ones you use and of course, this is important for people who've had treatment for cancer. They've had radiation treatments. They've had one of the many different chemotherapy drugs and so detoxifications even more important for these people.

Dr. Winters: And I think—I'm so glad you said that because you had a vulnerable population to begin with when they got cancer but now, you've added known mitochondrial poisons to the mix which are making those mitochondria even more vulnerable to become more susceptible to DNA damage which then can lead to cancer again. That's why the American Cancer Society states that over 70 percent will have a a recurrence. So that's why. Okay? That's probably the reason why, um, if that. So knowing that even things like Tylenol, they're like, "Oh, I have a little headache. I'm gonna take a Tylenol. Oh, I stubbed my toe. I'm gonna take a Tylenol," Tylenol is one of the biggest mitochondrial poisons out there and it's available over the count—counter.

You know? So we—they think that even it has to be a big hardcore pharmaceutical, um, chemotherapeutic agent but it doesn't have to be.

It can be something as simple as a NSAID. You know, an over the counter, um, Tylenol or an, uh, ibuprofen even has this effect. So when that's coming in, like, so we have to kinda keep taking out there garbage as much as possible. One of the things I hear in most of my cancer patients before, during, and after treatment is they don't sweat or it's very difficult to get them to sweat. And when you look at this beautiful, you know, cloak that we have, our skin, our largest organ of absorption and elimination, it is so important to get that tuned up. That is one of my favorite treatments of detoxification is sweat therapy. Whether it's in a sweat lodge, a sauna, *[unintelligible]* infrared sauna, *[unintelligible]* sauna, a biomat, a jog, sitting in your hot car in Arizona for ten minutes.

[Laughter]

I don't care. You wanna sweat. Um, those are really critical for taking out the garbage. And you wanna drink good water, good quality filtered water. My city water in Durango has seven known carcinogens. You can now put your zip code into the EWG water website and know what's in your water source and then do something about it.

So, you know, you wanna drink good filtered water to flush the tissues. You wanna, you know, just like you would wash a car. You're gonna rinse it down with water afterwards. Same type of thing. And then the other is a—is again one of the best strategies for cleansing is intermittent fasting. And that's where, again, we talked about the autophagy of just giving the body a break. So it's not gonna put all of its attention on digestion but it gets anywhere from a 13 to—to 24 hour break and it just gets to kinda dump out the debris that's in there and start afresh, start anew. That's why we called it breakfast.

Is historically, you know, you finish dinner and you wouldn't theoretically eat again for 13 to 16 hours. Well, most of us are having a late night snack and then we're up in the middle of the night and we're putting something in our mouth the second we get out of bed. We never get that phase of autophagy. So those three simple and free, you know, approaches, um, can be the most impactful and then of course, you said it perfectly.

There's 1 million tools in our toolbox to push it a little more assertively depending on the individual, their vital forces, if they're taking other pharmaceuticals and how to do it delicately. Because I've seen a lot of people cause harm by pushing too hard with detox, um, and if we don't know how their detox pathways work, we can backfire pretty terribly. Again, we don't have to guess anymore as we said early on. We really can be precise an even elegant with this now but those are kinda my three favorite tools that come to mind.

Dr. Stengler: That's excellent. Just a little bit more on the intermittent fasting. Uh, something simple most people can do. If you have cancer, it's very, very important. So an example would be you have an early dinner. Perhaps you, you know, have your dinner around 5:00PM and then just water only until breakfast the next morning. That would be an example you'd use with some of your patients. And as we know, there's been some recent research even on the risk for breast cancer, how you can greatly reduce your risk for breast cancer by just that simple technique.

Dr. Winters: Yeah. Yeah. It's crazy. So the risk of initial but also recurrence by—and they—and the—the study was only for 13 hours. 13 hours. You know? That's why I—I—in talking with other colleagues, that just blows my mind because it—we've become so metabolically inflexible. When I hear someone say, "I can't go the more than two hours without a snack," that is a huge red flag that they are metabolically un—unstable and that their mitochondria are really bogged down and really struggling and really sugar loaded and really sugar burning. That is an absolutely, "Woo," like, little red flag for me. When—when they don't sweat and they can't—and they have to eat every two hours, we're—we either have cancer already on board or it's working really hard to get on board.

Dr. Stengler: Right. And that's been one of the problems, I think, uh, similar to you. In nutritional medicine, there's been this concept for many decades. How people eat every two to three hours ... um, it's not normal. It's not natural. It makes no sense from adaptation. And, um, like you said before, we now know when you—

When you do eat food, you take a lot of energy for digestion and you will create some metabolic toxins. It's just a normal part of digestion, uh, cellular energy production. You will create some toxins. So like you're saying, you're taking that burden off, creating those toxins and the inner cellular changes. Um, if you're eating on a more regular pattern, not, like, so often, the typical, you know, two to

	three times a day kinda thing.
Dr. Winters:	Exactly. Exactly. And then we've ever seen folks like Dr. Longos work and others saying, you know, even a three to five day pass around your chemotherapy will absolutely enhance the efficacy of the therapy while protecting your healthy cells and then my patients who do that don't need the—the preload drugs. They're not needing the dexamethasone or the antihistamine or the antinausea meds because their own body is capable of leaning that out and dealing with that toxic burden of the chemotherapy. So it's so elegant to see that.
Dr. Stengler:	Right. So would you say with your patients, you like to see them, unless there's some health reason why they can't, some uncontrolled diabetes or something like that, uh, a minimal of 24 hours of water fasting minimum before the day of chemotherapy?
	Or what's your typical protocol?
Dr. Winters:	My minimum is to make sure they stopped eating at least at dinner. Um, before—so I like them to have at least a, uh, a 13 to 16 hours window prechemo of nothing—nothing on board but water. Then the day of chemo and if they can tolerate it, go the whole next day. So that's kind of like I try to kinda go for a, uh, a 20, you know, like a 36 to 48 hour fast but even Longo's work is taking people of starting to fast. Let's say you have chemo on Thursday. They're having their last meal on Monday night. They're not eating on Tuesday, Wednesday, day of chemo Thursday, Friday, and then they break the fast on Saturday morning.
	So that's basically a five day fast and that's what his research was shown on. Holy shmoly. Is it powerful for people who can do it? It's much more of psychological, um, process than it is a physical and once people get to that, the first time they do it, they're so empowered, they go and do it again, and again, and again.
	And those who've been, maybe have done the fast and go back to eating something around the time of chemo for whatever reason, they feel worse. They're like, "I felt much

better when I didn't eat." And now, because of Longo's work, they do have the prolong, you know, medi—medical food fasting mimicking diet which, frankly, is a lot of processed crap and even Longo says it's better just to go with water and at the very least, homemade bone broth. Um, but, you know, for those folks who are, uh, par—paralyzed in fear of missing that much food for that long of time, that's a really good strategy for—for many.

Dr. Stengler: Right. Well, we can [*unintelligible*] people just to get some confidence in it, they could pick a, just a day, do some—do a water fast, see how you do, and when it comes time for your chemo, it won't be such a, you know, a scary thing for you.

Dr. Winters: I think that's a really good strategy. Yeah.

Dr. Stengler: Just excellent. So again, Dr. Winters, thank you for all your time in this series and we greatly appreciate it.

Dr. Winters: Thank you so much. And—and be well.

Dr. Stengler: Thank you.

THE KEY TO BALANCING HORMONES

— DR. FRANK SHALLENBERGER —

Dr. Stengler: Well, hi, everyone. Welcome back to *Outside-the-Box Cancer Therapies*, in this series with all the different experts from around the country in terms of helping people treat cancer with integrative medicine, to recover from cancer, to prevent cancer. And today, I have Dr. Frank Shallenberger. He's been in practice for 45 years, and we're gonna address a very important topic, one that a lot of doctors, especially oncologists, don't address, and that's the issue of imbalanced stress hormones, which relate to your adrenal glands, as well as an imbalanced thyroid.

And these kinds of problems often occur long before people have cancer, which compromises their immune system or quality of life, and especially after people have had cancer treatments—chemotherapy, radiation, surgery—all the emotional stress with these types of things. So Dr. Shallenberger, thanks for coming on the series again.

Dr. Shallenberger: Okay. Great.

Dr. Stengler: And you're an expert in hormone balance.

In your newsletter, *Second Opinion*, you write

about this quite a bit. Let's talk about the adrenal glands and the effects of stress hormone imbalance on the immune system and all the things we're talking about today.

Dr. Shallenberger: Well, let me just start off this way and say that when I do lectures to doctors, and I'm talking to them about how they would diagnose whether their patients have adrenal insufficiency, I put the question, "How do you diagnose when the patient has adrenal insufficiency?" and the answer is, "They're in your office," because if their adrenal—the point is that when we get stressed out from an illness or whatever it is that is stressing us, as long as our adrenals can pump out the hormones, these hormones keep things steady. They keep us feeling pretty good.

It's when the adrenal gland gets exhausted, it can't pump out these hormones anymore, that things start to unravel, start to fall apart, and then we say, "Okay, it's time to go see the doctor now."

Dr. Stengler: Yeah.

Dr. Shallenberger: So realistically, most of—pretty much every patient that I'm gonna see that is challenged with a chronic condition, whether—especially chronic pain, but chronic—it could be something relatively minor like chronic insomnia, for example, or it could be major like cancer, but they almost always have adrenal insufficiency. They're almost always overburdened.

Dr. Stengler: Give us some of the classic symptoms for the viewers.

Dr. Shallenberger: Yeah—so first thing I wanna say is that blood tests, urine tests, saliva tests, whatever, are notoriously inaccurate in diagnosing these conditions. So this is—the best—the thing I found out is the best way to diagnose it is clinically. How is the patient feeling? The hallmark is exhaustion. So if you tell me, "Frank, my energy is pretty much good all day. I don't have a problem. I don't need coffee. I don't need anything. I'm pretty much okay." Especially in the afternoon, your energy level is holding up, I'm thinking your adrenal must be working pretty well. But that's not the case for most people.

You ask them, "How is your energy holding up?" That's the chief complaint, you know, everybody says, "Oh, I get tired." The hallmark of adrenal insufficiency is tiredness in the afternoon or even just symptoms in the afternoon, like, "I get my headache in the afternoon." "My back starts acting up in the afternoon." "My brain doesn't quite work right in the afternoon." Anything in the afternoon is kind of a hallmark.

Now, when it gets really bad, it's in the morning as well. But people will tell you, "Yeah, you know, I first started feeling tired and rundown in the afternoon. I'd have to go get a cup of coffee," or, "I'd have to really force it," and that's your classic example.

Dr. Stengler: And so someone who's going through cancer therapy, obviously—I mean, virtually 100 percent are gonna have some degree of problem with that—yeah.

Dr. Shallenberger: Exactly! Well, I had a woman come in the other day. She has had a couple rounds of conventional chemotherapy, and she's got an ovarian cancer. She came in, and her chief complaint is tiredness and fatigue.

She's too tired to get up and get around. Her last chemo was maybe five weeks ago. She's just adrenally exhausted. We gave her adrenal treatment, and in three or four days she's feeling lots better, and it had nothing to do with the cancer, per se. It just—this condition had worn her out.

Dr. Stengler: Yeah. So what kind of things do you like to use? Obviously, you're an expert in integrative medicine. You like to use nutrition and supplements and natural hormones. What kind of things do you find help your patients?

Dr. Shallenberger: Well, with adrenal, from a dietary perspective, you really wanna watch the stimulants carefully. Now, they can have a cup of coffee. They can have a little bit of stimulants, but they tend to overdo it. So you want to eliminate any excess stimulants. You wanna make sure that—typically, you wanna make sure they get a good, big breakfast—a good, very substantial breakfast. That sets the tone for the rest of the day. Many people—

Dr. Stengler: They've done studies on that.

Dr. Shallenberger: Yeah, and many people that are adrenally insufficient, for some reason, they choose to skip breakfast, which is not the best idea.

Then from an herbal perspective, I like licorice. Licorice works great. I like pantothenic acid. I like vitamin C. These are very powerful nutrients that can improve the way your adrenal works. And then we give the major adrenal hormones. There's two major adrenal hormones: hydrocortisone and DHEA. And we give those—give those—hydrocortisone and DHEA—to the patient along with the licorice, and it's three, four days—I mean, that's one way to make your diagnosis.

If the patient is tired, and you give them hydrocortisone, DHEA and licorice, and three days later they're not feeling a heck of a lot better, you probably missed your diagnosis. Maybe something else is going on.

Dr. Stengler: Yeah—very good.

Dr. Shallenberger: It works that fast.

Dr. Stengler: It's like a therapeutic trial.

Dr. Shallenberger: Yeah.

Dr. Stengler: You get to see—very good. So that's excellent. Now, there's also a big connection between stress and thyroid function and adrenal function and thyroid function. Talk to the viewers about how common it is, especially again with people under chronic stress and cancer and other illnesses, they start having thyroid problems.

Dr. Shallenberger: Hypothyroidism, low thyroid function, is the single-most undiagnosed condition in the United States, if not the world.

And the reason is because we're not using the right tests. In the old days—and I'm talking pre-'60s. We used metabolic functions—we used metabolic testing to determine what's going on with the patient's thyroid because thyroid regulates metabolism. If your metabolic rate is low, you need thyroid. If it's not—how much thyroid do you need? You need enough thyroid to bring your metabolic rate up to what it ought to be.

Then along came the '60s, came these blood tests, and doctors are trained to use them. I was trained when I went to medical school to diagnose low thyroid conditions with blood tests, and it's just inaccurate for most people.

Dr. Stengler: It's just very ballpark-ish, would you say?

Dr. Shallenberger: I wouldn't even say it's that good. I'd say probably there's a one-in-ten chance that the thyroid blood test will actually determine a low metabolic rate sort of hypothyroidism.

Dr. Stengler: And that's why the women and the men get frustrated. They've been to their conventional doctor. They got fatigue. They're chilly. They're gaining weight. They got poor cognitive function and said, "Well, my doctor ran some thyroid tests, and he said it's just—it's really good. But I have all these symptoms." I mean, you hear it every day in practice, but—

Dr. Shallenberger: Yeah, so if you actually check their metabolic rate, you'll find out they're low, and you can give them some thyroid.

Dr. Stengler: Now, you're unique in that.

Dr. Shallenberger: Yeah.

Dr. Stengler:	You wanna briefly just review how you do that?
Dr. Shallenberger:	Sure, sure—the technical term is "indirect calorimetry." That's the fancy name. What it amounts to is we check how your body is using oxygen. So we basically put a mask on, kind of like a SCUBA mask. As you're breathing through this device, we're measuring how you use oxygen. That determines your metabolism. So if you have an efficient metabolism, you're gonna use oxygen to a higher level.
	If you have an inefficient metabolism, you're gonna use it at the lower level. So by measuring the oxygen and what you're doing over time with the oxygen, I can tell you what your metabolism is. And what I've learned is—it's remarkable. Two things just stand out. One of those is that nine out of ten times, when the metabolic rate is incredibly depressed, the blood tests are totally normal. The other thing is when I go to the literature and I search the literature and I try to find somebody somewhere that has published a paper that shows some correlation between the blood tests and metabolism—
Dr. Stengler:	They don't exist or—
Dr. Shallenberger:	Sixty years of medicine, it's never been done. Nobody's actually tried to correlate these two, which is why doctors keep—continue to rely on this inaccurate way to diagnose the condition.
Dr. Stengler:	And you think part of the problem is there's probably just certain things you can't measure, of course, with a blood test.
	If you're measuring hormones circulating around the blood—but it's what attaches to the cell and gets—
Dr. Shallenberger:	There's so many other factors.
Dr. Stengler:	—affects the cell and—and other factors there.
Dr. Shallenberger:	Yeah, not to mention receptor sites, not to remember liver clearance, and enzymes like the iodinoase. There's so many other factors that come into play.

Dr. Stengler:	Right, right—so what kind of things do you use with your patients then, because this low thyroid is so common, which also, by the way, if you've got cancer affects your immune system?
Dr. Shallenberger:	Yeah, you know, one of the things that Max Gerson, who's very famous and published the book on 50 successful cases cured of cancer, no chemo, no radiation, nothing: just with his diet. One of the things he did, he gave everybody iodine. He gave everybody thyroid just across the board. And so when you stop and think about that, you start to realize at an early—just clinically, he understood that these people are—these people are hypothyroid. If you get cancer, you're probably hypothyroid. And if—and again, thyroid is what's driving the mitochondria.
	I don't think people appreciate how determinant to your mitochondrial function the thyroid is. It's probably the single-most important thing that's gonna determine your number of mitochondria and the ability for them to function, is your thyroid hormone levels. If you don't have them adequately, there's gonna be some problems.
Dr. Stengler:	Right—in terms of cancer, of course, there's this term being used a lot now, although it's been around for many decades: the Metabolic Theory.
Dr. Shallenberger:	Yes.
Dr. Stengler:	Like Warburg talked about.
Dr. Shallenberger:	Yeah.
Dr. Stengler:	And so how your mitochondria health is, like you said, influences kind of the environment of the cells and whether cancer cells can thrive better and all that. And like you said, the thyroid has a direct effect on that that important energy factory called the mitochondria.
Dr. Shallenberger:	Very definitely.

Dr. Stengler:	I've seen other studies where just giving thyroid you can see tremendous increases in just hours in white blood cell count.
Dr. Shallenberger:	Oh, yeah! It's just—it's so fundamental. These are one of those things that's fundamental, and fundamental things are like the foundation of a house.
	If you don't have that down, you're gonna have problems.
Dr. Stengler:	So with your patients, just in general, of course, especially the patients who have been through cancer or have cancer, I mean, really as part of the protocol, their adrenal glands and their thyroid, which we're talking about today, it just needs to be addressed.
Dr. Shallenberger:	If you don't address it, the quality of life isn't there. The patients don't feel as well. And they're probably not gonna get as good a result as they would have if you address it.
Dr. Stengler:	Right—and maybe just a few words on bioidentical thyroid. What's your experience with that, and there's a certain percent of patients you like to use the bioidentical thyroid with?
Dr. Shallenberger:	Mostly that's what I do, is I use bioidentical thyroid. Now, the thing is that everybody—I've found that everybody is different. And so, you know, for the listeners, we have T4, and we have T3, and actually there's something called T2. But primarily, most doctors are focused on T3 and T4.
	But the ratio of those two things is important to certain people. We typically will use a 4-to-1 ratio, T4 to T3. But for some people, a 3-to-1 ratio, a 2-to-2 ratio is gonna be a better ratio for them. So you have to be willing to actually look at their metabolic rates. If you give them a 4-to-1 ratio, and you're giving them a fairly substantial amount of the bioidentical thyroid, and you're not seeing their metabolism come up correspondingly, you've probably got the wrong ratio.

So now you've gotta go—this is where the blood test can actually be helpful in looking at those ratios.

Dr. Stengler: Well, in summary, there you've heard it, people. Adrenal problems, thyroid problems—problems just in the general population, but if you have cancer there's gonna be issues going on there. You need a good integrative doctor like Dr. Shallenberger to help you get these things balanced out. So Dr. Shallenberger, excellent information as always. Thank you.

Dr. Shallenberger: Yeah, thanks, Mark.

POST SURGERY REBUILD

— DR. MARK LABEAU —

Dr. Stengler: Hi, everyone. Welcome back to Outside the Box Cancer Therapies. And I'm here with Dr. LaBeau, who practice with me at the—at our clinic here in Encinitas, California and we have a very important topic we're going to cover, a unique topic, and that is the relationship between the structure of the human body and the functioning of the immune system for those of you trying to prevent cancer, are undergoing cancer treatment, uh, and so it's kind of a unique relationship between this and so Dr. LaBeau, thank you for coming on the program.

So why don't we start off talking about your background. You're an osteopathic doctor. Lot of viewers know what that is and some don't and I know we always get used to explaining what we do and how we've been trained, but give us a little bit of background as an osteopathic doctor: how you've been trained and... um, what's the difference between that and a medical doctor and how many years you've been practicing.

Dr. LaBeau: So as far as training: Same basic license as an MD, but we get additional training in physical medicine as a chiropractic physician, or a physical therapist.

Um, part of the, uh, difference, though, is, as far as our approach, as far as musculoskeletal medicine, is we're not looking at it just for treating back pain, we're looking at it for optimizing blood and nerve circulation.

	Um, lymphatic circulation which particularly applies to working with patients with cancer. Um, the, uh, I've been practicing for over 30 years.
Dr. Stengler:	Yeah.
Dr. LaBeau:	With 10 of those years being—working primarily with patients with, uh, cancer and, uh, uh, auto-immune type problems.
Dr. Stengler:	Mm-hmm. Yeah, you've had good experience in the field of cancer. Let's talk to the viewers a bit about their relationship between the structure of the body. You know, we've got the spine and the muscles and lymphatic systems all interconnected and of course this all affects the immune system. People are familiar with chiropractic, but let's talk about, uh, from the osteopathic viewpoint how this all interconnects and why It's so important.
Dr. LaBeau:	Well, part of the interconnection is, one of the things I've noticed over the years when I was working with the patients at, at the, oh, with cancer patients is that many of those patients had, um, history of trauma and some musculoskeletal injury before, either at the site of cancer, or at some key immune junction.
Dr. Stengler:	Mm-hmm and so people are somewhat surprised to find out, you know, depending on how the structure of the spine is and the m muscles; this affects the lymphatics and lymphatics are very important part of our immune system. Talk a bit more about that.
Dr. LaBeau:	Well, lymphatics are definitely a part, big part, of the immune system. You're, you're going to get large amounts of lymphatics in the shoulder area, chest area, and the groin area, so, uh, that's good in terms of it's spread out throughout the body to go and help as an early warning system and attack, uh, areas that are foreign, uh, infections and the like.
Dr. Stengler:	Mm-hmm.
Dr. LaBeau:	Uh, go after cancer, early cancer cells, uh, but on the negative side it can be overrun if there's local cancer and it can use those same viaducts to go and spread throughout the body.

Dr. Stengler:	Right. So as, as an osteopathic doctor what kind of things do you do to optimize the lymphatic system? I mean, you're working with, honestly, the spine and the muscles. Tell the viewers a bit more about how you, you know, help to improve lymphatic function.
Dr. LaBeau:	Well, I think it's helpful to understand, uh, circulation from a slightly—from a slightly different osteopathic perspective.
Dr. Stengler:	Mm.
Dr. LaBeau:	Commonly we think of circulation as the arterial blood going to the organs and the venous blood bringing it back, but that's really only part of the story.
	The arterial blood is definitely going to the organs, but on the return is a combination of venous and lymphatic circulation, so all—so the lymphatic circulation I look at it sort of like the venous circulation is like the highways and the lymphatic circulation is sort of going through the side streets and, and getting some of the delivery to the houses and homes or the individual cells in the body—case of the body.
	So, everything has to return back to the heart. So that part of circulation is, is vitally important.
Dr. Stengler:	Right. So, people who've had a history of cancer, or have cancer, um, they've heard of lymphatics, but again, you can't have an optimally functioning immune system if you have lymphatic problems. Do you like the term lymphatic congestion, and what's all happening with that concept?
Dr. LaBeau:	Well, part of our training is to look at areas that are, um, having either inflammation or areas that are restricted—and with that is you're going to have restriction of blood, nerve supply, and lymphatics.
Dr. Stengler:	Right.
Dr. LaBeau:	So that's part of the key aspect is looking at the underlying aspects. So, when, when I'm working with a patient with cancer I'm looking at any predisposing factors that might, um, oh, diminish lymphatic circulation and, uh, diminish overall healing them.

Dr. Stengler: And what were some of those things be obviously structural component, which we're going to talk more about, uh, maybe things like toxins, nutritional stash, you find that affects the lymphatics quite directly.

Dr. LaBeau: Well that, that's, you know, when I—and from an osteopathic perspective we're trained to look at the whole body, so you're right.

Dr. Stengler: Right.

Dr. LaBeau: So, part of the therapeutic approach is to do testing to evaluate for causes of what we're finding—what I'm, what I'm finding structurally.

Dr. Stengler: Right and then what's, uh, for the viewers, what's the connection between, let's say, having, you know, spinal misalignments, chiropractors call them, you know, subluxations.

Uh, problems with the spine and in terms of interfering with proper nerve flow, you know, to the organs. That all affects the immune system and how the body functions, too.

Dr. LaBeau: Well, anatomically by the nature of the beast, nerves and, uh, blood vessels are protected by being adjacent to the bony structure. So that's good in one sense, but if the bony structure is significantly out of line then that same protection lands it impeding this—the very circulation. So that's, that's why the spine is really one of the conduit areas and one of the prime areas to look for, for any imbalances.

Dr. Stengler: And its seems like just in medicine in general, um, especially in the terms of cancer, it's just not an area oncologists really look at. You don't hear much about oncologists recommending the patients, you know, uh, get a spinal-muscular assessment, you know, for improving lymphatic flow, nerve flow, and better immunity. You just don't find that happening. Has that been your experience?

Dr. LaBeau: Well, a part of the challenge, I think, in, in medicine, and oncology certainly is really the, uh, probably the best example for that, but in medicine in general the focus is often more disease and symptom, uh, focus rather than patient focused.

And I think that's one of the first things that I noticed in approaching patients form an osteopathic perspective; we're encouraged to look at the patient that has the disease, not the disease that happens to be layered on top of the patient.

Uh, so that, that patient focused approach is, is, I think, part of the key.

Dr. Stengler: Absolutely. What are some of the treatments, um, you would use with patients? Say maybe someone has a history of cancer, they got cancer, and you're, you know, one of the things, you know, your treatments are good for, besides helping the immune system, is just people in discomfort and pain.

Dr. LaBeau: Yes.

Dr. Stengler: Um, talk more about that.

Dr. LaBeau: Well, some of the pain is going to be from the cancer itself and it was one of the intriguing questions I looked into before, uh, as I was looking to transition and work primarily with cancer patients, because I pulled, uh, from some of the research, because I was in an academic, uh, environment prior to coming here to California.

And so, I asked my other colleagues I says, "Well, what was your thoughts as far as the role of physical medicine with patients for oncology?" And it really was, I found, greatly unknown.

Dr. Stengler: Yeah.

Dr. LaBeau: So, I basically took a, uh, logical approach that as long as any of the therapy I did was no more, um, vigorous than their daily activity I was going to do no more harm than their daily activity.

Dr. Stengler: Mm.

Dr. LaBeau: So that was, that was sort of the problem-solving approach as far as dosage in therapy. Because one of the things that I've always been interested in, in physical medicine, is the primary side effect for physical medicine is when there's over dosage of therapy.

Dr. Stengler: Mm.

Dr. LaBeau:	Where you're pushing things harder than they can be, and particularly with a cancer patient this is critical, because as you realize you're going to have some problems with metastatic disease, so you can actually have bones involved. They can be fractured.
	Uh you want to find that fine balance between getting the immune system going and, and getting circulation going.
	But you don't want to aggravate the exact site of cancer.
Dr. Stengler:	Right.
Dr. LaBeau:	Uh, because you don't want to go and, and, sort of stare up the, the bee hive if you would.
Dr. Stengler:	Right. And that's why training is so important. You know, as an osteopathic doctor you're trained to be able to analyze these things and give appropriate care. Um, you know, you've seen many cancer patients over the years. I mean, well over a decade of treatment now, um, you find, uh, the patients with cancer getting your treatments; it just helps them in terms of reducing pain and stress and, uh, just better overall movement and function? Better quality of life scores?
Dr. LaBeau:	Well, it, it certainly does that and I find particularly beneficial of integrating it along with, uh—take—I want to say take into consideration the therapy they're having.
Dr. Stengler:	Mm-hmm.
Dr. LaBeau:	For instance, uh, if they're having surgery; often times the side effects of surgery is going to be inflammation and you're going to have muscles that are traumatized from being cut into.
	Uh, so there's, uh, the irony is, is even though—say, for instance, if you had surgery to remove a cancer although the cancer might be removed you're creating an impaired immune system, because you've created al ot of restriction in, in the tissue. So part of the goal is, is to get the tissue movement back to normal.
Dr. Stengler:	Right.
Dr. LaBeau:	And, uh, another type of therapy that's often used, radiation therapy, by the nature of base causes fibrosis and

hardening a tissue, so once again you want to get, uh, you know, often times if it's a—

For instance, topically, you'll get, uh, more of a rubbery type sensation. One of the best examples of this was I had a patient, uh, not so long ago that actually had cancer of the breast, uh, a couple decades before and, uh, she was coming in for some back problems and I thought, "Okay, uh, you know, she's saying how this was a tender problem, bothering me on my ack and my shoulder blade for, you know, for quite a while."

And as I was working with her I was working on some of the ribs and by the nature of the beast I tend to look at some of the ribs from the front side of the chest as well as the back of the chest—

And she kinda jumped in pain and she says, "Boy" she says, "I can't even—the front of my breast, uh, or chest, uh, after I had the breast surgery I can't even go and take a shower, because even just a shower beating on them"— This was 20 years prior!

Dr. Stengler: Yeah.

Dr. LaBeau: So, I worked with her with several visits and we're able to remove that tension in through there and, and get that circulation. So that area, by that—all that time when, when there's pain there chronically like that, that area's still being compromised in terms of circulation, so any kind of disease, or recurrence, could potentially come into those areas.

Dr. Stengler: Yeah, they're more susceptible.

Dr. LaBeau: Yeah.

Dr. Stengler: Well, there's several different treatments that you do with people musculoskeletally. Maybe you can just briefly review them, um, that trigger-point work, cranial-sacral, The, uh, manipulation, acupuncture.

Maybe just review some of those, uh, briefly if you would.

Dr. LaBeau: Yeah. Well the, uh, um, usually the big thing I start out with in terms of diagnosis is trying to challenge the area at the range of motion.

So, what I've found particularly in most of the patients and what we've really seen in the field is most of the chronic musculoskeletal problems are in the soft tissue around the bones.

Dr. Stengler: Mm-hmm.

Dr. LaBeau: So, the big focus of my therapy is called myofascial therapy. Myo being derived from the word muscle and fascia from the connective tissue, which is the supportive tissue that, that envelopes the body.

Best example of fascia, because it's kind of hard for people to understand, is if you had a selective acid that could go and destroy all the bones and all the organs of the body the fascia is wrapped around every organ; you would be able to see the traces of every organ of the body just from the fascia.

Dr. Stengler: Mm.

Dr. LaBeau: So, it literally forms a network, a web, around, around the whole body. So, uh, a body stocking if you want.

Dr. Stengler: Yeah.

Dr. LaBeau: Uh, so that, that is really the tissue focus I focus on primarily.

And then once I loosen that—once I find that tissue is loosened up then you only have to just give a little nudge to bones and, and they will tend to go and, and go into place.

So, I tend to start out with the soft tissue and then I move more into the boney type articulations.

Dr. Stengler: Mm-hmm, mm-hmm.

Dr. LaBeau: And then, um, and then if I'm looking up in the head and neck area then that's where the cranial-sacral therapy comes in, because that' s- that is, in a sense, looking at myofascial therapy for the central nervous system.

Dr. Stengler: Okay.

Dr. LaBeau: Very similar type techniques, but you're working—focused—you're focus intent and, and therapeutic options as far as looking at the cranial bones.

And the cranium, uh, is actually made up of 22 boney plates that need to move ever so subtly about 8 to 10 times per minute. So in, in that situation if there's any head or neck, like, say for instance when I—often times when I've seen patients with, uh, neck, uh, cancer of the neck area, esophageal cancer, you'll get a lot of matting and scarring of that area from either the removal—because of the many muscles have been removed.

Dr. Stengler: Mm-hmm.

Dr. LaBeau: Or, again, because of radiation therapy.

Dr. Stengler: Wow. And then how about acupuncture? I know you do some acupuncture, too. How do you find that helpful?

Dr. LaBeau: Acupuncture is a—acupuncture's a great adjunct in terms of adding circulation, improving circulation on local point. So often times I like to finish off using some acupuncture in some of those areas that are key hot points, or where you want to try to get the energy or the circulation enhanced.

Dr. Stengler: Right. And probably last category would be you do some regenerative injections, too, where maybe joints have been damaged and loss of cartilage and pain and restricted motion.

Uh, talk a bit about that. Just some of the injection—natural injections.

Dr. LaBeau: Well regenerative therapy is—yeah. Regenerative therapy is kind of interesting therapy and it's something that I've gotten into tin the last few years, because I've found that, you know, there's certain limitations of what you can do with the physical medicine and I, uh, I initially had some patients that had chronic knee problems, uh, and, uh, finding that, uh, uh, this type of therapy has potential for actually healing, uh, the knee to the point and joints to the point that they can have a surgery.

So with the regenerative therapy you're using a combination of, uh, nutraceuticals, ozone, and you're injecting it both at a combination and a joints and locally around tender, trigger areas often times, uh, where tendons are connected into bones and you're helping regenerate and actually—you're reduplicating an injury, sort of a controlled injury if you want, so that the inflammation is coming into that area and, uh, um, basically stimulating a healing response.

Dr. Stengler:	Yeah and we see great results with that. Well, you know, in, in closing here. I mean, people have to realize; osteopathic doctors like you, I mean, we do a lot of similar things. Because when you see people with cancer and we see quite a few people at the clinic here with that, um, yeah, you're looking at their musculoskeletal balance and all that, but, you know, you're prescribing nutritional IVs and IV Vitamin C and supplements and pain medications when people need it and referring to specialists.
	So it really is more just musculoskeletal. It's very comprehensive.
Dr. LaBeau:	Yeah, it's really an integrative approach.
Dr. Stengler:	Yeah. Yeah, that's great. Well that's one of the reasons we work well together. Dr. LaBeau has, you know, extensive training in this field and, again, a unique approach on the connection between the musculoskeletal system, the lymphatics, the immune system, and why that's so important with cancer.
	So, Dr. LaBeau, thank you for your time.
Dr. LaBeau:	Thank you.